# Ayur-Vidya™ Therapeutic Guide

Vaidya Atreya Smith

Cover by: www.theresabarzyk.com

Sanskrit Sutra on the Cover:
"There is no substance in the world which cannot be used therapeutically on the condition that it is used rationally and with a specific objective."
CS.SU.26.12

**By Vaidya Atreya Smith, B.Sc.**

The name *Ayur-Vidya*™ is a trademark of the company Ayur-Vidya LLC

www.ayur-vidya.com

ISBN-13: 978-1540369109
ISBN-10: 1540369102

# DISCLAIMER

This book is a reference work on the traditional medical system of India, Āyurveda, and is not intended to treat, diagnose or prescribe food, herbs or medicine. The information contained herein is in no way to be considered as a substitute for consultation with a duly licensed health-care professional and can be dangerous for non-medical personnel. The author and publisher disclaim any responsibly for the misuse of this information.

**Books by Vaidya Atreya Smith:**

Prana the Secret of Yogic Healing, Samuel Weiser, 1996

Practical Ayurveda, Samuel Weiser, 1998

Ayurvedic Healing for Women, Samuel Weiser, 1999

Secrets of Ayurvedic Massage, Lotus Press, 2000

Perfect Balance, Avery Publishing, 2001

Ayurvedic Nutrition Course Textbook, Editions Turiya, 2001

Panchakarma - Shodhana Chikitsa Textbook, Editions Turiya, 2003

Ayurvedic Nutrition, CreateSpace, 2010

The Psychology of Transformation in Yoga, CreateSpace, 2013

Ayurvedic Medicine for Westerners, Vol. 1; Anatomy and Physiology in Ayurveda, CreateSpace, 2013

Ayurvedic Medicine for Westerners, Vol. 2; Pathology & Diagnosis in Ayurveda, CreateSpace, 2014

Ayurvedic Medicine for Westerners, Vol. 3; Clinical Protocols & Treatments in Ayurveda, CreateSpace, 2015

Ayurvedic Medicine for Westerners, Vol. 4; Dravyaguna for Westerners, CreateSpace, 2013

Ayurvedic Medicine for Westerners, Vol. 5; Application of Ayurvedic Treatments Throughout Life, CreateSpace, 2016

# DEDICATION

We at Ayur-Vidya™ would like to dedicate this reference manual and our work in general to humanity. We hope that our work helps to reduce the suffering in the world. May all beings be at peace.

# CONTENTS

# Introduction

The foundation of health is our diet and lifestyle. According to Ayurveda the human body is made up from five categories of matter. Likewise, our food is also composed of these same five categories of matter. Hence, in Ayurveda the physical body is often referred to as the "food body" as it is nothing more than the result of the nutrients we take into our bodies.

This idea is much more profound than it seems on the surface. On one hand, it means we could modify our body's function by modifying our food. On another hand, it means we should then be able to correct problems in tissues (to some extent) by using the appropriate diet for this purpose. Still pursuing this idea further, it could mean that if something is wrong (e.g., pollution, etc.) in our food chain we will eventually manifest problems in our bodies.

There are many different ways we can look at this general idea that changing our diet could change our health. Before exploring this avenue of thought it is important to realize that many people and organizations have vested interests in refuting diet as factor of health and disease prevention. Even more developed are those people who state that diet is important, but these pills (which they happen to sell) will make up the difference of a nutrient poor diet (e.g., 'you don't have to worry about food if you buy the right pill' mentality). Why would anyone want to refute that diet is helping to maintain health and prevent disease? Mainly for money; either to sell medicines, supplements, or a dietary system.

If we really explore the idea that our body is made of 'food' and 'food' makes our body it is empowering. Ayurveda sees this as empowering because it allows us to prevent disease, live healthy and happily. It is empowering to think that we have some control in a world where we are losing control of so many things so quickly and on so many levels.

The Ayurvedic view of food is that it is a pleasure to be enjoyed. The main concept in this vision is that we can eat whatever we want *if we can digest it*. This means if we can assimilate the nutrients in the food – assuming there are nutrients to absorb. So, we have two important concepts here:

1) not just swallowing food, actually being able to assimilate the nutrients in the food;

2) if we are unable to assimilate the nutrients, the food could stick around and putrefy in the digestive system.

These two concepts are opposites, when one works the other doesn't and vice versa. In Ayurveda, these two concepts are called *Agni* and *Ama*. Agni is the digestive ability to separate nutritive elements from non-nutritive elements and to be able to assimilate the nutritive ones into the body. These nutrients then go on to build and form tissues.

The opposite of Agni is Āma. Ama or (aama) is food that has not been assimilated as nutrients, nor evacuated as waste. It stays in the body and putrefies. The GI tract is a warm, humid, dark environment that favors purification of food that is stagnant. Ama is formed when Agni is not working well. When our digestive capacity, or Agni, is working well it is impossible for Ama (non-digested food) to form in the intestines. This is all well and good one may say, but who or what is controlling, or disturbing Agni and our capacity to assimilate nutrients and thus form rotting food masses in the body?

Through generations of observation Ayurveda noted that the body has three managers that control all the functions, or physiology, of the body. During the fetus formation, these same managers control how the structure of the body is formed, and they continue to do so until growth is finished at the end of adolescence. The nature of observation based health systems is functional in both orientation and vision. Historically traditional Greek, Persian, Chinese and Indian medical systems are all what we call now 'functional medicine'. This is because the function of the body is given precedence over the structure of the body; structure as the result of function. Hence, all of these ancient systems have 'managers' that control the functions of the body (e.g., physiology).

In Ayurveda, there are three managers that control the homeostasis or physiological processes of the body. Among their many tasks they also control the digestive function or Agni. Therefore, Ayurveda places a huge importance on the managers of the body because they control how the food is digested, nutrients absorbed and distributed. When the managers do not work well the result is Ama, or non-digested food accumulating in the body. To understand what Ama is I suggest opening up the drain underneath your kitchen sink. See that smelly, black, sticky, putrid stuff? That is more or less what Ama is in our bodies; a slow accumulation of rotting food.

This explains why Ayurveda views dietary rules according to function and the manager who controls those functions. In other words, Ayurveda bases the dietary advice according to the manager because they are the single most important factor in transforming the food or herbs into nutrients that can be assimilated into the body. This is due to the fact that the manager controls Agni, and Agni digests the food.

The three managers, or *Dosha* in Sanskrit, are called *Vāta*, *Pitta* and *Kapha*. Their names imply the functions that they carry out in the body, Vata as wind or movement; Pitta as fire or transformation; Kapha as water or cohesion. Obviously, the names are metaphorical and not as important as understanding that they control our digestion and capacity to either maintain health or become sick. This is why Ayurvedic theory is based on the *Tridosha*, or three Doshas (managers).

In conclusion, the Ayurvedic vision is based on the concept that the whole world (our bodies, our food, and everything else) is made up of five categories of matter (*Panchamahabhuta*). This means we can adjust or modify the body by changing the food we consume. All functions in the body are controlled by three managers (Tridosha) who also dictate how our body assimilates nutrients and evacuates waste in the digestive system. The digestion of nutrients is carried out by Agni which is controlled by the three Doshas. Hence, all dietary advice in Ayurveda is given according to how these three Doshas (managers) function, because they control Agni. If they do their work correctly we stay healthy, if they fail to function correctly we build up non-digested food (Ama) in the body and this gives rise to disease. In general, Ayurveda says seventy-five percent of disease is due to Ama accumulation in the body. Hence, when considering our health, the first step is to analyze our food quality, our diet and our lifestyle because these factors form the foundation of health according to Ayurveda.

# Chapter One
## About Diet & Lifestyle

Ayurvedic diets are based on the three Doshas, or managers, of the body. There is a clear choice of using a lifetime diet that is based on our overall Dosha dominance (*Prakriti*), or of using a short-term diet based on treating a Dosha that is malfunctioning (*Vikriti*).

Lifetime diets are more open and less strict than short-term diets. In other words, a Prakriti diet (long-term or lifetime) is more open and relaxed than a Vikriti diet (short-term) that is used to treat a problem or disorder. Prakrit diets are more open and relaxed because they are structured to maintain health and prevent disease. Vikriti diets are strict because they are used to correct a malfunction in Dosha (manager) and Agni (digestive power).

The first thing to do is decide what you or your patient needs, an open long-term diet (Prakriti) or a short-term diet (Vikriti). Do you need to maintain health? Or do you need to correct an imbalance in the body?

Once this choice is made the diet can be tighten up (stricter) for a short-term diet or loosened up for a long-term diet. For example, the same Vata diet (a diet that reduces or balances Vata) can be used for a short-term, strict diet to reduce Vata, or it can be used in a more relaxed way for the long-term maintenance of Vata.

Each person can decide how open or strict the diet needs to be for their situation. If you are a professional, you can advise the patient according to what you feel if appropriate as per their Dosha and Agni. The key factor is to choose a diet that you can actually digest and enjoy eating. Suffering through a diet is not going to help anyone in the long-run. The psychology also needs to be satisfied, not only the body. Typically, what happens if the mind is not satisfied with the diet the patient will start snacking all the time on snacks.

Classical Ayurveda recognizes seven constitutional types or Prakriti. These are listed as Vata, Pitta, Kapha, Vata/Pitta, Vata/Kapha, Pitta/Kapha, and Vata/Pitta/Kapha. The first three are called "pure" types and the other four "dual" or "mixed" types. Ayurveda does not make a distinction between Vata/Pitta or Pitta/Vata. Some people cite nine types which give importance to the exact mix, however this is not needed nor is it used traditionally. This means that Ayurveda has seven general diet plans.

## To find out your constitution take the test on www.ayur-vidya.com

Note that Ayurvedic diets are usually vegetarian with dairy, but these diets are easy to modify either towards adding more animal products or to be Vegan. The choice is up to the individual, how do they want to eat and live. A professional can advise the patient on what they feel is best for their situation, or view on life.

Another important factor in Ayurvedic diets is lifestyle. In traditional Ayurvedic texts diet is actually part of lifestyle. How we live on a daily basis can be even more important than what we eat. An example could be someone who eats very well, but overworks and gets run down. Diet and lifestyle should be given equal value as either one can nullify the other. For instance, someone who lives a very regular, structured life, but eats junk food.

Ayurveda insists on using a lifestyle and diet together. If this is done then the results are balanced and rapid. The most important example of this is when we are treating Vata Dosha. The most important factor with a Vata diet is eating regularly and at regular hours every day. The food is less important than the regularity because Vata gets increased and unstable by irregular eating times. Due to the light, unstable nature of Vata any food eaten will help to reduce Vata. This is one reason why many people snack all day long as an instinctive reflex to reduce Vata (e.g., reduce stress, anxiety, etc.). Hence, the following dietary advice is always given with lifestyle advice as well.

Each person has a different need of nutrients and a different capacity to absorb and assimilate those nutrients. A healthy food for one person can be a disease-causing factor for another. In order to use the Ayurvedic system we need to look at food and food classifications differently than we are used to in the biochemical nutritional model. The Ayurvedic view of food is based on our Agni and how well we can digest the food and access the nutrients inside.

First, we can begin to view foods not as separate categories per se. Instead we can shift our point of view to seeing food according to the person who is going to eat it. This requires a paradigm shift in the way we normally look at food. The prime difference is looking at food according to the metabolism (Dosha and Agni) of the person rather than according to the nutrient content in the food or broad food groups.

Instead of saying, "Eat an apple a day because it has vitamin X", the new viewpoint is, "What shall I eat today to keep my Doshas in balance." This is an individualistic approach that requires the person to have a minimum understanding and responsibility for their own health.

It should be clearly understood that people using Ayurvedic nutrition are doing so because they want to take control over their life, health and empowerment. Ayurveda is a patient friendly system that encourages participation. Only you are capable of restoring your own health because it is you who is lifting your hand to your mouth and putting in the basic supply of health (food) into your body. No one is force feeding you food. For the health care professional, this needs to be made clear to the patient, and then support or assist them in changing their diet and lifestyle in any way possible.

## Eat According to Your Metabolic Capacity (Agni)

In the following diets an effort has been made to distinguish between very aggravating and mildly aggravating foods as per constitution or Prakriti. This also applies to the opposite situation of very beneficial and mildly beneficial foods. In both cases an attempt has been made to show the variegated qualities of food in relation to an individual. The headings, **Best, Medium, Mixed, Sometimes, Rarely and Worst** have been chosen to give an indication of food actions on any given constitutional type. For the mathematical minded I have also included a percentage indication to show the percentage of use that is beneficial for any given type. This would mean that a food in the 'Best' column could be used 100% of the time by the person corresponding to the chart. By the same token a person choosing a food in the 'Rarely' column would use the food only 20% percent of the time.

The following chart will clarify the percentage idea. However, I have adjusted the number of times per week to correspond to the amount needed to aggravate a person. Hence, 20% is 1-2 times per week instead of four as eating a lemon four times a week is enough to aggravate a Pitta type, but not 1 or 2 times. The following chart can give you an idea as to the amount needed to disturb you. Note that almost no food is listed as 100% because it is possible to overeat or consume any food to the point of aggravation. Also note that almost no food is listed as 'Worst' or 0% because in most cases eating a food once per week will not aggravate your Doshas and Agni. Therefore, we see that the majority of foods fall into a general use area for all of the constitutions.

| 100% | 21 | times in the week |
|------|------|-------------------|
| 80% | 16-18 | times in the week |
| 60% | 8-10 | times in the week |
| 40% | 3-4 | times in the week |
| 20% | 1-2 | times in the week |
| 0% | 0 | times in the week |

It should be pointed out that a variety of foods need to be eaten in a week's time. If you eat a certain kind of food every day, day in and day out, it will have greater power to disturb you and cause disruption in your metabolism. It is far better to eat a variety of foods during the week.

**The Vata type of person** will tend to have a variable digestive capacity. This means that foods that are concentrated and hard to digest should be avoided or taken in small amounts. The Vata type is also sensitive to gas forming foods and foods that deplete the moisture content in the body. The astringency of some foods has a drying effect on the tissues and can deplete moisture content in tissues. The Vata type is the most prone to have food allergies due to their variable enzyme function. These people tend to binge and have both a variable appetite and digestion. Hence, they should consume food in moderate amounts and at regular intervals.

In the table below a summery is given on the effects of food groups on the Vata type of person. This is a general guide to show how groups of foods affect these people. The foods are grouped according to their general action on the metabolism of the Vata type and judge nutritional value accordingly.

## Summary of Vata Type Food Groups

| TYPE OF FOOD | Effect of food on constitution | | | | | |
|---|---|---|---|---|---|---|
| Percentage | 100% | 80% | 60% | 40% | 20% | 0% |
| | Best | Medium | Mixed | Some-times | Rarely | Worst |
| Fruits | | | X | | | |
| Vegetables | | | X | | | |
| Grains | | X | | | | |
| Beans | | | | | X | |
| Nuts & Seeds | | X | | | | |
| Dairy | | X | | | | |
| Oils | | X | | | | |
| Animal Products | | | X | | | |
| Sweeteners | | | X | | | |
| Spices | | X | | | | |
| Beverages | | X | | | | |
| Vitamins & Minerals | | | | X | | |

## Outline of Lifestyle (Dinacharya) for Vata Prakriti
- Wake up early in the morning, before sunrise when possible
- Go to the toilet to remove waste (stool, urine, etc.)
- Drink 750ml to 1 liter of warm/hot water
- Clean or scrape the tongue, then gargle with Sesame oil (Gandusa)
- Put 1 or 2 drops of oil in each nostril (Snehana Nasya)
- Do Abhyanga (apply sesame oil all over the body, or a Vata Massage oil)
- Do mild Yoga Asana or mild exercise for 10 to 20 minutes,

end with 5 minutes of Nadishodhana (alternate nostril breathing)
- Meditate for 5 to 10 minutes
- Take a hot shower or bath to remove oil from Abhyanga
- Get dressed
- Eat a light to medium Breakfast
- Go to work
- Eat a medium Lunch with some cooked food
- Take a short walk to digest and relax
- Go back to work
- Mild exercise (optional: depending if there was morning exercise)
- Eat a light to medium Dinner with mainly cooked food
- Relax
- Optional Abhyanga if needed, with optional 5 minutes of Nadishodhana (alternate nostril breathing); follow with hot shower. Do this if one has had a very stressful day
- Massage the bottoms of the feet with oil, put socks on (to protect the sheets).
- Go to bed by 10 pm and sleep by 11 pm

Vata Prakriti needs three meals a day. Breakfast, lunch and dinner should be about the same size. Vata type should not eat too much or too little; if they are hungry three hours after eating the meal was too light; if they are hungry six to seven hours later the meal was too heavy. Vata types can have a snack at 4 pm to 5 pm if they eat dinner later than 7.30 pm due to work; they should avoid sweets at this time – dried fruit, nuts, etc. are better in the afternoon. Snacking at other times should be avoided.

**The Pitta type of person** has the strongest digestive capacity and can digest most any food, junk food, or chemical food (soft drinks) for years without a hint of a problem. Around 37 years-old, give or take a few years, this begins to change. The Pitta type is the most sensitive to sour (fermented) and acidic foods that increase Pitta the body. They also may be attracted to hot spices, but these also pose problems in the long run. These kinds of foods tend to increase the bile production in the liver and pancreas which increases the acidic nature of both blood and plasma. Human cells are very sensitive to the pH level of the body and high Pitta or acidity ages cells or breaks down their normal metabolic function. The Pitta type has the strongest enzyme capacity unless too many spicy or acidic foods are eaten. These people have the greatest capacity for both the variety and quantity of food.

In the table below a summery is given on the effects of food groups on the Pitta type of person. This is a general guide to show how groups of foods affect these people. The foods are grouped according to their general action on the metabolism of the Pitta type of person and judge nutritional value accordingly.

## Summary of Pitta Type Food Groups

| TYPE OF FOOD | Effect of food on constitution | | | | | |
|---|---|---|---|---|---|---|
| Percentage | 100% | 80% | 60% | 40% | 20% | 0% |
| | Best | Medium | Mixed | Some-times | Rarely | Worst |
| Fruits | | X | | | | |
| Vegetables | | X | | | | |
| Grains | | X | | | | |
| Beans | | | X | | | |
| Nuts & Seeds | | | | X | | |
| Dairy | | | X | | | |
| Oils | | | | | X | |
| Animal Products | | | | | X | |
| Sweeteners | | | X | | | |
| Spices | | | | | X | |
| Beverages | | X | | | | |
| Vitamins & Minerals | | | | X | | |

## Outline of Lifestyle (Dinacharya) for Pitta Prakriti
- Wake up early in the day, before sunrise when possible
- Go to the toilet and remove waste (stool, urine, etc.)
- Drink 500ml of room temperature or cool water
- Clean or scrape the tongue, then gargle with Sesame oil (Gandusa)
- Do Jala Neti if needed (nasal wash)

- Add one drop of ghee to each nostril
- Do Abhyanga (apply sunflower oil all over the body, or a Pitta Massage Oil)
- Do Yoga Asana or exercise for 20 to 30 minutes, end with 5 minutes of Nadishodhana (alternate nostril breathing)
- Meditate 5 to 10 minutes
- Take a hot shower or bath to remove oil from Abhyanga
- Get dressed
- Eat a substantial Breakfast
- Go to work
- Eat a substantial Lunch; if tried or sleepy after eating the quantity was too much
- Take a short walk to digest and relax
- Go to work
- Exercise now if unable to exercise in the morning
- Eat a substantial Dinner
- Relax
- Optional 5 minutes of Nadishodhana (alternate nostril breathing) before bed if the day was very difficult or if there are problems sleeping
- Go to bed by 10 pm and sleep by 11 pm

Pitta Prakriti needs three meals a day. Breakfast, lunch and dinner should be roughly the same size. Pitta types need more food than the other types due to the strong Agni (digestion). They need to eat every four hours, longer periods of more than five hours without food create hyperacid and acid reflux conditions. Snacking should be avoided between meals. It is better to eat substantial meals and avoid snacking.

**The Kapha type of person** has the slowest digestive function. These people will be the most prone to weight gain and obesity due to the slower rate of metabolism. They will have to pay the closest attention to the quantities of food consumed and will have the most restrictive diet accordingly. They are the most sensitive to carbohydrates especially in simple sugars, yet all excess tends to clog and further slowdown the transformation of food. Dairy products due to their mucus forming properties and congestive qualities can also trouble them. The enzyme function of these people is lower than the other types, but is consistent. Hence, they can have stronger digestive power than the fluctuating Vata type. The Kapha type has the most restrictive diet in both quantity and variety of foods.

In the table below a summery is given on the effects of food groups on the Kapha type. This is a general guide to show how groups of foods affect these people. The foods are grouped according to their general action on the metabolism of the Kapha type of person and judge nutritional value accordingly.

## Summary of Kapha Type Food Groups

| TYPE OF FOOD | Effect of food on constitution | | | | | |
|---|---|---|---|---|---|---|
| Percentage | 100% | 80% | 60% | 40% | 20% | 0% |
|  | Best | Medium | Mixed | Some-times | Rarely | Worst |
| Fruits |  |  | X |  |  |  |
| Vegetables |  | X |  |  |  |  |
| Grains |  |  | X |  |  |  |
| Beans |  | X |  |  |  |  |
| Nuts & Seeds |  |  |  | X |  |  |
| Dairy |  |  |  |  | X |  |
| Oils |  |  |  |  | X |  |
| Animal Products |  |  |  |  | X |  |
| Sweeteners |  |  |  |  |  | X |
| Spices | X |  |  |  |  |  |
| Beverages |  |  |  | X |  |  |
| Vitamins & Minerals |  |  |  |  | X |  |

## Outline of Lifestyle (Dinacharya) for Kapha Prakriti

- Wake up early in the day, before sunrise when possible
- Go to the toilet and remove waste (stool, urine, etc.)
- Drink 250ml to 300ml of warm/hot water
- Start cooking Ginger tea (see recipe next chapter)
- Clean or scrape the tongue, then gargle with Sesame oil (Gandusa)
- Do Jala Neti (nasal wash) followed by one drop of sesame oil in each nostril

- Do Utvartana (or Udvartana powder massage), or luffa sponge massage
- Do strong Yoga Asana or strong exercise, end with 5 minutes of Nadishodhana (alternate nostril breathing)
- Meditate 10 to 15 minutes
- Take a hot shower or bath
- Get dressed
- Finish making Ginger tea, put in thermos to drink the whole day
- Skip breakfast or eat one piece of sour / acid fruit (Grapefruit, etc.)
- Go to work
- Eat a substantial Lunch; if tired or sleepy after eating the quantity was too much
- Take a short walk to digest and relax
- Go to work
- Mild Exercise (optional depending on morning exercise)
- Eat a light Dinner, no dessert
- Relax
- Optional 5 minutes of Nadishodhana (alternate nostril breathing) before bed if the day was very difficult or if there are problems sleeping
- Go to bed by 10 pm and sleep by 11 pm

Kapha Prakriti needs only two meals a day. Lunch should be the most nourishing meal and dinner should be lighter. Breakfast should be skipped, if needed sour or acidic fruit can be eaten at breakfast time. No solid foods should be eaten in the morning. Snacking should be avoided at all times of the day. If the desire to eat sweets and snacks happens in the evening after eating then the dinner meal was too light, or not nourishing.

**The Vata/Pitta type of person** will tend to have a light but regular digestive capacity. In general, this type does not have extreme digestive traits. They tend to be medium eaters with regular appetites. Having regular meals three times a day is very important and to avoid snacking between meals is also important. Their Pitta side can easily become disturbed by eating too much acidic, fermented and pungent foods; all of which are good for the Vata side in small amounts. Food in general is more important to favor their Pitta side and use the lifestyle and regularity to control more their Vata side. This type can favor a Vata diet from 1ˢᵗ of August to the end of January and favor a Pitta diet from the 1ˢᵗ of February to the end of July (Northern Hemisphere).

In the table below a summery is given on the effects of food groups on the Vata/Pitta type of person. This is a general guide to show how groups of foods affect these people. The foods are grouped according to their general action on the metabolism of the Vata Pitta type and judge nutritional value accordingly.

## Summary of Vata/Pitta Type Food Groups

| TYPE OF FOOD | Effect of food on constitution | | | | | |
|---|---|---|---|---|---|---|
| Percentage | 100% | 80% | 60% | 40% | 20% | 0% |
| | Best | Medium | Mixed | Some-times | Rarely | Worst |
| Fruits | | X | | | | |
| Vegetables | | X | | | | |
| Grains | | X | | | | |
| Beans | | | X | | | |
| Nuts & Seeds | | | X | | | |
| Dairy | | | X | | | |
| Oils | | | | X | | |
| Animal Products | | | | X | | |
| Sweeteners | | | X | | | |
| Spices | | | X | | | |
| Beverages | | | X | | | |
| Vitamins & Minerals | | | | | X | |

Generally dual types will tend to have some of both types and not have any clear-cut distinction between the two. The traditional way Ayurveda worked with these types was to have them change the kinds of foods they eat according to the seasonal changes in year.

## Outline of Lifestyle (Dinacharya) for Vata/Pitta Prakriti
- Wake up early in the morning, before sunrise when possible
- Go to the toilet to remove waste (stool, urine, etc.)

- Drink 500ml of warm water
- Clean or scrape the tongue, then gargle with Sesame oil (Gandusa)
- Put 1 or 2 drops of oil in each nostril (Snehana Nasya)
- Do Abhyanga (apply sesame oil all over the body, or a Vata Massage oil in the fall and winter and Pitta Massage oil in the spring and summer)
- Do Yoga Asana or exercise for 20 to 30 minutes, end with 5 minutes of Nadishodhana (alternate nostril breathing)
- Meditate for 5 to 10 minutes
- Take a hot shower or bath to remove oil from Abhyanga
- Get dressed
- Eat a medium Breakfast
- Go to work
- Eat a medium Lunch with some cooked food
- Take a short walk to digest and relax
- Go back to work
- Exercise (optional: depending if there was morning exercise)
- Eat a medium Dinner with mainly cooked food
- Relax
- Optional Abhyanga if needed, with optional 5 minutes of Nadishodhana (alternate nostril breathing); follow with hot shower. Do this if one has had a very stressful day
- Massage the bottoms of the feet with oil, put socks on (to protect the sheets).
- Go to bed by 10 pm and sleep by 11 pm

Vata/Pitta Prakriti needs three meals a day. Breakfast, lunch and dinner should be about the same size and this will vary from person to person; medium to large depending on age, sex and profession. The Vata/Pitta type should not eat too much or too little; if they are hungry three hours after eating the meal was too light; if they are hungry six hours later the meal was too heavy. Regular meals times is very important for this type. Snacking should be avoided between meals. It is better to eat substantial meals and avoid snacking altogether.

**The Vata/Kapha type of person** will tend to have a slow steady digestion with some periods in the autumn of a variable digestive capacity. There needs to be blending to some extent of the Vata/Kapha diets as this person is neither a pure Vata nor a pure Kapha type. So, removing extremes in the diet is good. For example, this type of person can eat a small breakfast if hungry. They can eat a small amount of sweet foods and they can also take some natural oils with their meals. All of these changes are needed to keep Vata in balance. However, if too much oil, sweets or heavy food is eaten their Kapha side will increase and they will gain weight. Regularity of meals is very important to keep the Vata side of this type in balance, while food choices are more important for the Kapha side. This type should eat a Vata diet from the 1st of June to the end of November and a Kapha diet from the 1st of December until the end of May (Northern Hemisphere).

In the table below a summery is given on the effects of food groups on the Vata/Kapha type of person. This is a general guide to show how groups of foods affect these people. The foods are grouped according to their general action on the metabolism of the Vata/Kapha type and judge nutritional value accordingly.

## Summary of Vata/Kapha Type Food Groups

| TYPE OF FOOD | Effect of food on constitution | | | | | |
|---|---|---|---|---|---|---|
| Percentage | 100% | 80% | 60% | 40% | 20% | 0% |
| | Best | Medium | Mixed | Some-times | Rarely | Worst |
| Fruits | | | X | | | |
| Vegetables | | X | | | | |
| Grains | | X | | | | |
| Beans | | | X | | | |
| Nuts & Seeds | | | | X | | |
| Dairy | | | X | | | |
| Oils | | | | X | | |
| Animal Products | | | | X | | |
| Sweeteners | | | | X | | |
| Spices | | X | | | | |
| Beverages | | | X | | | |
| Vitamins & Minerals | | | | X | | |

Generally dual types will tend to have some of both types and not have any clear-cut distinction between the two. The traditional way Ayurveda worked with these types was to have them change the kinds of foods they eat according to the seasonal changes in year.

## Outline of Lifestyle (Dinacharya) for Vata/Kapha Prakriti

- Wake up early in the morning, before sunrise when possible
- Go to the toilet to remove waste (stool, urine, etc.)
- Drink 500ml of warm/hot water
- Start cooking Ginger tea (see recipe next chapter)
- Clean or scrape the tongue, then gargle with Sesame oil (Gandusa)
- Put 1 or 2 drops of Sesame oil in each nostril (Snehana Nasya)
- Do Abhyanga every second day (apply sesame oil all over the body, or a Vata Massage oil)
- Do mild Yoga Asana or mild exercise for 20 to 30 minutes, end with 5 minutes of Nadishodhana (alternate nostril breathing)
- Meditate for 10 to 15 minutes
- Take a hot shower or bath to remove oil from Abhyanga
- Get dressed
- Finish making Ginger tea, put in thermos to drink the whole day
- Eat a light Breakfast that favors acidic fruit and warm drinks
- Go to work
- Eat a medium Lunch with some cooked food, dairy products are OK
- Take a short walk to digest and relax
- Go back to work
- Mild exercise (optional: depending if there was morning exercise)
- Eat a medium Dinner with mainly cooked food
- Relax
- Optional 5 minutes of Nadishodhana (alternate nostril breathing); follow with hot shower. Do this if one has had a very stressful day
- Go to bed by 10 pm and sleep by 11 pm

Vata/Kapha Prakriti needs three meals a day. Breakfast should be light and lunch and dinner should be about the same size. Lunch is fairly open with heavier foods. The Vata/Kapha type should not eat too much or too little; if they are hungry three hours after eating the meal was too light; if they are hungry six to seven hours later the meal was too heavy. Snacking should be avoided at all times of the day. If the desire to eat sweets and snacks happens in the evening after eating then the dinner meal was too light, or not nourishing.

**The Pitta/Kapha type of person** will tend to have a strong regular digestion. Often these people are able to eat and digest huge amounts of food. If they stay physically active they will keep their weight stable. Unfortunately, if these people do not remain very active physically they will gain weight rather quickly. Their diet is in-between a pure Pitta and pure Kapha type with less pungent, acidic food than a pure Kapha, and less food in general than a pure Pitta. This type needs to be careful with oily, heavy foods; favor a Kapha diet from September 21st to March 20th and favor a Pitta diet from the 21st of March to the 20th of September (Northern Hemisphere).

## Summary of Pitta/Kapha Type Food Groups

| TYPE OF FOOD | Effect of food on constitution | | | | | |
|---|---|---|---|---|---|---|
| Percentage | 100% | 80% | 60% | 40% | 20% | 0% |
| | Best | Medium | Mixed | Some-times | Rarely | Worst |
| Fruits | | X | | | | |
| Vegetables | | X | | | | |
| Grains | | | X | | | |
| Beans | | | X | | | |
| Nuts & Seeds | | | | X | | |
| Dairy | | | | X | | |
| Oils | | | | X | | |
| Animal Products | | | | X | | |
| Sweeteners | | | | X | | |
| Spices (mild) | | X | | | | |
| Beverages | | | X | | | |
| Vitamins & Minerals | | | | X | | |

In the table above a summery is given on the effects of food groups on the Pitta/Kapha type of person. This is a general guide to show how groups of foods affect these people. The foods are grouped according to their general action on the metabolism of the Pitta/Kapha type and judge nutritional value accordingly.

Generally dual types will tend to have some of both types and not have any clear-cut distinction between the two. The traditional way Ayurveda worked with these types was to have them change the kinds of foods they eat according to the seasonal changes in year.

## Outline of Lifestyle (Dinacharya) for Pitta/Kapha Prakriti
- Wake up early in the day, before sunrise when possible
- Go to the toilet and remove waste (stool, urine, etc.)
- Drink 300ml of warm water
- Start cooking Ginger tea (see recipe next chapter)
- Clean or scrape the tongue, then gargle with Sesame oil (Gandusa)
- Do Jala Neti if needed (nasal wash)
- Add one drop of ghee to each nostril
- Do Abhyanga every third day or two times per week (Sesame oil all over the body, or a Kapha Massage Oil)
- Do Yoga Asana or exercise for 20 to 30 minutes, end with 5 minutes of Nadishodhana (alternate nostril breathing)
- Meditate 10 to 15 minutes
- Take a hot shower or bath to remove oil from Abhyanga
- Get dressed
- Finish making Ginger tea, put in thermos to drink the whole day
- Eat a medium Breakfast with fresh fruits
- Go to work
- Eat a medium Lunch; if tired or sleepy after eating the quantity was too much
- Take a short walk to digest and relax
- Go to work
- Exercise now if unable to exercise in the morning
- Eat a medium Dinner
- Relax
- Go to bed by 10 pm and sleep by 11 pm

Pitta/Kapha Prakriti needs three meals a day. Breakfast, lunch and dinner should be roughly the same size from medium to fairly large. Pitta/Kapha types need more food than the other types due to the strong Agni (digestion) and larger bodies. They need to eat every five or six hours. Skipping meals should be avoided. Snacking should be avoided between meals. It is better to eat substantial meals and avoid snacking.

**The Equal type, or Vata/Pitta/Kapha type, of person** will tend to have a strong, regular digestive capacity. In general, this is the best constitution for health, but also the rarest. Most foods in moderation are good for this type. They are closer to the Pitta/Kapha type than any other mix with a strong, regular, slightly slow digestive metabolism. They should avoid too many sweets and too much fried or oily food as their Kapha side can increase. They should also avoid too much fermented or pungent food – such as avoid daily consumption – because their Pitta side can easily become aggravated. Lastly, regular meals are very important to keep their Vata side in balance and stable. Hence, they should consume food in moderate amounts and at regular intervals during the day. Seasonal foods are the best for everyone and this is also true for the Equal type. Note a seasonal diet of changing according to constitution is not usually required for the Vata/Pitta/Kapha type. However, if there is a sign of weight gain the person can eat a Kapha diet from the 1st of December to the end of March (Northern Hemisphere).

Note that the Vata/Pitta/Kapha or Equal type is considered to be rare. These types of people are by far the least common, representing less than five percent of the population. They have the strongest immunity and are rarely sick. If you have a doubt about your constitution or Prakriti it is better to start with the hypotheses that you are a Dual type rather than an Equal type.

In the table below a summery is given on the effects of food groups on the Equal type of person. This is a general guide to show how groups of foods affect these people. The foods are grouped according to their general action on the metabolism of the Equal type and judge nutritional value accordingly.

## Summary of Vata Pitta Kapha Type Food Groups

| TYPE OF FOOD | Effect of food on constitution | | | | | |
|---|---|---|---|---|---|---|
| Percentage | 100% | 80% | 60% | 40% | 20% | 0% |
| | Best | Medium | Mixed | Some-times | Rarely | Worst |
| Fruits | | X | | | | |
| Vegetables | | X | | | | |
| Grains | | X | | | | |
| Beans | | | X | | | |
| Nuts & Seeds | | | X | | | |
| Dairy | | | X | | | |
| Oils | | | X | | | |
| Animal Products | | | X | | | |
| Sweeteners | | | | X | | |
| Spices | | | X | | | |
| Beverages | | | X | | | |
| Vitamins & Minerals | | | | X | | |

Generally equal types will tend to have some of all types and not have any clear-cut distinction between the three. The traditional way Ayurveda worked with these types was to have them change the kinds of foods they eat according to the seasonal changes in year. This is less important for the equal type of person.

## Outline of Lifestyle (Dinacharya) for Vata/Pitta/Kapha Prakriti

- Wake up early in the day, before sunrise when possible
- Go to the toilet and remove waste (stool, urine, etc.)
- Drink 300ml of warm water
- Start cooking Ginger tea (see recipe next chapter)
- Clean or scrape the tongue, then gargle with Sesame oil (Gandusa)
- Do Jala Neti if needed (nasal wash)
- Add one drop of ghee to each nostril
- Do Abhyanga every second day or three times per week (Sesame oil all over the body, or a Vata Massage Oil)
- Do Yoga Asana or exercise for 20 to 30 minutes, end with 5

minutes of Nadishodhana (alternate nostril breathing)
- Meditate 10 to 15 minutes
- Take a hot shower or bath to remove oil from Abhyanga
- Get dressed
- Finish making Ginger tea, put in thermos to drink the whole day
- Eat a medium Breakfast with fresh fruits
- Go to work
- Eat a medium Lunch; if tired or sleepy after eating the quantity was too much
- Take a short walk to digest and relax
- Go to work
- Exercise now if unable to exercise in the morning
- Eat a medium Dinner
- Relax
- Go to bed by 10 pm and sleep by 11 pm

The Vata/Pitta/Kapha Prakriti needs three equal meals a day. Breakfast, lunch and dinner should be roughly the same size from medium to fairly large. Vata/Pitta/Kapha types need more food than the other types due to the strong Agni (digestion) and balanced bodies. They need to eat every five or six hours. Skipping meals should be avoided. Snacking should be avoided between meals. It is better to eat substantial meals and avoid snacking.

## Modifying a Prakriti diet to a Vikriti diet

The preceding dietary advice for Prakriti diets (lifetime or long-term diets) can be modified to a Vikriti diet (a short-term diet). When any kind of problem is present in the body or mind, it is advised to use a Vikriti diet to correct the problem. This is especially important when herbal products are used. This means if you have a bronchitis you could speed recovery by following a diet and lifestyle to reduce Kapha (mucus) and Pitta (inflammation) for several weeks until the disorder is gone.

In this example, the Pitta/Kapha diet and lifestyle could be adopted by any person for several weeks. With this logic, the diet should then become strict – avoid completely foods in the 40% column or "Sometimes" and focus on eating the foods indicated in the 60% and 80% columns. When this approach is followed the Doshas that are contributing to the disorder are reduced, this speeds up the natural healing processes of the body. If herbs are added to this then the results are even better.

How to modify a Prakriti diet into a Vikriti diet? Simply remove foods indicated in the 0%, 20%, and 40% columns. If the Vikriti diet is to be followed for more than a few weeks, then thirty percent of the 40% "Sometimes" foods can be taken. Vikriti diets may need to be followed for up to a year if a chronic disorder is being treated. Care needs to be taken to eat a balanced diet – using a variety of fresh foods and avoid eating the same foods all the time.

When a Vikriti diet is being followed the lifestyle should also become a bit stricter if possible. The combination of a more controlled lifestyle and diet gives quick results in most cases. We should always remember that a strict diet and lifestyle are used for short periods of time to correct a disorder and not to be followed for the whole life. This fact helps us psychologically to do a diet for a few months that is beneficial for our health.

For some disorders it may be indicated to start with a detoxifying diet or anti-Ama diet. This kind of diet is a special short-term diet to remove Ama or undigested food from the digestive system. As it has a number of contraindications this kind of diet is explained in the next chapter.

Fasting is also a traditional method used in Ayurveda to remove toxins or non-digested food from the body. Fasting also has a number of rules that follow the Prakriti of the individual. It has even more contraindications than the detoxifying diet. Hence, it is beyond this therapeutic guide. Please see the references at the end of this chapter for professionals who should be consulted for stronger therapies like fasting.

## Conclusion

In closing it is helpful to remember that the body does best with slow changes that last for long periods of time rather than radical changes in diet and lifestyle that last only for a few days or weeks.

It can also be helpful to note that not all changes need to be done at the same time, nor do they need to be followed strictly if the main goal is to prevent disorders and maintain health. A healthy dose of common sense (a disappearing commodity!) can be used when changing both diet and lifestyle. The following chart may help to show that not everything needs to be done at once. Even small changes give result! For example:

> 10% change will give 20% results
> 20% change will give 30% results
> 30% change will give 40% results
> 50% change will give 65% results
> 70% change will give 85% results
> 80% change will give 95% results

Therefore, our goal is to reach an eighty percent compliance with both diet and lifestyle as that will give a very positive therapeutic result. That will also allow us to function in society, go out with friends and family sometimes and generally enjoy life.

**For more information on diet and lifestyle:**

Professionals: Ayurvedic Medicine for Westerners, Vol. 3; *Clinical Protocols & Treatments in Ayurveda*, CreateSpace, 2015

Individuals: *Ayurvedic Nutrition*, CreateSpace, 2010

# Chapter Two
## Detoxifying Diet or Anti-Ama Diet

An anti-Ama diet is often needed before proceeding with a long-term nutritional program or herbal therapies. It is indicated whenever there is a covering on the tongue, or the stool sinks and/or has a strong smell. There are other signs of Ama accumulation such as chronic fatigue, etc. There are contraindications for a strongly reducing diet. This diet should not be given when there is any kind of wasting disease such as AIDS, tuberculosis, etc. It should not be given when the patient is young (under 10 years) or old (over 70), or recovering from a long illness. In other words, whenever a patient is weak it should not be used. It also should not be given to persons suffering from high Vata Vikriti, or a strong Vata imbalance.

Generally, all types can use this diet at the beginning of spring and at the end of summer to prevent disease on a seasonal basis. This kind of reducing diet should be avoided in winter if possible, especially in cold climates. In hot climates, it can be used year-round.

This diet has to be slightly adjusted for each constitution and according to their individual situation. Depending on their lifestyle and climate the following duration can be used:

- Vata not more than two weeks
- Pitta not more than four weeks
- Kapha not more than four months

## Percentage of Food Groups

| | | | |
|---|---|---|---|
| Fruit | 10% | Animal Products | 0% |
| Vegetables | 35% | Fish | 0% |
| Grains | 45% | Oils (ghee) | 1% |
| Beans | 3% | Sweeteners | 0% |
| Nuts/seeds | 0% | Spice | 5% |
| Dairy | 0% | Supplements | 1% |

## Anti-Ama Diet Guide for All Types

| Food Group | Kind of Food |
|---|---|
| Fruit | 1 Grapefruit or other sour fruit in the morning |
| Vegetables | 1/2 cup barley, alfalfa and wheat sprouts daily; NO nightshades, all other veggies steamed for lunch and dinner - use only one veggie per meal; veggie juices are excellent with mild spice or ginger. |
| Grains | 1/2 to 1 cup cooked whole grains per lunch and dinner as per constitution; NO white flour, bread or pastry; Khichari is good; Pitta types can take whole grain cereals in the morning. |
| Beans | No beans, except Khichari made with Mung beans |
| Nuts/Seeds | No, unless sprouted |
| Dairy | No |
| Animal Products | No (eggs included) |
| Fish/shell fish | No |
| Oils | No, only ghee should be used |
| Sweeteners | No, only raw honey can be used at 1/2 teaspoon per day when needed |
| Spices | Little or no Salt, all spices are good especially ginger and black pepper |

| Beverages | No cold drinks, alcohol, coffee or other stimulants; water is good and some mild herbal teas can be used |
|---|---|
| Supplements | Spirulina, chlorella can be used; blue green algae is strongly reducing, so it is not good for Vata types; all other supplements should be avoided during detox. |

Sprouts are strongly cleansing and are often enough on their own when combined with a simple diet to clear Ama. For old, chronic formations of Ama this kind of diet is highly recommended. The amount of raw foods used should follow the constitution, age, season and Agni. However, most people will benefit from using primarily raw foods during this diet supplemented with cooked whole grains, or cooked sprouted grains.

If any indications of high Vata or emaciation occur using this diet it should be stopped immediately. Signs of excessive use for an anti-Ama diet are:

- Insomnia
- Fainting
- Loss of appetite
- Emaciation
- Palpitations
- Lack of energy, motivation
- Listlessness
- Absence of menstruation
- Lack of concentration

This diet is quite "un-grounding" and is not good to use for people who are healers, psychics, construction workers, athletes, social workers, or have other physical or mentally demanding jobs. Also, note the psychological state of the client, as this diet needs a fairly stable mental state. I suggest to avoid using this diet when the client is undergoing major emotional changes.

If the body is detoxified too fast some problems can manifest. I do not consider this to be a good sign. Some practitioners say that these signs are part of a 'healing crisis'. It is true that the body will sometimes have worse symptoms before having a relief of all symptoms. *However, this is more the exception than the rule.*

In my clinical practice this happens less than 10% of the time.

The trick is to avoid detoxifying the body too fast. If the body is detoxified slowly then the increase of negative symptoms will not occur. Hence, introducing a cleansing, anti-Ama diet, slowly into a patient's program is *usually* best. My patients all have to work and take care of family, etc. Giving them a strong cleansing diet would force them to miss time working and perhaps create further psychological burdens. However, if the patient is very ill it may be better to go directly into using this cleansing diet.

Common signs of detoxifying the body too fast:
- Headaches
- Skin Rashes
- Diarrhea
- Nausea

Usually, if adequate spice is given to keep the Agni strong these signs will not manifest. By far the most common occurring sign of detoxification is the headache. My approach is to reduce the amounts of raw or cleansing foods until the symptoms disappear. Then I slowly increase the doses of these foods when the symptoms and metabolism stabilize.

When prescribing a detoxifying diet, it is important to see the patient more often - at least once per week. Pancha Karma, the Ayurvedic detoxifying program, is very good to accompany an anti-Ama diet. *Be very aware that a strongly detoxifying diet or Pancha Karma can reduce the Agni to a very problematic level.* Maintaining Agni is the most important consideration in reducing Ama and detoxifying therapies. It should be stressed that simply eating a few raw or healing foods alone is not enough to change a disease or the beginning stages of pathology. The client must use the whole Ayurvedic methodology and diet together to be successful.

In order the keep Agni strong it is recommended to use a ginger root decoction tea during the anti-Ama diet. This tea can be used at any time, even with a normal diet, when Agni needs to be supported or increased. In Ayurveda, fresh ginger root is considered to be balanced for all types of persons. It is important to adjust the amount of ginger root to fit your tastes. If ginger is disliked by you, or the patient, use the following spices alone without ginger.

## Instructions on how to make ginger tea

This is a standard formula to increase Agni and remove Ama (toxins).

The basic idea is to cook the fresh ginger root and then to add the following spices into the tea to infuse. The combination of the spices and ginger root increases Agni and helps remove Ama from the digestive system. In the list below a "1" means one part, and a "0" means nothing. For example, for a Vata mix of spices use equal parts of Cumin, Cardamom, Fenugreek and Fennel seeds. Leave out the other spices. If you do not have, or cannot find the spices, simple use what you can get.

| V | P | K | Latin | Common Name |
|---|---|---|---|---|
| 1 | 1 | 1 | Cumimum cyminum | Cumin |
| 1 | 1 | 1 | Elettaria cardamomum | Cardamom |
| 0 | 1 | 0 | Coriandrum sativum | Coriander |
| 1 | 0 | 1 | Trigonella foenum-graecum | Fenugreek |
| 0 | 1 | 1 | Cinnamomum zeylanicum | Cinnamon |
| 1 | 1 | 1 | Foeniculum vulgare | Fennel |

Dosage:  2-4 grams per 1 quart (32 fluid ounces) or 1 liter of water

### Instructions:

Take ¼ to ½ inch (7 to 14 mm) of peeled, diced fresh ginger and bring it to a boil in 1 quart (32 fluid ounces) or 1 liter (33.8 fluid ounces) of filtered (drinkable) water. Simmer the ginger root for 10 minutes then turn off the heat (gas, electricity, etc.). Now add 4 grams (2 level teaspoons) of the powdered spices listed above (the mix of spices indicated by your Ayurvedic practitioner or the test). The whole seeds or spices should be crushed or broken a bit if they are not in powder. Cover the saucepan and wait 20 minutes as the spices infuse. Drink this tea in 100 ml doses (3.4 fluid ounce) throughout the day; this is ten equal doses in the day. Total amount should be 1 quart or 1 liter per day.

This tea is safe for long term use to remove Ama, but should be stopped after one year in most cases.

## Khichari recipe

Khichari is a nutrient balanced rice dish that balances the three Doshas and helps to detoxify the body. It is considered to be very easy to digest and highly nutritive.

Instructions:
Ingredients: 1 cup white basmati rice and ½ cup of mung dal (split mung beans without skin – they are yellow). 6 cups hot water, 1 tsp of ghee, ¼ tsp. cumin seeds, ¼ tsp. ground cumin, ¼ tsp. ground coriander, ½ tsp. powdered turmeric, 1 pinch of asafetida powder (optional), ½ inch of ginger fresh, peeled and finely chopped or grated, 1 pinch of salt, fresh coriander chopped or lime

Wash the rice and mung dal together several times. Add the ghee to a saucepan and heat with medium heat. Sauté the cumin seeds in the ghee until they burst or pop. Add the remaining spices and ginger while stirring. Immediately, add the rice and mung beans while stirring constantly for 5 minutes. Add the water and salt after removing from the heat. Cover and bring to a boil for 10 minutes. Then reduce the heat and cook slowly for 30 minutes at a low heat until soft; adding water if needed. Khichari is not a dry preparation, it is humid and moist.
Note: for Vegans use cold pressed sesame oil instead of ghee

Traditionally, the preparation of Khichari can be modified for each Dosha by changing the ratio of rice to mung dal:
Vata – 1 cup rice to ½ cup dal
Pitta – 1 cup rice to 1 cup dal
Kapha – ½ cup rice to 1 cup dal

## Khichari (faster variant)
Use the same ingredients, but instead of cooking the spices in ghee, put all ingredients directly in cold water. Bring to a boil and cook for 30 minutes over low heat. Serve with a little bit of ghee, or sesame oil for Vegans.

# Chapter Three
## About Using Herbs

There are many common misunderstandings about using herbs to promote health today.

One common misconception is that herbs work like modern medicines in that they target specific places in the body. Medicinal plants, or herbs, have a long history as both medicine and promotors of health in human history. There is little doubt that – when used correctly – herbs can help people recover their health. This being said, it is important to understand that plants do not work in the same way as chemical medicines. Herbs work on homeostasis and metabolism generally. When the whole plant (e.g., the part of the plant traditionally used therapeutically) is used the therapeutic action is general and less specific. This is exactly why using the whole plant is safe, because its action is general and working more on homeostasis than a specific place in the body.

There is trend to change the way that herbs work by making concentrated extracts of the plant and either adding it back into the plant or marketing the extract itself as a product. People wrongly think that the extract is the same as the original herb and is as safe as using the whole plant. This is simply not true. In September 2016, I had the good fortune to meet and hear a lecture from Dr. Rama Jayasundar, who has a PhD from Cambridge in nuclear science. She is using Nuclear Magnetic Resonance (NMR) spectroscopy to understand medicinal plants as per Ayurveda. She has found that the whole plant in water solutions correspond perfectly with traditional

Ayurvedic classification of taste, action, etc. However, when plant extracts were used the classification changed; when alcohol extracts were tested, they also changed. In fact, she found through repeated experimentation that only water solution based preparations of the whole plant (e.g., part of the plant used traditionally for a therapeutic result) matched the classical texts and classifications of the herbs. Dr. Jayasundar is also an Ayurvedic physician and works for the Indian government in research; she is the only person to date with a doctorate in both nuclear physics and Ayurveda.

Traditional healing systems like TCM or Ayurveda have always understood that herbs work in a broad, nonspecific manner. They also have developed many low-tech pharmacological methods to make extracts and increase the potency of herbs. In spite of having the knowledge and skill to do this the main way traditional systems of herbal medicine increased potency was by combining whole plants in formulas. The ancients found this to be a safer, more balanced method of administering herbs. This in turn means that they accepted that herbs should be combined with other herbs in order to target specific locations in the body. This is the approach we use at Ayur-Vidya and the approach I have used in my clinical practice over the last thirty years.

Another misconception is that herbs treat specific diseases. This misunderstanding is much like the first in that modern man is conditioned to think of disease as a fixed set of symptoms. This implies that the absence of symptoms indicates health.

Herbs rarely, if ever, treat specific diseases because a fixed set of symptoms (e.g., disease) is the result of some underlying malfunction of homeostasis or metabolism. In other words, the "disease" is simply what we can see, the cause of the symptoms is often due to a number of factors. Herbs do work very well to help restore health by working on 'homeostasis' (i.e., t*he tendency of the body to seek and maintain a condition of balance or equilibrium within its internal environment, even when faced with external changes*).

According to Ayurvedic medicine the managers of homeostasis are the cause of disease – the three Doshas, or Vata, Pitta and Kapha. When these managers do their job correctly the body stays healthy; when they function poorly, or are disrupted in their work then the homeostasis of the body is disrupted and disease results. Hence, traditional systems of functional health care tended to focus on the underlying causes of disorders rather than on the symptoms. The current obsession with symptoms is a very recent development in medicine and the history of human health care. The unfortunate problem is that people want to use herbs according to the modern trend of medicine and herbs simply do not work well on a set group of symptoms, or 'disease'. That is to say that herbs don't work well as symptomatic medicines. This is why modern studies rarely show medicinal plants as being effective treatments for diseases. Herbs work best when the cause of the disorder is addressed, not the apparent fixed symptoms.

Another misconception common today concerns dosage and the adage that 'more is better'. This is especially a problem in the United States where we see excess as normal.

Most herbs work better in lower doses taken over longer periods of time. Plants are safest when used in lower doses and they also work better to regulate or correct the homeostasis when given in low doses. As I was born in California I have had to work consciously on using lower doses professionally with my patients and with myself. For many years, I followed the trend to use high doses thinking that larger amounts of herbs are going to give 'larger' results. The more I studied Ayurveda the more I noticed that Indians typically use very low doses compared to, say Americans from the USA. Over the last ten years I have slowly been reducing the doses I use professionally. The clinical results are better with lower doses. There are less reactions, less issues concerning digestive problems, and there is an overall better response to correcting homeostasis. I have noted that the Doshas (managers) become disturbed much less when using lower doses vs using high doses of herbs.

Another plus side of using low doses is that it is less expensive and the patients save money. I am constantly indicating doses of 'over the shelf' products (e.g., spirulina, etc.) that are one eighth to one fourth what is indicated on the label. Lower doses are easier to digest and assimilate than higher doses. An old dictum in Ayurveda says, "it is not what you eat, it is what you can digest that gives health".

Still another misunderstanding is that herbs, or herbal preparations, will work well without changing diet and lifestyle. This in itself is the reason many treatments with herbs fail. It is related to the first two misconceptions that 'herbs treat specific locations' and that 'herbs treat disease'.

As noted before herbs work generally in the body to correct underlying disturbances. Whenever possible it is best to treat these disturbances before they manifest as diseases with fixed symptoms. As Benjamin Franklin so aptly put it, "an ounce of prevention is worth a pound of cure". So, using herbs to treat the underlying state, or foundation, of the body is the traditional approach of using herbs. Still further, all traditional forms of health care emphasis diet and lifestyle as the main source of health. Sadly, the symptomatic approach of the 'magic bullet to cure every disease' actively denounces any relation of diet and lifestyle to health. This was (and is) needed to remove the possibility that an individual could actually prevent or cure a disorder by their own effort to eat and live right. As symptomatic medicine is economics based it was / is important to remove the very idea that a patient can improve their health with diet, lifestyle and self-effort. Symptomatic medicine needs unhealthy people to sell pills to; for many years pharmaceutical companies have invested millions in "anti-obesity" medications because it is seen as the next multi-billion-dollar medical gold mine (after HRT).

The fact is that herbs and herbal preparations are not chemicals; they are more like concentrated food. They are not strong enough to overcome a poor diet, or a lifestyle that is not suited to the individual. In order for herbs to work well they need support. We need to make an effort to live in a balanced manner and to eat real food that we can digest. When we support the herbal treatment with diet and lifestyle the results are often incredible; likewise, when we do not change our diet and lifestyle the failure of herbs to make any significant change is often disappointing.

Knowledge is power. Knowing what we want and starting to achieve that goal is empowering. Keeping this in mind we should start where we can. If we are a professional, then we can help the patient to understand that they do not need to change their diet and lifestyle radically in order to take herbs. Or they do not need herbs in order to begin to change diet and lifestyle. The best changes are those made slowly and consciously because we want to feel better. A little change in diet, or a small change in lifestyle is enough to give noticeable results.

Begin with what is possible, if taking herbs is where you can start, start with that. But know also that the more you support the herbal preparations with dietary changes and simple lifestyle changes the better results you will get. If herbs are not your thing, work on diet, or lifestyle, or both. Professionals need to communicate and find out what the patient is able to do and support them. Remember that herbs are not 'magic bullets' and will do their job slowly, but surely if supported.

# Chapter Four
# List of Disorders

This section is the main part of this book on how to use and understand the formulas Ayur-Vidya™ offers to both practitioners and the public. If you have not already read the early parts of this book I strongly suggest doing so before trying to use the following formulas. Remember that herbs are not 'magic bullets' and need diet and lifestyle changes to work correctly.

There are over 200 disorders which are common today listed in the following pages. The idea in Ayurveda is to try and discover the Dosha that is causing the disorder. Hence, for almost all disorders there are three formulas, one for Vata, Pitta, or Kapha. It is common that two or even three Doshas are involved in the problem. Protocol is to try and treat the first Dosha to become disrupted. If the treatment does not work it is because we have not targeted the 'right' Dosha, or Dosha that started the pathology. If after one month of treatment no significant change is noted, then try the second Dosha involved in the pathology.

If you feel that there are two Doshas in the pathology equally I suggest using a diet / lifestyle for the two Doshas, or for Mixed Types. For example, if you feel you have a Vata and Kapha disorder use the diet and lifestyle for the Vata / Kapha Dual or Mixed Type – a strict diet if symptoms are strong, or a more open Prakriti diet if symptoms are mild. Then use the herbal formulas for the stronger of the two Doshas; usually this is Vata if Vata is one of the two Doshas, followed by Pitta, and then Kapha.

In Ayurveda, a Dosha that causes a disorder has "ja" added to it. This means a "Vataja" blend will treat Vata Dosha as the cause of the disorder; Pittaja as the cause; Kaphaja as the cause.

## Understanding the logic of Ayur-Vidya™ formulas

Ayur-Vidya™ formulas as based on classical pharmacology in Ayurveda. Most Ayurvedic formulas use equal amounts of herbs, sometimes favoring the major herb or primary with greater ratios in the formula.

The formulas presented by Ayur-Vidya™ follow this logic, mainly an equal quantity of herbs in each formula. This means when you use the blend of 401 plus 406 you are getting an equal amount of six herbs (i.e., 16.66% of each herb). Sometimes, in order to better target the causal Dosha, a primary herb is used with a blend. For example, the single herb 201 with the blend 405 would target Pachaka Pitta more than 405 alone, because this mix would give 50% of 201 and 16.66% of the three herbs in 405.

While at first glance these formulas may seem simplistic or illogical they are based on a 29-year study of classic Ayurvedic formulas. The main difference in these formulas is not the logic, nor the ratio blends; it is the use of Western herbs in the series 400. Every effort has been made to use the maximum amount of local (North American) botanicals in the Ayur-Vidya™ blends. This is because classical Ayurvedic texts tell us to use food and herbs from our local environment because they are better adapted to our body's needs. This is what we are presenting to you as an individual or as a professional health care provider: an Ayurvedic treatment approach adapted to North American people.

NOTE: As with all herbal remedies, allergic reactions are possible. If there are signs of allergic reactions, stop treatment and seek medical advice. Ayur-Vidya™ does not recommend the use of our formulas without medical supervision if pregnant, breast-feeding or when giving to children under the age of sixteen. Do not mix Ayur-Vidya™ preparations with medications; consult your doctor if unsure.

All blends of herbs can be found on our website:
www.ayur-vidya.com

## Abdominal distention

| Dosha | Code | Common Name | Latin Name |
|-------|------|-------------|------------|
| Vataja | 401 | Cumin | Cumimum cyminum |
| | | Fennel | Foeniculum vulgare |
| | | Cardamom | Elettaria cardamomum |
| | 407 | Turmeric | Curcuma longa |
| | | Barberry | Berberis vulgaris |
| | | Dandelion | Taraxacum officinale |
| Pittaja | 402 | Coriander | Coriandrum sativum |
| | | Cumin | Cumimum cyminum |
| | | Fennel | Foeniculum vulgare |
| | 407 | Turmeric | Curcuma longa |
| | | Barberry | Berberis vulgaris |
| | | Dandelion | Taraxacum officinale |
| Kaphaja | 403 | Ginger | Zingiber officinale |
| | | Cumin | Cumimum cyminum |
| | | Fenugreek | Trigonella foenum-graecum |
| | 407 | Turmeric | Curcuma longa |
| | | Barberry | Berberis vulgaris |
| | | Dandelion | Taraxacum officinale |

| Dosha | Low Dose | High Dose |
|-------|----------|-----------|
| Vata | 1 of each X2 per day before meals | 2 of each X2 per day before meals |
| Pitta | 1 of each X2 per day with meals | 2 of each X2 per day with meals |
| Kapha | 2 of each X2 per day after meals | 3 of each X2 per day after meals |

## Description:

Abdominal distention is Vataja by function and Kaphaja by location. It can also be Pittaja if there are signs of acidity or heat. The bloating or distention is Vata Roga, therefore all formulas work on Samana Vayu and the causal Dosha.

Use the Vataja herbs if Vata is predominant in the Vikriti (imbalance) with a Vata Vikriti diet / lifestyle.

Use the Pittaja herbs if Pitta is predominant in the Vikriti (imbalance) with a Pitta Vikriti diet / lifestyle.

Use the Kaphaja herbs if Kapha is predominant in the Vikriti (imbalance) with a Kapha Vikriti diet / lifestyle.

## Abdominal pain

| Dosha | Code | Common Name | Latin Name |
|---|---|---|---|
| **Vataja** | 404 | Angelica | Angelica archangelica |
| | | Wild yam | Dioscorea villosa |
| | | Valerian | Valeriana officinalis |
| | 301 | Amalaki | Emblica officinalis |
| | | Bibhitaki | Terminalia belerica |
| | | Haritaki | Terminalia chebula |
| **Pittaja** | 405 | Burdock | Arctium lappa |
| | | Yellow dock | Rumex crispus |
| | | Milk Thistle | Silybum marianum |
| | 301 | Amalaki | Emblica officinalis |
| | | Bibhitaki | Terminalia belerica |
| | | Haritaki | Terminalia chebula |
| **Kaphaja** | 405 | Burdock | Arctium lappa |
| | | Yellow dock | Rumex crispus |
| | | Milk Thistle | Silybum marianum |
| | 301 | Amalaki | Emblica officinalis |
| | | Bibhitaki | Terminalia belerica |
| | | Haritaki | Terminalia chebula |

| Dosha | Low Dose | High Dose |
|---|---|---|
| **Vata** | 1 of each X2 per day before meals | 2 of each X2 per day before meals |
| **Pitta** | 1 of each X2 per day with meals | 2 of each X2 per day with meals |
| **Kapha** | 2 of each X2 per day after meals | 3 of each X2 per day after meals |

## Description:

Abdominal pain is Vataja by function. Depending on where the pain is located it can be Kaphaja (stomach), Pittaja (small intestine), or Vataja (colon) by location. The main goal of this formula is to reduce Apana Vayu, secondary Samana Vayu and then the causal Dosha. This disorder is classified as a Vata Roga condition.

Use the Vataja herbs if Vata is predominant in the Vikriti (imbalance) with a Vata Vikriti diet / lifestyle.

Use the Pittaja herbs if Pitta is predominant in the Vikriti (imbalance) with a Pitta Vikriti diet / lifestyle.

Use the Kaphaja herbs if Kapha is predominant in the Vikriti (imbalance) with a Kapha Vikriti diet / lifestyle.

## Acidity (heart burn)

| Dosha | Code | Common Name | Latin Name |
|---|---|---|---|
| Vataja | 201 | Amalaki | Emblica officinalis |
| | 210 | Shankhpushpi | Convolvulus pluricaulis |
| | 211 | Shatavari | Asparagus racemosus |
| Pittaja | 201 | Amalaki | Emblica officinalis |
| | 405 | Burdock | Arctium lappa |
| | | Yellow dock | Rumex crispus |
| | | Milk Thistle | Silybum marianum |
| Kaphaja | 201 | Amalaki | Emblica officinalis |
| | 407 | Turmeric | Curcuma longa |
| | | Barberry | Berberis vulgaris |
| | | Dandelion | Taraxacum officinale |

| Dosha | Low Dose | High Dose |
|---|---|---|
| Vata | 1 of each X2 per day before meals | 2 of each X2 per day before meals |
| Pitta | 1 of each X2 per day with meals | 2 of each X2 per day with meals |
| Kapha | 2 of each X2 per day after meals | 3 of each X2 per day after meals |

## Description:

Acidity is a Pitta Roga disorder by function and location. Pitta be aggravated by itself (Pittaja) or the acidity can be Vataja or Kaphaja through stress or congestion respectively. This formula works on Pachaka Pitta and the causal Dosha. Avoid fried, pungent, acidic and fermented foods during the first two weeks of treatment, a Pitta diet, then follow the diet as per Vikriti.

Use the Vataja herbs if Vata is predominant in the Vikriti (imbalance) with a Vata Vikriti diet / lifestyle.

Use the Pittaja herbs if Pitta is predominant in the Vikriti (imbalance) with a Pitta Vikriti diet / lifestyle.

Use the Kaphaja herbs if Kapha is predominant in the Vikriti (imbalance) with a Kapha Vikriti diet / lifestyle.

## Acne

| Dosha | Code | Common Name | Latin Name |
|---|---|---|---|
| **Vataja** | 401 | Cumin | Cumimum cyminum |
| | | Fennel | Foeniculum vulgare |
| | | Cardamom | Elettaria cardamomum |
| | 407 | Turmeric | Curcuma longa |
| | | Barberry | Berberis vulgaris |
| | | Dandelion | Taraxacum officinale |
| | 408 | Vitex | Vitex agnus-castus |
| | | Black cohosh | Cimicifuga racemosa |
| | | Cramp bark | Viburnum opulus |
| **Pittaja** | 402 | Coriander | Coriandrum sativum |
| | | Cumin | Cumimum cyminum |
| | | Fennel | Foeniculum vulgare |
| | 405 | Burdock | Arctium lappa |
| | | Yellow dock | Rumex crispus |
| | | Milk Thistle | Silybum marianum |
| | 208 | Manjishta | Rubia cordifolia |
| **Kaphaja** | 403 | Ginger | Zingiber officinale |
| | | Cumin | Cumimum cyminum |
| | | Fenugreek | Trigonella foenum-graecum |
| | 408 | Vitex | Vitex agnus-castus |
| | | Black cohosh | Cimicifuga racemosa |
| | | Cramp bark | Viburnum opulus |
| | 209 | Punarnava | Boerhaavia diffusa |

| Dosha | Low Dose | High Dose |
|---|---|---|
| **Vata** | 1 of each X2 per day before meals | 2 of each X2 per day before meals |
| **Pitta** | 1 of each X2 per day with meals | 2 of each X2 per day with meals |
| **Kapha** | 2 of each X2 per day after meals | 3 of each X2 per day after meals |

## Description:

There are many causes to Acne, from diet to endocrine imbalance. Any Dosha can cause this disorder, use the formula as per Vikriti.

Use the Vataja herbs if Vata is predominant in the Vikriti (imbalance) with a Vata Vikriti diet / lifestyle.

Use the Pittaja herbs if Pitta is predominant in the Vikriti (imbalance) with a Pitta Vikriti diet / lifestyle.

Use the Kaphaja herbs if Kapha is predominant in the Vikriti (imbalance) with a Kapha Vikriti diet / lifestyle.

## Adrenal weakness

| Dosha | Code | Common Name | Latin Name |
|---|---|---|---|
| **Vataja** | 205 | Gokshura | Tribulus terrestris |
| | 301 | Amalaki | Emblica officinalis |
| | | Bibhitaki | Terminalia belerica |
| | | Haritaki | Terminalia chebula |
| | 409 | Marshmallow | Althaea officinalis |
| | | Gotu kola | Centella asiatica |
| | | Stinging nettles | Urtica dioica |
| **Pittaja** | 205 | Gokshura | Tribulus terrestris |
| | 208 | Manjishta | Rubia cordifolia |
| | 402 | Coriander | Coriandrum sativum |
| | | Cumin | Cumimum cyminum |
| | | Fennel | Foeniculum vulgare |
| | 409 | Marshmallow | Althaea officinalis |
| | | Gotu kola | Centella asiatica |
| | | Stinging nettles | Urtica dioica |
| **Kaphaja** | 208 | Manjishta | Tribulus terrestris |
| | 209 | Punarnava | Boerhaavia diffusa |
| | 403 | Ginger | Zingiber officinale |
| | | Cumin | Cumimum cyminum |
| | | Fenugreek | Trigonella foenum-graecum |
| | 409 | Marshmallow | Althaea officinalis |
| | | Gotu kola | Centella asiatica |
| | | Stinging nettles | Urtica dioica |

| Dosha | Low Dose | High Dose |
|---|---|---|
| **Vata** | 1 of each X2 per day before meals | 2 of each X2 per day before meals |
| **Pitta** | 1 of each X2 per day with meals | 2 of each X2 per day with meals |
| **Kapha** | 2 of each X2 per day after meals | 3 of each X2 per day after meals |

## Description:

The Adrenal glands are part of Meda Dhatu so Kapha Roga by structure and Vata by function. These formulas treat the causal Dosha.

Use the Vataja herbs if Vata is predominant in the Vikriti (imbalance) with a Vata Vikriti diet / lifestyle.

Use the Pittaja herbs if Pitta is predominant in the Vikriti (imbalance) with a Pitta Vikriti diet / lifestyle.

Use the Kaphaja herbs if Kapha is predominant in the Vikriti (imbalance) with a Kapha Vikriti diet / lifestyle.

## Agni (imbalanced)

| Dosha | Code | Common Name | Latin Name |
|---|---|---|---|
| Vataja | 401 | Cumin | Cumimum cyminum |
| | | Fennel | Foeniculum vulgare |
| | | Cardamom | Elettaria cardamomum |
| | 404 | Angelica | Angelica archangelica |
| | | Wild yam | Dioscorea villosa |
| | | Valerian | Valeriana officinalis |
| Pittaja | 402 | Coriander | Coriandrum sativum |
| | | Cumin | Cumimum cyminum |
| | | Fennel | Foeniculum vulgare |
| | 405 | Burdock | Arctium lappa |
| | | Yellow dock | Rumex crispus |
| | | Milk Thistle | Silybum marianum |
| Kaphaja | 403 | Ginger | Zingiber officinale |
| | | Cumin | Cumimum cyminum |
| | | Fenugreek | Trigonella foenum-graecum |
| | 406 | Myrrh | Commiphora myrrha |
| | | Elecampane | Inula helenium |
| | | Yellow dock | Rumex crispus |

| Dosha | Low Dose | High Dose |
|---|---|---|
| Vata | 1 of each X2 per day before meals | 2 of each X2 per day before meals |
| Pitta | 1 of each X2 per day with meals | 2 of each X2 per day with meals |
| Kapha | 2 of each X2 per day after meals | 3 of each X2 per day after meals |

## Description:

Any Dosha can disrupt Agni function. Agni is controlled by Pachaka Pitta, Samana Vayu and Kledaka Kapha. When there is Vishama Agni use the Vataja blend; there is Tikshna Agni use the Pittaja blend; and when there is Munda Agni use the Kaphaja blend of herbs. This will target the correct sub-Dosha and balance Agni. (see Ama)

Use the Vataja herbs if Vata is predominant in the Vikriti (imbalance) with a Vata Vikriti diet / lifestyle.

Use the Pittaja herbs if Pitta is predominant in the Vikriti (imbalance) with a Pitta Vikriti diet / lifestyle.

Use the Kaphaja herbs if Kapha is predominant in the Vikriti (imbalance) with a Kapha Vikriti diet / lifestyle.

## AIDS (or Cachexia)

| Dosha | Code | Common Name | Latin Name |
|---|---|---|---|
| Vataja | 203 | Ashwagandha | Withania somnifera |
| | 206 | Guduchi | Tinospora cordifolia |
| | 212 | Pau d'arco | Tabebuia impetiginosa |
| | 301 | Amalaki | Emblica officinalis |
| | | Bibhitaki | Terminalia belerica |
| | | Haritaki | Terminalia chebula |
| Pittaja | 201 | Amalaki | Emblica officinalis |
| | 206 | Guduchi | Tinospora cordifolia |
| | 212 | Pau d'arco | Tabebuia impetiginosa |
| | 301 | Amalaki | Emblica officinalis |
| | | Bibhitaki | Terminalia belerica |
| | | Haritaki | Terminalia chebula |
| Kaphaja | 206 | Guduchi | Tinospora cordifolia |
| | 209 | Punarnava | Boerhaavia diffusa |
| | 212 | Pau d'arco | Tabebuia impetiginosa |
| | 301 | Amalaki | Emblica officinalis |
| | | Bibhitaki | Terminalia belerica |
| | | Haritaki | Terminalia chebula |

| Dosha | Low Dose | High Dose |
|---|---|---|
| Vata | 1 of each X2 per day before meals | 2 of each X2 per day before meals |
| Pitta | 1 of each X2 per day with meals | 2 of each X2 per day with meals |
| Kapha | 2 of each X2 per day after meals | 3 of each X2 per day after meals |

## Description:

Acquired immune deficiency syndrome or acquired immunodeficiency syndrome (AIDS) is a set of symptoms and infections resulting from the damage to the human immune system caused by the human immunodeficiency virus (HIV). This condition progressively reduces the effectiveness of the immune system and leaves individuals susceptible to opportunistic infections. HIV is transmitted through direct contact of a mucous membrane or the bloodstream with a bodily fluid containing HIV, such as blood, semen, vaginal fluid, pre-seminal fluid, and breast milk. Antiretroviral treatment reduces both the mortality and the morbidity of HIV infection, but these drugs are expensive and routine access to antiretroviral medication is not available in all countries. Due to the difficulty in treating HIV infection, preventing infection is a key aim in controlling AIDS.

Cachexia or wasting syndrome is loss of weight, muscle atrophy, fatigue, weakness, and significant loss of appetite in someone who is not actively trying to lose weight. The formal definition of cachexia is the loss of body mass that cannot be reversed nutritionally: Even if the affected patient eats more calories, lean body mass will be lost, indicating a primary pathology is in place. Cachexia can be seen in patients with cancer, AIDS, chronic obstructive lung disease, multiple sclerosis, congestive heart failure, tuberculosis, familial amyloid polyneuropathy, mercury poisoning, heavy metal poisoning and hormonal deficiency.

In Ayurvedic medicine these kinds of disorders are related to poor lifestyle choices, poor diets and low immunity, or Ojas. Usually all Doshas are implicated in this kind of pathology, therefore it is advised to follow the Prakriti of the patient; if this is not known treat the dominate Dosha of Vikriti. These blends can be used as a starting point for building immunity and increasing nutrient absorption in the intestines. These herbal blends build Ojas and Shukra Dhatu as per Prakriti.

Care needs to be given regarding Agni and Ama formation when using these blends as they are heavy to digest. It is best to begin with a low dose and work up to the higher dose over one month. These blends can be used when there is a small amount of Ama present on the tongue as there are enough digestives to help remove Ama. These blends are safe to use for several years, the minimum time for treatment would be three months.

Use the Vataja herbs if Vata is predominant in the Prakriti with a Vata Prakriti diet / lifestyle.

Use the Pittaja herbs if Pitta is predominant in the Prakriti with a Pitta Prakriti diet / lifestyle.

Use the Kaphaja herbs if Kapha is predominant in the Prakriti with a Kapha Prakriti diet / lifestyle.

## Alzheimer's

| Dosha | Code | Common Name | Latin Name |
|---|---|---|---|
| Vataja | 203 | Ashwagandha | Withania somnifera |
| | 206 | Guduchi | Tinospora cordifolia |
| | 211 | Shatavari | Asparagus racemosus |
| | 301 | Amalaki | Emblica officinalis |
| | | Bibhitaki | Terminalia belerica |
| | | Haritaki | Terminalia chebula |
| Pittaja | 203 | Ashwagandha | Withania somnifera |
| | 206 | Guduchi | Tinospora cordifolia |
| | 208 | Manjishta | Rubia cordifolia |
| | 301 | Amalaki | Emblica officinalis |
| | | Bibhitaki | Terminalia belerica |
| | | Haritaki | Terminalia chebula |
| Kaphaja | 203 | Ashwagandha | Withania somnifera |
| | 206 | Guduchi | Tinospora cordifolia |
| | 209 | Punarnava | Boerhaavia diffusa |
| | 301 | Amalaki | Emblica officinalis |
| | | Bibhitaki | Terminalia belerica |
| | | Haritaki | Terminalia chebula |

| Dosha | Low Dose | High Dose |
|---|---|---|
| Vata | 1 of each X2 per day before meals | 2 of each X2 per day before meals |
| Pitta | 1 of each X2 per day with meals | 2 of each X2 per day with meals |
| Kapha | 2 of each X2 per day after meals | 3 of each X2 per day after meals |

## Description:

In Ayurveda, there are two clear causes of Alzheimer's disease. One of them is related to Vata Dosha and the other to Pitta Dosha. An additional factor is the presence of Ama and a general malfunction of Agni.

When there is chronic Vata Vriddhi Majja Dhatu is dried out and becomes weakened by the dry attributes of Vata. Majja Pāka is reduced by this dryness; this is a major contributor to neuron and synapse loss in the brain and the development of plaque accumulation. The biochemistry is controlled by Pitta and Agni on both a general and specific level. The malfunction of Majja Dhatu Agni will cause the amyloid precursor protein (APP) to be divided. This results directly in the formation of plaque in the brain tissue. Ayurvedic protocol indicates that if the Majja Dhatu Agni is not functioning correctly then the primary, or Jathar Agni, is also compromised; this would result in the formation of Ama in both the digestive level and Dhatu level.

Ama accumulation in the Dhatus is a primary causal factor of tissue degeneration and plaque formation. Modern medicine notes that poor diet is a contributing factor, but has been unable to understand exactly why or how it accelerates this disorder. Unhealthy diets are linked to poorly educated populations and this also reflects in the rates of Alzheimer's among the under privileged. Therefore, diet and lifestyle are the main therapies for Alzheimer's disease both in prevention and treatment.

If there is no real apparent Vikriti, of if the Vikriti seems relatively minor, treatment can follow the Prakriti of the person. The first approach would be to treat any Vikriti manifestations if there are any. If you remain unclear and have no clear indications through the text or through observation then treat Vata with the Vataja blend of herbs, diet and lifestyle as Vata Dosha controls old age and aging in general.

Use the Vataja herbs if Vata is predominant in the Vikriti (imbalance) with a Vata Vikriti diet / lifestyle.

Use the Pittaja herbs if Pitta is predominant in the Vikriti (imbalance) with a Pitta Vikriti diet / lifestyle.

Use the Kaphaja herbs if Kapha is predominant in the Vikriti (imbalance) with a Kapha Vikriti diet / lifestyle.

## Ama (to remove undigested food)

| Dosha | Code | Common Name | Latin Name |
|---|---|---|---|
| Vataja | 401 | Cumin | Cumimum cyminum |
| | | Fennel | Foeniculum vulgare |
| | | Cardamom | Elettaria cardamomum |
| | 407 | Turmeric | Curcuma longa |
| | | Barberry | Berberis vulgaris |
| | | Dandelion | Taraxacum officinale |
| Pittaja | 402 | Coriander | Coriandrum sativum |
| | | Cumin | Cumimum cyminum |
| | | Fennel | Foeniculum vulgare |
| | 407 | Turmeric | Curcuma longa |
| | | Barberry | Berberis vulgaris |
| | | Dandelion | Taraxacum officinale |
| Kaphaja | 403 | Ginger | Zingiber officinale |
| | | Cumin | Cumimum cyminum |
| | | Fenugreek | Trigonella foenum-graecum |
| | 407 | Turmeric | Curcuma longa |
| | | Barberry | Berberis vulgaris |
| | | Dandelion | Taraxacum officinale |

| Dosha | Low Dose | High Dose |
|---|---|---|
| Vata | 1 of each X2 per day before meals | 2 of each X2 per day before meals |
| Pitta | 1 of each X2 per day with meals | 2 of each X2 per day with meals |
| Kapha | 2 of each X2 per day after meals | 3 of each X2 per day after meals |

## Description:

Ama is the result of poor Agni function, which is the result of poor Dosha function. Hence, any Dosha can cause Ama to form in the body. When there is Vishama Agni use the Vataja blend; there is Tikshna Agni use the Pittaja blend; and when there is Munda Agni use the Kaphaja blend of herbs. This will target the correct sub-Dosha and balance Agni. These blends will also remove the Ama that has accumulated in the digestive system. Modifying diet and reducing heavy foods during treatment is needed to achieve good results.

These formulas can also be used when there is low energy, Chronic Fatigue Syndrome (CFS), low immunity due to toxins, headaches due to toxins, gas, bloating, indigestion due to Ama, food allergies and any other kind of Ama problem. This formula will also have a secondary effect to clear and clean Rasa Dhatu and Meda

Dhatu and will help to remove Ama from these locations and their Srotas over time. It is also good idea to use the digestive tea made with fresh ginger to increase the effectiveness of this formula. Use this blend from one to three months on the average and not more than six months at one time.

According to Ayurveda roughly eighty percent of disease are due to the accumulation of Ama in the body. If we imagine that our body is able to digest ninety-nine percent of our food, what happens to the other one percent? Using the image of one drop of water as the one percent we do not digest can be useful to visualize the Ayurvedic point of view. One drop of water per meal per week (3 x 7 = 21) times 52 weeks in a year (21 x 52 = 1092) is 1092 drops of water. As a quart of water has 18,927.06 drops (or 20,000 drops per liter) it only takes 17.33 years for us to build up a quart of 'water'. Using this analogy of a drop of water we can see that if our digestion is strong and healthy, e.g., digesting ninety-nine percent of our food, we still end up accumulating a quart of Ama after seventeen years.

It does not take much to figure out that if we have weak or chronic digestive problems that the rate of accumulating Ama can be much faster than seventeen years. Hence, many ancient cultures throughout the world have suggested fasting once or twice a year to remove this undigested food.

Use the Vataja herbs if Vata is predominant in the Vikriti (imbalance) with a Vata Vikriti diet / lifestyle.

Use the Pittaja herbs if Pitta is predominant in the Vikriti (imbalance) with a Pitta Vikriti diet / lifestyle.

Use the Kaphaja herbs if Kapha is predominant in the Vikriti (imbalance) with a Kapha Vikriti diet / lifestyle.

## Amenorrhea

| Dosha | Code | Common Name | Latin Name |
|-------|------|-------------|------------|
| Vataja | 211 | Shatavari | Asparagus racemosus |
| | 401 | Cumin | Cumimum cyminum |
| | | Fennel | Foeniculum vulgare |
| | | Cardamom | Elettaria cardamomum |
| | 408 | Vitex | Vitex agnus-castus |
| | | Black cohosh | Cimicifuga racemosa |
| | | Cramp bark | Viburnum opulus |
| Pittaja | 208 | Manjishta | Rubia cordifolia |
| | 402 | Coriander | Coriandrum sativum |
| | | Cumin | Cumimum cyminum |
| | | Fennel | Foeniculum vulgare |
| | 405 | Burdock | Arctium lappa |
| | | Yellow dock | Rumex crispus |
| | | Milk Thistle | Silybum marianum |
| | 408 | Vitex | Vitex agnus-castus |
| | | Black cohosh | Cimicifuga racemosa |
| | | Cramp bark | Viburnum opulus |
| Kaphaja | 208 | Manjishta | Rubia cordifolia |
| | 403 | Ginger | Zingiber officinale |
| | | Cumin | Cumimum cyminum |
| | | Fenugreek | Trigonella foenum-graecum |
| | 406 | Myrrh | Commiphora myrrha |
| | | Elecampane | Inula helenium |
| | | Yellow dock | Rumex crispus |
| | 408 | Vitex | Vitex agnus-castus |
| | | Black cohosh | Cimicifuga racemosa |
| | | Cramp bark | Viburnum opulus |

| Dosha | Low Dose | High Dose |
|-------|----------|-----------|
| Vata | 1 of each X2 per day before meals | 2 of each X2 per day before meals |
| Pitta | 1 of each X2 per day with meals | 2 of each X2 per day with meals |
| Kapha | 2 of each X2 per day after meals | 3 of each X2 per day after meals |

## Description:

These formulas work well in short term conditions (six months or less) for Secondary Amenorrhea. This disorder is usually either Vataja or Kaphaja; e.g., by function or location. Ayurveda sees one cause of amenorrhea as being a constriction, or lack of movement, of Apana

Vayu in Artavavahasrota. Prana Vayu may also be involved if there is a hormone imbalance. The constriction of Apana Vayu will stop the flow of Artava in Artavavahasrota. While promoting menstrual flow (Artava or *Rajah*) is good, herbs that move Apana Vayu and reduce Vata Vriddhi should be the main focus. Also, one should try to determine why Vata (Apana Vayu) has become increased and disturbed in the first place.

As Kapha controls Rasa Dhatu and the menstrual fluid is the Upadhatu of Rasa Dhatu Amenorrhea can be due to low levels of Rasa Dhatu. Verify the state of Kapha and Rasa Dhatu. If Kapha is not working properly there could be an insufficiency of Rasa Dhatu. This is common for women who are too thin for their body height / weight ratio (for example professional athletes). In other words, women with low Rasa often suffer from Amenorrhea as there is no Upadhatu to make the menstrual fluid.

There are occasionally Pittaja types of Amenorrhea in which Pitta has increased in Rakta Dhatu and causes acidic types of congestion. Because the uterus and vagina are part of Rakta Dhatu this congestion in Rakta Dhatu can cause acidic congestion in the uterus preventing Artava from flowing through and out of the vagina. This is rarer and the woman would show signs of excess heat and possible inflammation in the pelvic area.

Amenorrhea can be the symptom of another more serious problem. Correct diagnosis is important and it is strongly suggested that women consult their gynecologist to know what the cause may be before trying Ayurvedic treatments. This is especially true for Primary Amenorrhea.

Use the Vataja herbs if Vata is predominant in the Vikriti (imbalance) with a Vata Vikriti diet / lifestyle.
Use the Pittaja herbs if Pitta is predominant in the Vikriti (imbalance) with a Pitta Vikriti diet / lifestyle.
Use the Kaphaja herbs if Kapha is predominant in the Vikriti (imbalance) with a Kapha Vikriti diet / lifestyle.

## Anemia

| Dosha | Code | Common Name | Latin Name |
|---|---|---|---|
| Vataja | 209 | Punarnava | Boerhaavia diffusa |
| | 301 | Amalaki | Emblica officinalis |
| | | Bibhitaki | Terminalia belerica |
| | | Haritaki | Terminalia chebula |
| | 404 | Angelica | Angelica archangelica |
| | | Wild yam | Dioscorea villosa |
| | | Valerian | Valeriana officinalis |
| Pittaja | 208 | Manjishta | Rubia cordifolia |
| | 301 | Amalaki | Emblica officinalis |
| | | Bibhitaki | Terminalia belerica |
| | | Haritaki | Terminalia chebula |
| | 405 | Burdock | Arctium lappa |
| | | Yellow dock | Rumex crispus |
| | | Milk Thistle | Silybum marianum |
| Kaphaja | 209 | Punarnava | Boerhaavia diffusa |
| | 301 | Amalaki | Emblica officinalis |
| | | Bibhitaki | Terminalia belerica |
| | | Haritaki | Terminalia chebula |
| | 406 | Myrrh | Commiphora myrrha |
| | | Elecampane | Inula helenium |
| | | Yellow dock | Rumex crispus |

| Dosha | Low Dose | High Dose |
|---|---|---|
| Vata | 1 of each X2 per day before meals | 2 of each X2 per day before meals |
| Pitta | 1 of each X2 per day with meals | 2 of each X2 per day with meals |
| Kapha | 2 of each X2 per day after meals | 3 of each X2 per day after meals |

## Description:

Anemia is a Pitta Roga problem by location; Rakta Dhatu (liver). Functionally it can be Vataja, Pittaja or Kaphaja so use the blend as per Vikriti.

Use the Vataja herbs if Vata is predominant in the Vikriti (imbalance) with a Vata Vikriti diet / lifestyle.

Use the Pittaja herbs if Pitta is predominant in the Vikriti (imbalance) with a Pitta Vikriti diet / lifestyle.

Use the Kaphaja herbs if Kapha is predominant in the Vikriti (imbalance) with a Kapha Vikriti diet / lifestyle.

## Angina

| Dosha | Code | Common Name | Latin Name |
|---|---|---|---|
| Vataja | 202 | Arjuna | Terminalia arjuna |
| | 203 | Ashwagandha | Withania somnifera |
| | 401 | Cumin | Cumimum cyminum |
| | | Fennel | Foeniculum vulgare |
| | | Cardamom | Elettaria cardamomum |
| Pittaja | 202 | Arjuna | Terminalia arjuna |
| | 208 | Manjishta | Rubia cordifolia |
| | 402 | Coriander | Coriandrum sativum |
| | | Cumin | Cumimum cyminum |
| | | Fennel | Foeniculum vulgare |
| Kaphaja | 202 | Arjuna | Terminalia arjuna |
| | 209 | Punarnava | Boerhaavia diffusa |
| | 403 | Ginger | Zingiber officinale |
| | | Cumin | Cumimum cyminum |
| | | Fenugreek | Trigonella foenum-graecum |

| Dosha | Low Dose | High Dose |
|---|---|---|
| Vata | 1 of each X2 per day before meals | 2 of each X2 per day before meals |
| Pitta | 1 of each X2 per day with meals | 2 of each X2 per day with meals |
| Kapha | 2 of each X2 per day after meals | 3 of each X2 per day after meals |

## Description:

Angina is caused by reduced blood flow to the heart muscle. The most common cause of reduced blood flow to the heart is Coronary Artery Disease (CAD). The heart muscle is controlled by Kapha, the heart function is controlled by Pitta, and the nervous plexus is controlled by Vata. The heart is part of Rakta Dhatu and any Dosha can cause this problem functionally. It is best to understand why the problem is expressing itself. These blends work best in early stages.

Use the Vataja herbs if Vata is predominant in the Vikriti (imbalance) with a Vata Vikriti diet / lifestyle.

Use the Pittaja herbs if Pitta is predominant in the Vikriti (imbalance) with a Pitta Vikriti diet / lifestyle.

Use the Kaphaja herbs if Kapha is predominant in the Vikriti (imbalance) with a Kapha Vikriti diet / lifestyle.

## Anorexia

| Dosha | Code | Common Name | Latin Name |
|-------|------|-------------|------------|
| Vataja | 211 | Shatavari | Asparagus racemosus |
| | 401 | Cumin | Cumimum cyminum |
| | | Fennel | Foeniculum vulgare |
| | | Cardamom | Elettaria cardamomum |
| | 404 | Angelica | Angelica archangelica |
| | | Wild yam | Dioscorea villosa |
| | | Valerian | Valeriana officinalis |
| Pittaja | 201 | Amalaki | Emblica officinalis |
| | 211 | Shatavari | Asparagus racemosus |
| | 402 | Coriander | Coriandrum sativum |
| | | Cumin | Cumimum cyminum |
| | | Fennel | Foeniculum vulgare |
| Kaphaja | 203 | Ashwagandha | Withania somnifera |
| | 403 | Ginger | Zingiber officinale |
| | | Cumin | Cumimum cyminum |
| | | Fenugreek | Trigonella foenum-graecum |

| Dosha | Low Dose | High Dose |
|-------|----------|-----------|
| Vata | 1 of each X2 per day before meals | 2 of each X2 per day before meals |
| Pitta | 1 of each X2 per day with meals | 2 of each X2 per day with meals |
| Kapha | 2 of each X2 per day after meals | 3 of each X2 per day after meals |

## Description:

The exact cause of anorexia nervosa is unknown in modern medicine. As with many diseases, it may be a combination of biological, psychological and sociological factors. Ayurveda classifies this disorder as Vataja functionally and capable of damaging any or all structures (Dhatu) of the body. Left untreated it can result in death. It is strongly recommended for the person to consult a psychologist specialized in eating disorders as this problem requires individualized attention and support. Use the blend as per Vikriti.

Use the Vataja herbs if Vata is predominant in the Vikriti (imbalance) with a Vata Vikriti diet / lifestyle.

Use the Pittaja herbs if Pitta is predominant in the Vikriti (imbalance) with a Pitta Vikriti diet / lifestyle.

Use the Kaphaja herbs if Kapha is predominant in the Vikriti (imbalance) with a Kapha Vikriti diet / lifestyle.

## Anxiety

| Dosha | Code | Common Name | Latin Name |
|-------|------|-------------|------------|
| **Vataja** | 207 | Haritaki | Terminalia chebula |
| | 210 | Shankhpushpi | Convolvulus pluricaulis |
| | 404 | Angelica | Angelica archangelica |
| | | Wild yam | Dioscorea villosa |
| | | Valerian | Valeriana officinalis |
| | 410 | Passion flower | Passiflora incarnata |
| | | Skullcap | Scutellaria lateriflora |
| | | Gotu kola | Centella asiatica |
| **Pittaja** | 204 | Bramhi | Bacopa monnieri |
| | 402 | Coriander | Coriandrum sativum |
| | | Cumin | Cumimum cyminum |
| | | Fennel | Foeniculum vulgare |
| | 410 | Passion flower | Passiflora incarnata |
| | | Skullcap | Scutellaria lateriflora |
| | | Gotu kola | Centella asiatica |
| **Kaphaja** | 204 | Bramhi | Bacopa monnieri |
| | 403 | Ginger | Zingiber officinale |
| | | Cumin | Cumimum cyminum |
| | | Fenugreek | Trigonella foenum-graecum |
| | 410 | Passion flower | Passiflora incarnata |
| | | Skullcap | Scutellaria lateriflora |
| | | Gotu kola | Centella asiatica |

| Dosha | Low Dose | High Dose |
|-------|----------|-----------|
| **Vata** | 1 of each X2 per day before meals | 2 of each X2 per day before meals |
| **Pitta** | 1 of each X2 per day with meals | 2 of each X2 per day with meals |
| **Kapha** | 2 of each X2 per day after meals | 3 of each X2 per day after meals |

## Description:

Anxiety is Vata Roga caused by any of the Doshas. Treatment should follow the dominant Vikriti.

Use the Vataja herbs if Vata is predominant in the Vikriti (imbalance) with a Vata Vikriti diet / lifestyle.

Use the Pittaja herbs if Pitta is predominant in the Vikriti (imbalance) with a Pitta Vikriti diet / lifestyle.

Use the Kaphaja herbs if Kapha is predominant in the Vikriti (imbalance) with a Kapha Vikriti diet / lifestyle.

## Aphrodisiac

| Dosha | Code | Common Name | Latin Name |
|---|---|---|---|
| Vataja | 203 | Ashwagandha | Withania somnifera |
| | 205 | Gokshura | Tribulus terrestris |
| | 211 | Shatavari | Asparagus racemosus |
| | 301 | Amalaki | Emblica officinalis |
| | | Bibhitaki | Terminalia belerica |
| | | Haritaki | Terminalia chebula |
| Pittaja | 201 | Amalaki | Emblica officinalis |
| | 203 | Ashwagandha | Withania somnifera |
| | 211 | Shatavari | Asparagus racemosus |
| | 402 | Coriander | Coriandrum sativum |
| | | Cumin | Cumimum cyminum |
| | | Fennel | Foeniculum vulgare |
| Kaphaja | 201 | Amalaki | Emblica officinalis |
| | 203 | Ashwagandha | Withania somnifera |
| | 206 | Guduchi | Tinospora cordifolia |
| | 403 | Ginger | Zingiber officinale |
| | | Cumin | Cumimum cyminum |
| | | Fenugreek | Trigonella foenum-graecum |

| Dosha | Low Dose | High Dose |
|---|---|---|
| Vata | 1 of each X2 per day before meals | 2 of each X2 per day before meals |
| Pitta | 2 of each X2 per day before meals | 3 of each X2 per before meals |
| Kapha | 2 of each X2 per day before meals | 4 of each X2 per day before meals |

## Description:

Aphrodisiac in Ayurveda means to 'promote health of the reproductive system'. Treatment should follow the Prakriti of the person as this is a *Vajikarana* therapy, not a disease treatment. The blends above strengthen Shukra Dhatu and help develop healthy sperm and ovum.

Use the Vataja herbs if Vata is predominant in the Prakriti with a Vata Prakriti diet / lifestyle.

Use the Pittaja herbs if Pitta is predominant in the Prakriti with a Pitta Prakriti diet / lifestyle.

Use the Kaphaja herbs if Kapha is predominant in the Prakriti with a Kapha Prakriti diet / lifestyle.

## Arteriosclerosis

| Dosha | Code | Common Name | Latin Name |
|---|---|---|---|
| Vataja | 202 | Arjuna | Terminalia arjuna |
| | 207 | Haritaki | Terminalia chebula |
| | 401 | Cumin | Cumimum cyminum |
| | | Fennel | Foeniculum vulgare |
| | | Cardamom | Elettaria cardamomum |
| Pittaja | 202 | Arjuna | Terminalia arjuna |
| | 402 | Coriander | Coriandrum sativum |
| | | Cumin | Cumimum cyminum |
| | | Fennel | Foeniculum vulgare |
| | 407 | Turmeric | Curcuma longa |
| | | Barberry | Berberis vulgaris |
| | | Dandelion | Taraxacum officinale |
| Kaphaja | 202 | Arjuna | Terminalia arjuna |
| | 403 | Ginger | Zingiber officinale |
| | | Cumin | Cumimum cyminum |
| | | Fenugreek | Trigonella foenum-graecum |
| | 407 | Turmeric | Curcuma longa |
| | | Barberry | Berberis vulgaris |
| | | Dandelion | Taraxacum officinale |

| Dosha | Low Dose | High Dose |
|---|---|---|
| Vata | 1 of each X2 per day before meals | 2 of each X2 per day before meals |
| Pitta | 1 of each X2 per day with meals | 2 of each X2 per day with meals |
| Kapha | 2 of each X2 per day after meals | 3 of each X2 per day after meals |

## Description:

Arteriosclerosis is a general term describing any hardening (and loss of elasticity) of medium or large arteries. It is generally Vataja by function and Pittaja by structure. Any Dosha can cause this problem which is mainly due to poor diet and lifestyle. Any Dosha can either cause Vata to increase, or Pitta to reduce in the arteries.

Use the Vataja herbs if Vata is predominant in the Vikriti (imbalance) with a Vata Vikriti diet / lifestyle.

Use the Pittaja herbs if Pitta is predominant in the Vikriti (imbalance) with a Pitta Vikriti diet / lifestyle.

Use the Kaphaja herbs if Kapha is predominant in the Vikriti (imbalance) with a Kapha Vikriti diet / lifestyle.

## Arthritis

| Dosha | Code | Common Name | Latin Name |
|-------|------|-------------|------------|
| **Vataja** | 401 | Cumin | Cumimum cyminum |
| | | Fennel | Foeniculum vulgare |
| | | Cardamom | Elettaria cardamomum |
| | 404 | Angelica | Angelica archangelica |
| | | Wild yam | Dioscorea villosa |
| | | Valerian | Valeriana officinalis |
| | 407 | Turmeric | Curcuma longa |
| | | Barberry | Berberis vulgaris |
| | | Dandelion | Taraxacum officinale |
| **Pittaja** | 402 | Coriander | Coriandrum sativum |
| | | Cumin | Cumimum cyminum |
| | | Fennel | Foeniculum vulgare |
| | 405 | Burdock | Arctium lappa |
| | | Yellow dock | Rumex crispus |
| | | Milk Thistle | Silybum marianum |
| | 407 | Turmeric | Curcuma longa |
| | | Barberry | Berberis vulgaris |
| | | Dandelion | Taraxacum officinale |
| **Kaphaja** | 403 | Ginger | Zingiber officinale |
| | | Cumin | Cumimum cyminum |
| | | Fenugreek | Trigonella foenum-graecum |
| | 406 | Myrrh | Commiphora myrrha |
| | | Elecampane | Inula helenium |
| | | Yellow dock | Rumex crispus |
| | 407 | Turmeric | Curcuma longa |
| | | Barberry | Berberis vulgaris |
| | | Dandelion | Taraxacum officinale |

| Dosha | Low Dose | High Dose |
|-------|----------|-----------|
| **Vata** | 1 of each X2 per day before meals | 2 of each X2 per day before meals |
| **Pitta** | 1 of each X2 per day with meals | 2 of each X2 per day with meals |
| **Kapha** | 2 of each X2 per day after meals | 3 of each X2 per day after meals |

## Description:

Arthritis is a group of conditions involving damage to the joints of the body. There are different forms of arthritis and each has a different cause. This formula can be used for any kind of joint / muscle / tendon / ligament disorder in which Ama is a primary cause. In Ayurveda, most of the many forms of arthritis are due to the accumulation of Ama in the body. As Vata controls the bones this is considered to be a Vata Roga problem. Any Dosha can cause this problem and is due to poor dietary choices and lifestyle.

These formulas target the digestive system and specifically the colon (*Asthidharakala*) that nourishes Asthi Dhatu. It reduces Ama and inflammation in Asthi Dhatu. It works slowly so the person needs at least six to twelve months of treatment before having a major change in pathology. Symptomatic relief can manifest after a few weeks of use. Choose the formula according to Vikriti indication on the test.

After changing the diet and lifestyle the whole process of healing can be accelerated dramatically by Ayurvedic external therapies. These are called Snehana and Svedhana in general terms. Exact treatments need to be done by an Ayurvedic therapist and adapted to the individual. These entail the use of medicated oils (not essential oils) and the application of heat. This liquefies and removes Ama from the joints.

Use the Vataja herbs if Vata is predominant in the Vikriti (imbalance) with a Vata Vikriti diet / lifestyle.

Use the Pittaja herbs if Pitta is predominant in the Vikriti (imbalance) with a Pitta Vikriti diet / lifestyle.

Use the Kaphaja herbs if Kapha is predominant in the Vikriti (imbalance) with a Kapha Vikriti diet / lifestyle.

## Asthma

| Dosha | Code | Common Name | Latin Name |
|---|---|---|---|
| **Vataja** | 210 | Shankhpushpi | Convolvulus pluricaulis |
| | 401 | Cumin | Cumimum cyminum |
| | | Fennel | Foeniculum vulgare |
| | | Cardamom | Elettaria cardamomum |
| | 410 | Passion flower | Passiflora incarnata |
| | | Skullcap | Scutellaria lateriflora |
| | | Gotu kola | Centella asiatica |
| **Pittaja** | 201 | Amalaki | Emblica officinalis |
| | 402 | Coriander | Coriandrum sativum |
| | | Cumin | Cumimum cyminum |
| | | Fennel | Foeniculum vulgare |
| | 410 | Passion flower | Passiflora incarnata |
| | | Skullcap | Scutellaria lateriflora |
| | | Gotu kola | Centella asiatica |
| **Kaphaja** | 209 | Punarnava | Boerhaavia diffusa |
| | 403 | Ginger | Zingiber officinale |
| | | Cumin | Cumimum cyminum |
| | | Fenugreek | Trigonella foenum-graecum |
| | 406 | Myrrh | Commiphora myrrha |
| | | Elecampane | Inula helenium |
| | | Yellow dock | Rumex crispus |

| Dosha | Low Dose | High Dose |
|---|---|---|
| **Vata** | 1 of each X2 per day before meals | 2 of each X2 per day before meals |
| **Pitta** | 1 of each X2 per day with meals | 2 of each X2 per day with meals |
| **Kapha** | 2 of each X2 per day after meals | 3 of each X2 per day after meals |

## Description:

Asthma is a very common chronic disease involving the respiratory system in which the airways constrict, become inflamed, and are lined with excessive amounts of mucus. It is Kapha Roga by structure and Vata Roga by function; any Dosha can cause this disorder.

Use the Vataja herbs if Vata is predominant in the Vikriti (imbalance) with a Vata Vikriti diet / lifestyle.

Use the Pittaja herbs if Pitta is predominant in the Vikriti (imbalance) with a Pitta Vikriti diet / lifestyle.

Use the Kaphaja herbs if Kapha is predominant in the Vikriti (imbalance) with a Kapha Vikriti diet / lifestyle.

## Atheroma

| Dosha | Code | Common Name | Latin Name |
|---|---|---|---|
| Vataja | 202 | Arjuna | Terminalia arjuna |
| | 301 | Amalaki | Emblica officinalis |
| | | Bibhitaki | Terminalia belerica |
| | | Haritaki | Terminalia chebula |
| | 404 | Angelica | Angelica archangelica |
| | | Wild yam | Dioscorea villosa |
| | | Valerian | Valeriana officinalis |
| Pittaja | 202 | Arjuna | Terminalia arjuna |
| | 301 | Amalaki | Emblica officinalis |
| | | Bibhitaki | Terminalia belerica |
| | | Haritaki | Terminalia chebula |
| | 405 | Burdock | Arctium lappa |
| | | Yellow dock | Rumex crispus |
| | | Milk Thistle | Silybum marianum |
| | 407 | Turmeric | Curcuma longa |
| | | Barberry | Berberis vulgaris |
| | | Dandelion | Taraxacum officinale |
| Kaphaja | 202 | Arjuna | Terminalia arjuna |
| | 209 | Punarnava | Boerhaavia diffusa |
| | 301 | Amalaki | Emblica officinalis |
| | | Bibhitaki | Terminalia belerica |
| | | Haritaki | Terminalia chebula |
| | 407 | Turmeric | Curcuma longa |
| | | Barberry | Berberis vulgaris |
| | | Dandelion | Taraxacum officinale |

| Dosha | Low Dose | High Dose |
|---|---|---|
| Vata | 1 of each X2 per day before meals | 2 of each X2 per day before meals |
| Pitta | 1 of each X2 per day with meals | 2 of each X2 per day with meals |
| Kapha | 2 of each X2 per day after meals | 3 of each X2 per day after meals |

## Description:

Atheroma is the degeneration of the inner layer of artery walls caused by accumulated fatty deposits and scar tissue, which can lead to restriction of circulation and a risk of thrombosis. Patches of atheroma are often called plaques of atheroma. Over months or years, patches of atheroma can become larger and thicker. In time, a patch of atheroma can make an artery narrower, which can restrict and reduce the blood flow through the artery.

Atheroma is the root cause of a number of cardiovascular diseases - that is, diseases of the heart or blood vessels. Atheroma can also mean an abnormal mass of fat or lipids, as in a sebaceous cyst, or in deposits in an arterial wall. Patches of atheroma can be formed of other matter than fat (lipid), for example, cholesterol, connective tissue, and white blood cells.

In Ayurveda, deposits in arteries are often linked to Ama or non-digested food. Other causes can be the over production of certain fluids or lipids by the body which are Kaphaja by nature. High heat, or mild inflammatory conditions in the arteries from Pittaja disorders will cause Kapha Dosha to increase and form plaques. Excess dryness in the arteries (from eating a no-fat diet for example) will cause Vataja forms of Atheroma manifesting as dry tissue accumulation. This disorder is Pitta Roga by structure and Kapha Roga by function, but any Dosha can cause this disorder which is the cause of many other cardiovascular disorders such as Atherosclerosis. Treatment should follow the Vikriti of the person.

Use the Vataja herbs if Vata is predominant in the Vikriti (imbalance) with a Vata Vikriti diet / lifestyle.

Use the Pittaja herbs if Pitta is predominant in the Vikriti (imbalance) with a Pitta Vikriti diet / lifestyle.

Use the Kaphaja herbs if Kapha is predominant in the Vikriti (imbalance) with a Kapha Vikriti diet / lifestyle.

## Atherosclerosis

| Dosha | Code | Common Name | Latin Name |
|---|---|---|---|
| **Vataja** | 202 | Arjuna | Terminalia arjuna |
| | 301 | Amalaki | Emblica officinalis |
| | | Bibhitaki | Terminalia belerica |
| | | Haritaki | Terminalia chebula |
| | 404 | Angelica | Angelica archangelica |
| | | Wild yam | Dioscorea villosa |
| | | Valerian | Valeriana officinalis |
| **Pittaja** | 202 | Arjuna | Terminalia arjuna |
| | 301 | Amalaki | Emblica officinalis |
| | | Bibhitaki | Terminalia belerica |
| | | Haritaki | Terminalia chebula |
| | 405 | Burdock | Arctium lappa |
| | | Yellow dock | Rumex crispus |
| | | Milk Thistle | Silybum marianum |
| | 407 | Turmeric | Curcuma longa |
| | | Barberry | Berberis vulgaris |
| | | Dandelion | Taraxacum officinale |
| **Kaphaja** | 202 | Arjuna | Terminalia arjuna |
| | 209 | Punarnava | Boerhaavia diffusa |
| | 301 | Amalaki | Emblica officinalis |
| | | Bibhitaki | Terminalia belerica |
| | | Haritaki | Terminalia chebula |
| | 407 | Turmeric | Curcuma longa |
| | | Barberry | Berberis vulgaris |
| | | Dandelion | Taraxacum officinale |

| Dosha | Low Dose | High Dose |
|---|---|---|
| **Vata** | 1 of each X2 per day before meals | 2 of each X2 per day before meals |
| **Pitta** | 1 of each X2 per day with meals | 2 of each X2 per day with meals |
| **Kapha** | 2 of each X2 per day after meals | 3 of each X2 per day after meals |

## Description:
Atherosclerosis is a specific form of arteriosclerosis – see Atheroma.

Use the Vataja herbs if Vata is predominant in the Vikriti (imbalance) with a Vata Vikriti diet / lifestyle.

Use the Pittaja herbs if Pitta is predominant in the Vikriti (imbalance) with a Pitta Vikriti diet / lifestyle.

Use the Kaphaja herbs if Kapha is predominant in the Vikriti (imbalance) with a Kapha Vikriti diet / lifestyle.

## Autoimmune disorders

| Dosha | Code | Common Name | Latin Name |
|---|---|---|---|
| Vataja | 203 | Ashwagandha | Withania somnifera |
| | 206 | Guduchi | Tinospora cordifolia |
| | 212 | Pau d'arco | Tabebuia impetiginosa |
| | 301 | Amalaki | Emblica officinalis |
| | | Bibhitaki | Terminalia belerica |
| | | Haritaki | Terminalia chebula |
| Pittaja | 201 | Amalaki | Emblica officinalis |
| | 206 | Guduchi | Tinospora cordifolia |
| | 212 | Pau d'arco | Tabebuia impetiginosa |
| | 301 | Amalaki | Emblica officinalis |
| | | Bibhitaki | Terminalia belerica |
| | | Haritaki | Terminalia chebula |
| Kaphaja | 206 | Guduchi | Tinospora cordifolia |
| | 209 | Punarnava | Boerhaavia diffusa |
| | 212 | Pau d'arco | Tabebuia impetiginosa |
| | 301 | Amalaki | Emblica officinalis |
| | | Bibhitaki | Terminalia belerica |
| | | Haritaki | Terminalia chebula |

| Dosha | Low Dose | High Dose |
|---|---|---|
| Vata | 1 of each X2 per day before meals | 2 of each X2 per day before meals |
| Pitta | 1 of each X2 per day with meals | 2 of each X2 per day with meals |
| Kapha | 2 of each X2 per day after meals | 3 of each X2 per day after meals |

## Description:

Autoimmune diseases arise from an overactive immune response of the body against substances and tissues normally present in the body. In other words, the body attacks its own cells. This may be restricted to certain organs (e.g., Hashimoto's disease) or involve a particular tissue, or tissues in different places (e.g., Multiple sclerosis, Rheumatoid arthritis, Goodpasture's disease, etc.). The treatment of autoimmune diseases is typically done with immunosuppression – medication which decreases the immune response.

These formulas can be used as a general treatment when the patient has been diagnosed with an autoimmune disorder and work on strengthening and correcting immune function. There are immunomodulating herbs in these blends to help restore the intelligence of the body. Ayurveda considers autoimmune disorders as a malfunction of prana often combined with Ama conditions. Therefore, the patient is advised to do Pranayama in conjunction with diet, lifestyle and herbal treatments. There are no restrictions for the length of time to take this formula so long as Agni is strong enough to digest the herbs.

Any Dosha cause autoimmune disorders by going into an excess state, deranging Agni, causing Ama and either hyper or hypo functions in their tissues or systems. There are many diseases that are suspected autoimmune disorders by modern medicine, but are not yet proved to be autoimmune. Ayurveda views these kinds of disorders as multi causal and can be triggered by emotional or mental shock, trauma, physical or psychological abuse, vaccines, accidents or environment. In all of these examples the Doshas are increased and disrupt Agni function in different area of the body. According to the individual situation various autoimmune disorders can result. While Ama is often present, it is not a prerequisite for an autoimmune disorder.

Note that if Ama is present in the body it is best to begin by using the 'Ama' herbal blends with an anti-Ama reducing diet. Normally treatment should follow Vikriti.

Use the Vataja herbs if Vata is predominant in the Vikriti (imbalance) with a Vata Vikriti diet / lifestyle.

Use the Pittaja herbs if Pitta is predominant in the Vikriti (imbalance) with a Pitta Vikriti diet / lifestyle.

Use the Kaphaja herbs if Kapha is predominant in the Vikriti (imbalance) with a Kapha Vikriti diet / lifestyle.

## Bacterial infections

| Dosha | Code | Common Name | Latin Name |
|-------|------|-------------|------------|
| Vataja | 207 | Haritaki | Terminalia chebula |
| | 407 | Turmeric | Curcuma longa |
| | | Barberry | Berberis vulgaris |
| | | Dandelion | Taraxacum officinale |
| Pittaja | 201 | Amalaki | Emblica officinalis |
| | 407 | Turmeric | Curcuma longa |
| | | Barberry | Berberis vulgaris |
| | | Dandelion | Taraxacum officinale |
| Kaphaja | 406 | Myrrh | Commiphora myrrha |
| | | Elecampane | Inula helenium |
| | | Yellow dock | Rumex crispus |
| | 407 | Turmeric | Curcuma longa |
| | | Barberry | Berberis vulgaris |
| | | Dandelion | Taraxacum officinale |

| Dosha | Low Dose | High Dose |
|-------|----------|-----------|
| Vata | 1 of each X2 per day before meals | 2 of each X2 per day before meals |
| Pitta | 1 of each X2 per day with meals | 2 of each X2 per day with meals |
| Kapha | 2 of each X2 per day after meals | 3 of each X2 per day after meals |

## Description:

Bacterial infections are facilitated by low immunity, disturbed Agni and the formation of Ama in the body. Any Dosha can cause this problem therefore treatments should follow Vikriti. If reoccurring infections are a problem use the "Low immunity" blend after one or two months of this blend.

Use the Vataja herbs if Vata is predominant in the Vikriti (imbalance) with a Vata Vikriti diet / lifestyle.

Use the Pittaja herbs if Pitta is predominant in the Vikriti (imbalance) with a Pitta Vikriti diet / lifestyle.

Use the Kaphaja herbs if Kapha is predominant in the Vikriti (imbalance) with a Kapha Vikriti diet / lifestyle.

## Blood clots

| Dosha | Code | Common Name | Latin Name |
|-------|------|-------------|------------|
| **Vataja** | 205 | Gokshura | Tribulus terrestris |
| | 208 | Manjishta | Rubia cordifolia |
| | 403 | Ginger | Zingiber officinale |
| | | Cumin | Cumimum cyminum |
| | | Fenugreek | Trigonella foenum-graecum |
| | 407 | Turmeric | Curcuma longa |
| | | Barberry | Berberis vulgaris |
| | | Dandelion | Taraxacum officinale |
| **Pittaja** | 208 | Manjishta | Rubia cordifolia |
| | 402 | Coriander | Coriandrum sativum |
| | | Cumin | Cumimum cyminum |
| | | Fennel | Foeniculum vulgare |
| | 405 | Burdock | Arctium lappa |
| | | Yellow dock | Rumex crispus |
| | | Milk Thistle | Silybum marianum |
| | 407 | Turmeric | Curcuma longa |
| | | Barberry | Berberis vulgaris |
| | | Dandelion | Taraxacum officinale |
| **Kaphaja** | 202 | Arjuna | Terminalia arjuna |
| | 208 | Manjishta | Rubia cordifolia |
| | 403 | Ginger | Zingiber officinale |
| | | Cumin | Cumimum cyminum |
| | | Fenugreek | Trigonella foenum-graecum |
| | 407 | Turmeric | Curcuma longa |
| | | Barberry | Berberis vulgaris |
| | | Dandelion | Taraxacum officinale |

| Dosha | Low Dose | High Dose |
|-------|----------|-----------|
| **Vata** | 1 of each X2 per day before meals | 2 of each X2 per day before meals |
| **Pitta** | 1 of each X2 per day with meals | 2 of each X2 per day with meals |
| **Kapha** | 2 of each X2 per day after meals | 3 of each X2 per day after meals |

## Description:

Blood clots form when platelets and plasma proteins thicken, forming a semisolid mass. Once these clots form, they can travel to other parts of your body, causing harm. A number of possible disorders caused by blood clots are:

-*Thrombosis* is the formation of a blood clot (thrombus) inside a blood vessel, obstructing the flow of blood through the circulatory system.

When a blood vessel is injured, the body uses platelets and fibrin to form a blood clot, because the first step in repairing it (hemostasis) is to prevent loss of blood. If that mechanism causes too much clotting, and the clot breaks free, an embolus is formed.

-*Thrombophlebitis* is phlebitis (vein inflammation) related to a blood clot or thrombus. When it occurs repeatedly in different locations, it is known as "Thrombophlebitis migrants" or "migrating thrombophlebitis".

-*Peripheral vascular disease* (PVD), also known as Peripheral Artery Disease (PAD) or peripheral artery occlusive disease (PAOD), includes all diseases caused by the obstruction of large arteries in the arms and legs.

These formulas can be used for all forms of blood clotting problems such as thrombosis, phlebitis, thrombophlebitis, or peripheral vascular diseases. These blends work to remove blood clots from Raktavaha Srota and normalize blood chemistry in Rasa and Rakta Dhatus. They can be used for prevention of these problems as well. These formulas correct blood circulation in terms of movement (Vata) and quality (Pitta) mainly in deeper veins. If you wish to improve peripheral circulation use the Mother Tincture of *Ginkgo biloba* at 20 drops X 3 per day with this blend. The herbal blends should be used for a minimum of three months and are safe to use for periods of up to one year.

According to Ayurveda the solidifying of blood (Rasa / Rakta) is caused by Vata Dosha. Pitta who controls blood circulation in Raktavaha Srota is disturbed by the clotting and generates more heat causing inflammation. Depending the disorder the causal Dosha can change; any Dosha can cause this disorder, use the blend as per Vikriti.

NOTE: These blends are CONTRAINDICATED with blood thinners or anticoagulants such as warfarin (e.g., Coumadin, Jantoven, Marevan, Uniwarfin) and fluindione (Previscan).

Use the Vataja herbs if Vata is predominant in the Vikriti (imbalance) with a Vata Vikriti diet / lifestyle.

Use the Pittaja herbs if Pitta is predominant in the Vikriti (imbalance) with a Pitta Vikriti diet / lifestyle.

Use the Kaphaja herbs if Kapha is predominant in the Vikriti (imbalance) with a Kapha Vikriti diet / lifestyle.

## Blood disorders

| Dosha | Code | Common Name | Latin Name |
|---|---|---|---|
| **Vataja** | 208 | Manjishta | Rubia cordifolia |
| | 301 | Amalaki | Emblica officinalis |
| | | Bibhitaki | Terminalia belerica |
| | | Haritaki | Terminalia chebula |
| | 404 | Angelica | Angelica archangelica |
| | | Wild yam | Dioscorea villosa |
| | | Valerian | Valeriana officinalis |
| | 407 | Turmeric | Curcuma longa |
| | | Barberry | Berberis vulgaris |
| | | Dandelion | Taraxacum officinale |
| **Pittaja** | 208 | Manjishta | Rubia cordifolia |
| | 301 | Amalaki | Emblica officinalis |
| | | Bibhitaki | Terminalia belerica |
| | | Haritaki | Terminalia chebula |
| | 405 | Burdock | Arctium lappa |
| | | Yellow dock | Rumex crispus |
| | | Milk Thistle | Silybum marianum |
| | 407 | Turmeric | Curcuma longa |
| | | Barberry | Berberis vulgaris |
| | | Dandelion | Taraxacum officinale |
| **Kaphaja** | 208 | Manjishta | Rubia cordifolia |
| | 301 | Amalaki | Emblica officinalis |
| | | Bibhitaki | Terminalia belerica |
| | | Haritaki | Terminalia chebula |
| | 406 | Myrrh | Commiphora myrrha |
| | | Elecampane | Inula helenium |
| | | Yellow dock | Rumex crispus |
| | 407 | Turmeric | Curcuma longa |
| | | Barberry | Berberis vulgaris |
| | | Dandelion | Taraxacum officinale |

| Dosha | Low Dose | High Dose |
|---|---|---|
| **Vata** | 1 of each X2 per day before meals | 2 of each X2 per day before meals |
| **Pitta** | 1 of each X2 per day with meals | 2 of each X2 per day with meals |
| **Kapha** | 2 of each X2 per day after meals | 3 of each X2 per day after meals |

## Description:

These blends work to reduce the causal Dosha behind blood disorders. Both Kapha and Pitta form blood; Kapha is responsible for the formation of blood plasma in Rasa Dhatu and Pitta is responsible for the formation of hemoglobin in Rakta Dhatu. Kapha is also responsible for the formation of blood cells in bone marrow, or Majja Dhatu. Pitta is creating heat by the transformation of nutrients and stores this heat in Rakta Dhatu. Vata Dosha is responsible to circulate the blood in the channels of Pitta, or Raktavaha Srota.

Because all three Doshas have important roles in blood formation, metabolism and circulation any of them can cause disorders of the blood. Therefore, use the herbal blend according to the Vikriti dominant Dosha when treating blood disorders.

This vary depending on what kind of pathology is manifesting for the patient. It could be a specific problem or a non-specific problem. These blends will remove Ama from the blood and restore correct blood metabolism. They will also help to remove virus or other pathogens from the blood.

NOTE: These blends are CONTRAINDICATED with blood thinners or anticoagulants such as warfarin (e.g., Coumadin, Jantoven, Marevan, Uniwarfin) and fluindione (Previscan).

Use the Vataja herbs if Vata is predominant in the Vikriti (imbalance) with a Vata Vikriti diet / lifestyle.

Use the Pittaja herbs if Pitta is predominant in the Vikriti (imbalance) with a Pitta Vikriti diet / lifestyle.

Use the Kaphaja herbs if Kapha is predominant in the Vikriti (imbalance) with a Kapha Vikriti diet / lifestyle.

## Boils

| Dosha | Code | Common Name | Latin Name |
|-------|------|-------------|------------|
| **Vataja** | 208 | Manjishta | Rubia cordifolia |
| | 212 | Pau d'arco | Tabebuia impetiginosa |
| | 404 | Angelica | Angelica archangelica |
| | | Wild yam | Dioscorea villosa |
| | | Valerian | Valeriana officinalis |
| | 407 | Turmeric | Curcuma longa |
| | | Barberry | Berberis vulgaris |
| | | Dandelion | Taraxacum officinale |
| **Pittaja** | 208 | Manjishta | Rubia cordifolia |
| | 212 | Pau d'arco | Tabebuia impetiginosa |
| | 405 | Burdock | Arctium lappa |
| | | Yellow dock | Rumex crispus |
| | | Milk Thistle | Silybum marianum |
| | 407 | Turmeric | Curcuma longa |
| | | Barberry | Berberis vulgaris |
| | | Dandelion | Taraxacum officinale |
| **Kaphaja** | 208 | Manjishta | Rubia cordifolia |
| | 212 | Pau d'arco | Tabebuia impetiginosa |
| | 406 | Myrrh | Commiphora myrrha |
| | | Elecampane | Inula helenium |
| | | Yellow dock | Rumex crispus |
| | 407 | Turmeric | Curcuma longa |
| | | Barberry | Berberis vulgaris |
| | | Dandelion | Taraxacum officinale |

| Dosha | Low Dose | High Dose |
|-------|----------|-----------|
| **Vata** | 1 of each X2 per day before meals | 2 of each X2 per day before meals |
| **Pitta** | 1 of each X2 per day with meals | 2 of each X2 per day with meals |
| **Kapha** | 2 of each X2 per day after meals | 3 of each X2 per day after meals |

## Description:

Boils are a toxic blood condition due to Ama. These blends remove Ama and cleanse Rasa and Rakta Dhatus; any Dosha can cause boils.

Use the Vataja herbs if Vata is predominant in the Vikriti (imbalance) with a Vata Vikriti diet / lifestyle.

Use the Pittaja herbs if Pitta is predominant in the Vikriti (imbalance) with a Pitta Vikriti diet / lifestyle.

Use the Kaphaja herbs if Kapha is predominant in the Vikriti (imbalance) with a Kapha Vikriti diet / lifestyle.

## Brain tonic

| Dosha | Code | Common Name | Latin Name |
|---|---|---|---|
| **Vataja** | 204 | Bramhi | Bacopa monnieri |
| | 210 | Shankhpushpi | Convolvulus pluricaulis |
| | 301 | Amalaki | Emblica officinalis |
| | | Bibhitaki | Terminalia belerica |
| | | Haritaki | Terminalia chebula |
| **Pittaja** | 204 | Bramhi | Bacopa monnieri |
| | 210 | Shankhpushpi | Convolvulus pluricaulis |
| | 402 | Coriander | Coriandrum sativum |
| | | Cumin | Cumimum cyminum |
| | | Fennel | Foeniculum vulgare |
| | 407 | Turmeric | Curcuma longa |
| | | Barberry | Berberis vulgaris |
| | | Dandelion | Taraxacum officinale |
| **Kaphaja** | 204 | Bramhi | Bacopa monnieri |
| | 210 | Shankhpushpi | Convolvulus pluricaulis |
| | 403 | Ginger | Zingiber officinale |
| | | Cumin | Cumimum cyminum |
| | | Fenugreek | Trigonella foenum-graecum |
| | 407 | Turmeric | Curcuma longa |
| | | Barberry | Berberis vulgaris |
| | | Dandelion | Taraxacum officinale |

| Dosha | Low Dose | High Dose |
|---|---|---|
| **Vata** | 1 of each X2 per day before meals | 2 of each X2 per day before meals |
| **Pitta** | 1 of each X2 per day with meals | 2 of each X2 per day with meals |
| **Kapha** | 2 of each X2 per day after meals | 3 of each X2 per day after meals |

## Description:

Use these blends as per Prakriti to strengthen the brain and mental functions. Useful during periods of intense intellectual work / study. NOTE: There are possible interaction with psychoactive medicines or antidepressants, large doses may cause dizziness and disorientation.

Use the Vataja herbs if Vata is predominant in the Prakriti (imbalance) with a Vata Prakriti diet / lifestyle.

Use the Pittaja herbs if Pitta is predominant in the Prakriti (imbalance) with a Pitta Prakriti diet / lifestyle.

Use the Kaphaja herbs if Kapha is predominant in the Prakriti (imbalance) with a Kapha Prakriti diet / lifestyle.

## Breast disorders (women)

| Dosha | Code | Common Name | Latin Name |
|---|---|---|---|
| **Vataja** | 211 | Shatavari | Asparagus racemosus |
| | 401 | Cumin | Cumimum cyminum |
| | | Fennel | Foeniculum vulgare |
| | | Cardamom | Elettaria cardamomum |
| | 407 | Turmeric | Curcuma longa |
| | | Barberry | Berberis vulgaris |
| | | Dandelion | Taraxacum officinale |
| | 408 | Vitex | Vitex agnus-castus |
| | | Black cohosh | Cimicifuga racemosa |
| | | Cramp bark | Viburnum opulus |
| **Pittaja** | 402 | Coriander | Coriandrum sativum |
| | | Cumin | Cumimum cyminum |
| | | Fennel | Foeniculum vulgare |
| | 405 | Burdock | Arctium lappa |
| | | Yellow dock | Rumex crispus |
| | | Milk Thistle | Silybum marianum |
| | 407 | Turmeric | Curcuma longa |
| | | Barberry | Berberis vulgaris |
| | | Dandelion | Taraxacum officinale |
| **Kaphaja** | 403 | Ginger | Zingiber officinale |
| | | Cumin | Cumimum cyminum |
| | | Fenugreek | Trigonella foenum-graecum |
| | 406 | Myrrh | Commiphora myrrha |
| | | Elecampane | Inula helenium |
| | | Yellow dock | Rumex crispus |
| | 407 | Turmeric | Curcuma longa |
| | | Barberry | Berberis vulgaris |
| | | Dandelion | Taraxacum officinale |

| Dosha | Low Dose | High Dose |
|---|---|---|
| **Vata** | 1 of each X2 per day before meals | 2 of each X2 per day before meals |
| **Pitta** | 1 of each X2 per day with meals | 2 of each X2 per day with meals |
| **Kapha** | 2 of each X2 per day after meals | 3 of each X2 per day after meals |

## Description:

Breast tissue is part of Rasa Dhatu and can be easily disturbed by diet and lifestyle. Hence, the basic treatment is to remove all carbonated drinks, all manufactured beverages and drink only water or herbal teas. The best plant to clear the breast channels in a tea is Dandelion root, (*Taraxacum officinale*). Diet is also very important to clear the breast tissues of Ama or congestion. A vegan diet as per Prakriti is the most efficient diet to cleanse breast tissues.

Any disorder of the breast is under the control of Kapha Dosha by structure, Rasa Dhatu, and Vata Dosha by function. Vyana Vayu (Vata) is responsible to cleanse and circulate lymph fluids and tissues. If this is not done, then the lymph nodes accumulate waste (Mala) materials and become congested. This congestion gives rise to a number of problems, so these blends are mainly concerned with cleansing Rasa Dhatu and breast tissues. Any Dosha can cause problems in the breasts. Vata creates problems of circulation and dryness; Pitta inflammations in the breast lymph tissues; and Kapha creates congestions in the breasts. When two Doshas are mixed, it is prudent to treat any inflammations (Pitta) first as this creates problems faster and of a more serious nature. Follow this treatment with the other Dosha involved in the problem.

Note that prevention is the best treatment. By keeping the breast tissues clean and flowing it should reduce the formation of cysts and tumors. Exercise is also an important aspect of lymph health as there is no 'pump' in the lymphatic system – it requires physical activity to circulate lymph fluids.

Use the Vataja herbs if Vata is predominant in the Vikriti (imbalance) with a Vata Prakriti diet / lifestyle.

Use the Pittaja herbs if Pitta is predominant in the Vikriti (imbalance) with a Pitta Prakriti diet / lifestyle.

Use the Kaphaja herbs if Kapha is predominant in the Vikriti (imbalance) with a Kapha Prakriti diet / lifestyle.

## Bronchitis

| Dosha | Code | Common Name | Latin Name |
|---|---|---|---|
| Vataja | 211 | Shatavari | Asparagus racemosus |
| | 406 | Myrrh | Commiphora myrrha |
| | | Elecampane | Inula helenium |
| | | Yellow dock | Rumex crispus |
| | 407 | Turmeric | Curcuma longa |
| | | Barberry | Berberis vulgaris |
| | | Dandelion | Taraxacum officinale |
| Pittaja | 402 | Coriander | Coriandrum sativum |
| | | Cumin | Cumimum cyminum |
| | | Fennel | Foeniculum vulgare |
| | 406 | Myrrh | Commiphora myrrha |
| | | Elecampane | Inula helenium |
| | | Yellow dock | Rumex crispus |
| | 407 | Turmeric | Curcuma longa |
| | | Barberry | Berberis vulgaris |
| | | Dandelion | Taraxacum officinale |
| Kaphaja | 403 | Ginger | Zingiber officinale |
| | | Cumin | Cumimum cyminum |
| | | Fenugreek | Trigonella foenum-graecum |
| | 406 | Myrrh | Commiphora myrrha |
| | | Elecampane | Inula helenium |
| | | Yellow dock | Rumex crispus |
| | 407 | Turmeric | Curcuma longa |
| | | Barberry | Berberis vulgaris |
| | | Dandelion | Taraxacum officinale |

| Dosha | Low Dose | High Dose |
|---|---|---|
| Vata | 1 of each X2 per day before meals | 2 of each X2 per day before meals |
| Pitta | 1 of each X2 per day with meals | 2 of each X2 per day with meals |
| Kapha | 2 of each X2 per day after meals | 3 of each X2 per day after meals |

## Description:

Bronchitis is an inflammation of the air passages within the lungs. It occurs when the trachea (windpipe) and the large and small bronchi (airways) within the lungs become inflamed because of infection or other causes. This is a Kapha Roga disorder by structure, Rasa Dhatu, and a Vataja disorder by function (Pranavaha Srota). Inflammation is due to an increase of Pitta in the lungs and can be due to pathogens, Ama or both.

Acute bronchitis, caused by secondary infection of the bronchi/viruses or bacteria and lasting several days or weeks. It is usually preceded by a common cold (Coryza) or influenza (flu). Some complications from contracting bronchitis affect measles and whooping coughs in children due to the virus depressing the body's normal defense mechanisms.

Chronic bronchitis, caused by prolonged irritation of the bronchial epithelium, is a persistent, productive cough lasting at least three months in two consecutive years. Certified definition of chronic bronchitis: 'When an individual has had a cough with sputum for three months (or more) in two consecutive years'.

In bronchitis, the membranes lining the larger air passages (bronchi) become inflamed (Fibrosis) and an excessive amount of mucus is produced. The person with bronchitis develops a bad cough to get rid of the mucus due to the reduction in number of and efficiency of the remaining ciliated cells. This increases the likelihood that a viral infection will be contracted by patients and sometimes it can lead to pneumonia. Airflow into and out of the lungs is partly blocked because of the swelling and extra mucus in the bronchi.

Early treatment is needed for herbs to cure this kind of acute problem. If the pathology has moved into the 5th or 6th stage of Kriyakala then herbs alone may not be enough. Regardless if the patient has used antibiotics or not the blends here should be used to clear and strengthen the lung tissues.

The effectiveness of the herbal blends here would be greatly increased if the patient uses herbal inhalations of aromic herbs. Classically, Ayurveda uses Camphor (*Cinnamomum camphora*) essential oil in hot water and the patient inhales the steam of the evaporating water / camphor mix. Other useful herbs for inhalations are Thyme (*Thymus vulgaris*) or Eucalyptus (*Eucalyptus globulus*). Note that essential oils should never be used internally or externally; inhalations are the only safe way to use essential oils.

Use the Vataja herbs if Vata is predominant in the Vikriti (imbalance) with a Vata Vikriti diet / lifestyle.

Use the Pittaja herbs if Pitta is predominant in the Vikriti (imbalance) with a Pitta Vikriti diet / lifestyle.

Use the Kaphaja herbs if Kapha is predominant in the Vikriti (imbalance) with a Kapha Vikriti diet / lifestyle.

## Candida

| Dosha | Code | Common Name | Latin Name |
|---|---|---|---|
| **Vataja** | 211 | Shatavari | Asparagus racemosus |
| | 207 | Haritaki | Terminalia chebula |
| | 401 | Cumin | Cumimum cyminum |
| | | Fennel | Foeniculum vulgare |
| | | Cardamom | Elettaria cardamomum |
| | 407 | Turmeric | Curcuma longa |
| | | Barberry | Berberis vulgaris |
| | | Dandelion | Taraxacum officinale |
| **Pittaja** | 211 | Shatavari | Asparagus racemosus |
| | 212 | Pau d'arco | Tabebuia impetiginosa |
| | 402 | Coriander | Coriandrum sativum |
| | | Cumin | Cumimum cyminum |
| | | Fennel | Foeniculum vulgare |
| | 407 | Turmeric | Curcuma longa |
| | | Barberry | Berberis vulgaris |
| | | Dandelion | Taraxacum officinale |
| **Kaphaja** | 207 | Haritaki | Terminalia chebula |
| | 212 | Pau d'arco | Tabebuia impetiginosa |
| | 403 | Ginger | Zingiber officinale |
| | | Cumin | Cumimum cyminum |
| | | Fenugreek | Trigonella foenum-graecum |
| | 407 | Turmeric | Curcuma longa |
| | | Barberry | Berberis vulgaris |
| | | Dandelion | Taraxacum officinale |

| Dosha | Low Dose | High Dose |
|---|---|---|
| **Vata** | 1 of each X2 per day before meals | 2 of each X2 per day before meals |
| **Pitta** | 1 of each X2 per day with meals | 2 of each X2 per day with meals |
| **Kapha** | 2 of each X2 per day after meals | 3 of each X2 per day after meals |

## Description:

Candida is a genus of yeasts. Many species of this genus are endosymbionts of animal hosts including humans. While usually living together with humans, some Candida species have the potential to cause disease. Clinically, the most significant member of the genus is *Candida albicans*, which can cause infections (called candidiasis or thrush) in humans, especially in immunocompromised patients. Many Candida species are members of gut flora in humans, including *C.*

*albicans.* The last decade has seen the sustained medical importance of opportunistic infections due to different Candida species mainly due to the worldwide increase in the number of immunocompromised patients, who are highly susceptible to opportunistic infections.

These formulas can be used for all types of digestive imbalances that implicate the digestive flora. In most cases Candida is an Ama condition that has been caused by a long-term disturbance of Agni that imbalances the bacteria, viruses and fungi that live in the intestines. This Ama condition can be caused by any Dosha. This formula will balance the flora and lower Ama levels in the digestive tract. The removal of Ama from the digestive system will tend to increase immunity as the body is not having to fight off a constant level of pathogens in the GI tract. These blends are safe to use from three to six months.

The diet should be changed to an anti-Ama diet appropriate for the Prakriti of the person. Coffee, carbonated drinks, alcohol and sugar should be removed from the diet as well as red meat. A vegan diet would be the best if possible. Lifestyle and diet should follow the Vikriti of the patient after the Anti-Ama diet has been completed.

Note for Thrush or vaginal candida that these blends are also helpful. Often chronic or reoccurring cases of thrush are due to an intestinal imbalance of the Candida yeasts that migrate to the vagina. This disrupts the vaginal flora and promotes the manifestation of vagina candida or thrush.

Use the Vataja herbs if Vata is predominant in the Vikriti (imbalance) with a Vata Vikriti diet / lifestyle.

Use the Pittaja herbs if Pitta is predominant in the Vikriti (imbalance) with a Pitta Vikriti diet / lifestyle.

Use the Kaphaja herbs if Kapha is predominant in the Vikriti (imbalance) with a Kapha Vikriti diet / lifestyle.

## Cardiac edema

| Dosha | Code | Common Name | Latin Name |
|---|---|---|---|
| Vataja | 202 | Arjuna | Terminalia arjuna |
| | 209 | Punarnava | Boerhaavia diffusa |
| | 404 | Angelica | Angelica archangelica |
| | | Wild yam | Dioscorea villosa |
| | | Valerian | Valeriana officinalis |
| Pittaja | 202 | Arjuna | Terminalia arjuna |
| | 209 | Punarnava | Boerhaavia diffusa |
| | 405 | Burdock | Arctium lappa |
| | | Yellow dock | Rumex crispus |
| | | Milk Thistle | Silybum marianum |
| Kaphaja | 202 | Arjuna | Terminalia arjuna |
| | 209 | Punarnava | Boerhaavia diffusa |
| | 406 | Myrrh | Commiphora myrrha |
| | | Elecampane | Inula helenium |
| | | Yellow dock | Rumex crispus |

| Dosha | Low Dose | High Dose |
|---|---|---|
| Vata | 1 of each X2 per day before meals | 2 of each X2 per day before meals |
| Pitta | 1 of each X2 per day with meals | 2 of each X2 per day with meals |
| Kapha | 2 of each X2 per day after meals | 3 of each X2 per day after meals |

### Description:

Cardiac edema is a Kapha Roga disorder by function and a Pitta disorder by location. Any Dosha can cause this problem when Avalambaka Kapha increases in the chest area including the lungs and heart. Kapha will cause congestion in the lungs or heart that can provoke this disorder; Pitta can cause congestion by provoking inflammation in the lungs or heart; and Vata can congestion by excessive dryness, or movement in the chest region. The patient should have exams to find out the cause of this disorder as it often a symptom of a more serious underlying problem.

Use the Vataja herbs if Vata is predominant in the Vikriti (imbalance) with a Vata Vikriti diet / lifestyle.

Use the Pittaja herbs if Pitta is predominant in the Vikriti (imbalance) with a Pitta Vikriti diet / lifestyle.

Use the Kaphaja herbs if Kapha is predominant in the Vikriti (imbalance) with a Kapha Vikriti diet / lifestyle.

## Cardiovascular Disease (CVD)

| Dosha | Code | Common Name | Latin Name |
|---|---|---|---|
| Vataja | 202 | Arjuna | Terminalia arjuna |
| | 301 | Amalaki | Emblica officinalis |
| | | Bibhitaki | Terminalia belerica |
| | | Haritaki | Terminalia chebula |
| | 404 | Angelica | Angelica archangelica |
| | | Wild yam | Dioscorea villosa |
| | | Valerian | Valeriana officinalis |
| Pittaja | 202 | Arjuna | Terminalia arjuna |
| | 301 | Amalaki | Emblica officinalis |
| | | Bibhitaki | Terminalia belerica |
| | | Haritaki | Terminalia chebula |
| | 405 | Burdock | Arctium lappa |
| | | Yellow dock | Rumex crispus |
| | | Milk Thistle | Silybum marianum |
| | 407 | Turmeric | Curcuma longa |
| | | Barberry | Berberis vulgaris |
| | | Dandelion | Taraxacum officinale |
| Kaphaja | 202 | Arjuna | Terminalia arjuna |
| | 209 | Punarnava | Boerhaavia diffusa |
| | 301 | Amalaki | Emblica officinalis |
| | | Bibhitaki | Terminalia belerica |
| | | Haritaki | Terminalia chebula |
| | 407 | Turmeric | Curcuma longa |
| | | Barberry | Berberis vulgaris |
| | | Dandelion | Taraxacum officinale |

| Dosha | Low Dose | High Dose |
|---|---|---|
| Vata | 1 of each X2 per day before meals | 2 of each X2 per day before meals |
| Pitta | 1 of each X2 per day with meals | 2 of each X2 per day with meals |
| Kapha | 2 of each X2 per day after meals | 3 of each X2 per day after meals |

## Description:

Cardiovascular Disease (CVD) kills almost three times as many people as cancer in the Western world. The term 'heart disease' is often used interchangeably with the term 'cardiovascular disease'. Cardiovascular disease generally refers to conditions that involve narrowed or blocked blood vessels that can lead to a heart attack (MI), chest pain (angina) or stroke. Other heart conditions, such as those that affect the heart's muscle, valves or rhythm, also are considered forms of heart disease. Diseases under the CVD umbrella include coronary artery disease (CAD), heart rhythm problems (arrhythmias), congestive heart disorders, congestive heart failure (CHF), ischemic heart disease (IHD), stroke, hypertensive heart disease, rheumatic heart disease (RHD), aortic aneurysms, cardiomyopathy, atrial fibrillation, and congenital heart defects.

The main treatment in Ayurveda for heart disorders or CVD is diet and lifestyle. Both diet and lifestyle should start with Vikriti indications and after basic stability is achieved then diet and lifestyle should be changed over to follow Prakriti. For mixed types this means seasonal diets and lifestyles. Stability means the patient is subjectively feeling better and objectively the symptomology that existed before treatment has reduced and is stable. In modern medicine, it is estimated that ninety percent of CVD is preventable.

Any Dosha can cause CVD as they are also disrupted from poor diet and lifestyle choices made by the patient. Agni gets disrupted which in turn disrupts the Dosha controlling the Agni; this may follow the Prakriti or Vikriti of the patient. Hence, it is important to understand that Doshas get deranged by poor diet and lifestyle as well as Dosha being able to cause heart disease on their own.

The guidelines can be used with the test: Vataja CVD gives variable onset, variable symptoms, shortness of breath; Pittaja CVD gives sudden onset, burning symptoms, strong & burning pain; Kaphaja CVD gives slow onset, congestive, regular symptoms. The treatment of diet, lifestyle and herbal blends should follow these indications and the indications of Vikriti from the test. The blends work to strengthen the heart, blood circulation, regulate cholesterol, remove Ama or plaque, and improve evacuation of wastes.

NOTE: These herbal blends may interfere with blood thinners or anticoagulants such as warfarin (e.g., Coumadin, Jantoven, Marevan, Uniwarfin) and fluindione (Previscan).

Use the Vataja herbs if Vata is predominant in the Vikriti (imbalance) with a Vata Vikriti diet / lifestyle.

Use the Pittaja herbs if Pitta is predominant in the Vikriti (imbalance) with a Pitta Vikriti diet / lifestyle.

Use the Kaphaja herbs if Kapha is predominant in the Vikriti (imbalance) with a Kapha Vikriti diet / lifestyle.

## Cholesterol

| Dosha | Code | Common Name | Latin Name |
|---|---|---|---|
| Vataja | 202 | Arjuna | Terminalia arjuna |
| | 301 | Amalaki | Emblica officinalis |
| | | Bibhitaki | Terminalia belerica |
| | | Haritaki | Terminalia chebula |
| | 404 | Angelica | Angelica archangelica |
| | | Wild yam | Dioscorea villosa |
| | | Valerian | Valeriana officinalis |
| Pittaja | 202 | Arjuna | Terminalia arjuna |
| | 301 | Amalaki | Emblica officinalis |
| | | Bibhitaki | Terminalia belerica |
| | | Haritaki | Terminalia chebula |
| | 405 | Burdock | Arctium lappa |
| | | Yellow dock | Rumex crispus |
| | | Milk Thistle | Silybum marianum |
| | 407 | Turmeric | Curcuma longa |
| | | Barberry | Berberis vulgaris |
| | | Dandelion | Taraxacum officinale |
| Kaphaja | 202 | Arjuna | Terminalia arjuna |
| | 209 | Punarnava | Boerhaavia diffusa |
| | 301 | Amalaki | Emblica officinalis |
| | | Bibhitaki | Terminalia belerica |
| | | Haritaki | Terminalia chebula |
| | 407 | Turmeric | Curcuma longa |
| | | Barberry | Berberis vulgaris |
| | | Dandelion | Taraxacum officinale |

| Dosha | Low Dose | High Dose |
|---|---|---|
| Vata | 1 of each X2 per day before meals | 2 of each X2 per day before meals |
| Pitta | 1 of each X2 per day with meals | 2 of each X2 per day with meals |
| Kapha | 2 of each X2 per day after meals | 3 of each X2 per day after meals |

## Description:

These blends regulate cholesterol, use as per Vikriti.

Use the Vataja herbs if Vata is predominant in the Vikriti (imbalance) with a Vata Vikriti diet / lifestyle.

Use the Pittaja herbs if Pitta is predominant in the Vikriti (imbalance) with a Pitta Vikriti diet / lifestyle.

Use the Kaphaja herbs if Kapha is predominant in the Vikriti (imbalance) with a Kapha Vikriti diet / lifestyle.

## Chronic Fatigue Syndrome (CFS)

| Dosha | Code | Common Name | Latin Name |
|-------|------|-------------|------------|
| Vataja | 203 | Ashwagandha | Withania somnifera |
| | 206 | Guduchi | Tinospora cordifolia |
| | 212 | Pau d'arco | Tabebuia impetiginosa |
| | 301 | Amalaki | Emblica officinalis |
| | | Bibhitaki | Terminalia belerica |
| | | Haritaki | Terminalia chebula |
| Pittaja | 201 | Amalaki | Emblica officinalis |
| | 206 | Guduchi | Tinospora cordifolia |
| | 212 | Pau d'arco | Tabebuia impetiginosa |
| | 301 | Amalaki | Emblica officinalis |
| | | Bibhitaki | Terminalia belerica |
| | | Haritaki | Terminalia chebula |
| Kaphaja | 206 | Guduchi | Tinospora cordifolia |
| | 209 | Punarnava | Boerhaavia diffusa |
| | 212 | Pau d'arco | Tabebuia impetiginosa |
| | 301 | Amalaki | Emblica officinalis |
| | | Bibhitaki | Terminalia belerica |
| | | Haritaki | Terminalia chebula |

| Dosha | Low Dose | High Dose |
|-------|----------|-----------|
| Vata | 1 of each X2 per day before meals | 2 of each X2 per day before meals |
| Pitta | 1 of each X2 per day with meals | 2 of each X2 per day with meals |
| Kapha | 2 of each X2 per day after meals | 3 of each X2 per day after meals |

### Description:

Chronic fatigue syndrome (CFS) is also commonly known as myalgic encephalomyelitis or ME. Symptoms of CFS include widespread muscle and joint pain, cognitive difficulties, chronic mental and physical exhaustion. The main cause in Ayurveda is a combination of Ama with low Ojas. These blends work to reduce Ama and increase Ojas. Any Dosha can cause this disorder, follow Vikriti indications.

Use the Vataja herbs if Vata is predominant in the Vikriti (imbalance) with a Vata Vikriti diet / lifestyle.

Use the Pittaja herbs if Pitta is predominant in the Vikriti (imbalance) with a Pitta Vikriti diet / lifestyle.

Use the Kaphaja herbs if Kapha is predominant in the Vikriti (imbalance) with a Kapha Vikriti diet / lifestyle.

## Cirrhosis of the Liver

| Dosha | Code | Common Name | Latin Name |
|---|---|---|---|
| **Vataja** | 401 | Cumin | Cumimum cyminum |
| | | Fennel | Foeniculum vulgare |
| | | Cardamom | Elettaria cardamomum |
| | 407 | Turmeric | Curcuma longa |
| | | Barberry | Berberis vulgaris |
| | | Dandelion | Taraxacum officinale |
| **Pittaja** | 402 | Coriander | Coriandrum sativum |
| | | Cumin | Cumimum cyminum |
| | | Fennel | Foeniculum vulgare |
| | 405 | Burdock | Arctium lappa |
| | | Yellow dock | Rumex crispus |
| | | Milk Thistle | Silybum marianum |
| | 407 | Turmeric | Curcuma longa |
| | | Barberry | Berberis vulgaris |
| | | Dandelion | Taraxacum officinale |
| **Kaphaja** | 208 | Manjishta | Rubia cordifolia |
| | 403 | Ginger | Zingiber officinale |
| | | Cumin | Cumimum cyminum |
| | | Fenugreek | Trigonella foenum-graecum |
| | 407 | Turmeric | Curcuma longa |
| | | Barberry | Berberis vulgaris |
| | | Dandelion | Taraxacum officinale |

| Dosha | Low Dose | High Dose |
|---|---|---|
| **Vata** | 1 of each X2 per day before meals | 2 of each X2 per day before meals |
| **Pitta** | 1 of each X2 per day with meals | 2 of each X2 per day with meals |
| **Kapha** | 2 of each X2 per day after meals | 3 of each X2 per day after meals |

## Description:

Cirrhosis is a late stage of scarring (fibrosis) of the liver caused by many forms of liver diseases and conditions, such as hepatitis and chronic alcoholism. It is a Pitta Roga disorder by both function and location.

Use the Vataja herbs if Vata is predominant in the Vikriti (imbalance) with a Vata Vikriti diet / lifestyle.

Use the Pittaja herbs if Pitta is predominant in the Vikriti (imbalance) with a Pitta Vikriti diet / lifestyle.

Use the Kaphaja herbs if Kapha is predominant in the Vikriti (imbalance) with a Kapha Vikriti diet / lifestyle.

# Cold (common)

| Dosha | Code | Common Name | Latin Name |
|-------|------|-------------|------------|
| **Vataja** | 401 | Cumin | Cumimum cyminum |
| | | Fennel | Foeniculum vulgare |
| | | Cardamom | Elettaria cardamomum |
| | 405 | Burdock | Arctium lappa |
| | | Yellow dock | Rumex crispus |
| | | Milk Thistle | Silybum marianum |
| | 406 | Myrrh | Commiphora myrrha |
| | | Elecampane | Inula helenium |
| | | Yellow dock | Rumex crispus |
| **Pittaja** | 402 | Coriander | Coriandrum sativum |
| | | Cumin | Cumimum cyminum |
| | | Fennel | Foeniculum vulgare |
| | 405 | Burdock | Arctium lappa |
| | | Yellow dock | Rumex crispus |
| | | Milk Thistle | Silybum marianum |
| | 406 | Myrrh | Commiphora myrrha |
| | | Elecampane | Inula helenium |
| | | Yellow dock | Rumex crispus |
| **Kaphaja** | 403 | Ginger | Zingiber officinale |
| | | Cumin | Cumimum cyminum |
| | | Fenugreek | Trigonella foenum-graecum |
| | 405 | Burdock | Arctium lappa |
| | | Yellow dock | Rumex crispus |
| | | Milk Thistle | Silybum marianum |
| | 406 | Myrrh | Commiphora myrrha |
| | | Elecampane | Inula helenium |
| | | Yellow dock | Rumex crispus |

| Dosha | Low Dose | High Dose |
|-------|----------|-----------|
| **Vata** | 1 of each X2 per day before meals | 2 of each X2 per day before meals |
| **Pitta** | 1 of each X2 per day with meals | 2 of each X2 per day with meals |
| **Kapha** | 2 of each X2 per day after meals | 3 of each X2 per day after meals |

## Description:

The Common Cold is a viral infectious disease of the upper respiratory tract which primarily affects the nose and sinuses. Signs and symptoms include coughing, sore throat, runny nose, sneezing, and sometimes fever which usually resolves in seven to ten days. Well over 200 virus strains are implicated in the cause of the common cold; the rhinoviruses are the most common. With children colds, can appear from three to six times a year – depending on their age and season. Ayurveda classifies a cold as Kapha Roga by both location and function as it is an increase of Avalambaka and Bodhaka Kapha in Rasa Dhatu. Any number of reasons can be behind Kapha increasing – foremost is Ama accumulation in the body from incorrect diet, food combinations or habits.

Rest with lots of fluids and avoiding Kapha increasing foods is the main treatment. Thyme (*Thymus vulgaris*) is the best single herb to use as it is antiviral and works to reduce both Vata and Kapha strongly. Thyme can be used as an infusion or inhalation, or both together. The inhalation of Thyme is an excellent treatment X3 to X4 per day when possible. If it is not available, then Camphor or Eucalyptus leaves can be used instead for inhalations. Echinacea tincture (*Echinacea angustifolia*) can also be used internally in combination with the inhalations at a dose appropriate for the age of the patient. Infusions of Sage (*Salvia officinalis*) are also very useful.

These blends are very effective to reduce Ama and Kapha in both Rasa Dhatu and specifically the respiratory system. Both Avalambaka and Bodhaka Kapha are reduced and controlled by these blends which combine well with all of the other treatments suggested above. After treatment of the Cold it is suggested to continue the use of these blends for another seven to ten days to assure the health of Rasa Dhatu. This treatment can be followed by several months of the 'Low immunity' blends to strengthen the person.

Use the Vataja herbs if Vata is predominant in the Vikriti (imbalance) with a Vata Vikriti diet / lifestyle.

Use the Pittaja herbs if Pitta is predominant in the Vikriti (imbalance) with a Pitta Vikriti diet / lifestyle.

Use the Kaphaja herbs if Kapha is predominant in the Vikriti (imbalance) with a Kapha Vikriti diet / lifestyle.

## Colic (Adult)

| Dosha | Code | Common Name | Latin Name |
|---|---|---|---|
| Vataja | 207 | Haritaki | Terminalia chebula |
| | 401 | Cumin | Cumimum cyminum |
| | | Fennel | Foeniculum vulgare |
| | | Cardamom | Elettaria cardamomum |
| | 404 | Angelica | Angelica archangelica |
| | | Wild yam | Dioscorea villosa |
| | | Valerian | Valeriana officinalis |
| Pittaja | 201 | Amalaki | Emblica officinalis |
| | 402 | Coriander | Coriandrum sativum |
| | | Cumin | Cumimum cyminum |
| | | Fennel | Foeniculum vulgare |
| | 407 | Turmeric | Curcuma longa |
| | | Barberry | Berberis vulgaris |
| | | Dandelion | Taraxacum officinale |
| Kaphaja | 207 | Haritaki | Terminalia chebula |
| | 403 | Ginger | Zingiber officinale |
| | | Cumin | Cumimum cyminum |
| | | Fenugreek | Trigonella foenum-graecum |
| | 407 | Turmeric | Curcuma longa |
| | | Barberry | Berberis vulgaris |
| | | Dandelion | Taraxacum officinale |

| Dosha | Low Dose | High Dose |
|---|---|---|
| Vata | 1 of each X2 per day before meals | 2 of each X2 per day before meals |
| Pitta | 1 of each X2 per day with meals | 2 of each X2 per day with meals |
| Kapha | 2 of each X2 per day after meals | 3 of each X2 per day after meals |

## Description:

Adult colic is a broad range of gastrointestinal disorders in which the main symptom is abdominal pain. This is a generally a Vata disorder, but any Dosha can cause colic pain, bloating and gas by aggravating Vata. Use the diet and herbal blends as per Vikriti.

Use the Vataja herbs if Vata is predominant in the Vikriti (imbalance) with a Vata Vikriti diet / lifestyle.

Use the Pittaja herbs if Pitta is predominant in the Vikriti (imbalance) with a Pitta Vikriti diet / lifestyle.

Use the Kaphaja herbs if Kapha is predominant in the Vikriti (imbalance) with a Kapha Vikriti diet / lifestyle.

## Colitis (IBD)

| Dosha | Code | Common Name | Latin Name |
|---|---|---|---|
| Vataja | 211 | Shatavari | Asparagus racemosus |
| | 301 | Amalaki | Emblica officinalis |
| | | Bibhitaki | Terminalia belerica |
| | | Haritaki | Terminalia chebula |
| | 407 | Turmeric | Curcuma longa |
| | | Barberry | Berberis vulgaris |
| | | Dandelion | Taraxacum officinale |
| Pittaja | 206 | Guduchi | Tinospora cordifolia |
| | 301 | Amalaki | Emblica officinalis |
| | | Bibhitaki | Terminalia belerica |
| | | Haritaki | Terminalia chebula |
| | 407 | Turmeric | Curcuma longa |
| | | Barberry | Berberis vulgaris |
| | | Dandelion | Taraxacum officinale |
| Kaphaja | 206 | Guduchi | Tinospora cordifolia |
| | 301 | Amalaki | Emblica officinalis |
| | | Bibhitaki | Terminalia belerica |
| | | Haritaki | Terminalia chebula |
| | 407 | Turmeric | Curcuma longa |
| | | Barberry | Berberis vulgaris |
| | | Dandelion | Taraxacum officinale |

| Dosha | Low Dose | High Dose |
|---|---|---|
| Vata | 1 of each X2 per day before meals | 2 of each X2 per day before meals |
| Pitta | 1 of each X2 per day with meals | 2 of each X2 per day with meals |
| Kapha | 2 of each X2 per day after meals | 3 of each X2 per day after meals |

## Description:

Ulcerative colitis is an inflammatory bowel disease (IBD) that causes inflammation and sores (ulcers) in the lining of the large intestine. It is a Pitta disorder by function and can be mixed with either Vata or Kapha. Ama is usually the cause, use as per Vikriti.

Use the Vataja herbs if Vata is predominant in the Vikriti (imbalance) with a Vata Vikriti diet / lifestyle.

Use the Pittaja herbs if Pitta is predominant in the Vikriti (imbalance) with a Pitta Vikriti diet / lifestyle.

Use the Kaphaja herbs if Kapha is predominant in the Vikriti (imbalance) with a Kapha Vikriti diet / lifestyle.

## Congestive heart disorders

| Dosha | Code | Common Name | Latin Name |
|---|---|---|---|
| **Vataja** | 202 | Arjuna | Terminalia arjuna |
| | 301 | Amalaki | Emblica officinalis |
| | | Bibhitaki | Terminalia belerica |
| | | Haritaki | Terminalia chebula |
| | 404 | Angelica | Angelica archangelica |
| | | Wild yam | Dioscorea villosa |
| | | Valerian | Valeriana officinalis |
| **Pittaja** | 202 | Arjuna | Terminalia arjuna |
| | 301 | Amalaki | Emblica officinalis |
| | | Bibhitaki | Terminalia belerica |
| | | Haritaki | Terminalia chebula |
| | 405 | Burdock | Arctium lappa |
| | | Yellow dock | Rumex crispus |
| | | Milk Thistle | Silybum marianum |
| | 407 | Turmeric | Curcuma longa |
| | | Barberry | Berberis vulgaris |
| | | Dandelion | Taraxacum officinale |
| **Kaphaja** | 202 | Arjuna | Terminalia arjuna |
| | 209 | Punarnava | Boerhaavia diffusa |
| | 301 | Amalaki | Emblica officinalis |
| | | Bibhitaki | Terminalia belerica |
| | | Haritaki | Terminalia chebula |
| | 407 | Turmeric | Curcuma longa |
| | | Barberry | Berberis vulgaris |
| | | Dandelion | Taraxacum officinale |

| Dosha | Low Dose | High Dose |
|---|---|---|
| **Vata** | 1 of each X2 per day before meals | 2 of each X2 per day before meals |
| **Pitta** | 1 of each X2 per day with meals | 2 of each X2 per day with meals |
| **Kapha** | 2 of each X2 per day after meals | 3 of each X2 per day after meals |

## Description:
See Cardiovascular Disease (CVD)

Use the Vataja herbs if Vata is predominant in the Vikriti (imbalance) with a Vata Vikriti diet / lifestyle.

Use the Pittaja herbs if Pitta is predominant in the Vikriti (imbalance) with a Pitta Vikriti diet / lifestyle.

Use the Kaphaja herbs if Kapha is predominant in the Vikriti (imbalance) with a Kapha Vikriti diet / lifestyle.

## Constipation

| Dosha | Code | Common Name | Latin Name |
|---|---|---|---|
| **Vataja** | 207 | Haritaki | Terminalia chebula |
| | 301 | Amalaki | Emblica officinalis |
| | | Bibhitaki | Terminalia belerica |
| | | Haritaki | Terminalia chebula |
| **Pittaja** | 301 | Amalaki | Emblica officinalis |
| | | Bibhitaki | Terminalia belerica |
| | | Haritaki | Terminalia chebula |
| | 407 | Turmeric | Curcuma longa |
| | | Barberry | Berberis vulgaris |
| | | Dandelion | Taraxacum officinale |
| **Kaphaja** | 207 | Haritaki | Terminalia chebula |
| | 403 | Ginger | Zingiber officinale |
| | | Cumin | Cumimum cyminum |
| | | Fenugreek | Trigonella foenum-graecum |
| | 406 | Myrrh | Commiphora myrrha |
| | | Elecampane | Inula helenium |
| | | Yellow dock | Rumex crispus |

| Dosha | Low Dose | High Dose |
|---|---|---|
| **Vata** | 1 of each X2 per day before meals | 2 of each X2 per day before meals |
| **Pitta** | 1 of each X2 per day with meals | 2 of each X2 per day with meals |
| **Kapha** | 2 of each X2 per day after meals | 3 of each X2 per day after meals |

## Description:

These blends are best used for constipation due to Kaphaja or Pittaja. I suggest using castor oil (*Ricinus communis*) for Vataja constipation for Vata Prakriti patients. Any dryness associated with constipation should be treated as Vataja. Constipation is a derangement of Agni, it is important to study Agni and find out what is disturbing Agni and treat that. There are two main types of constipation: 1) dry, hard stool – Vataja; 2) congested type – Pittaja / Kaphaja. Laxative herbs will tend to increase chronic constipation and should be avoided.

Use the Vataja herbs if Vata is predominant in the Vikriti (imbalance) with a Vata Vikriti diet / lifestyle.

Use the Pittaja herbs if Pitta is predominant in the Vikriti (imbalance) with a Pitta Vikriti diet / lifestyle.

Use the Kaphaja herbs if Kapha is predominant in the Vikriti (imbalance) with a Kapha Vikriti diet / lifestyle.

## Convalescence

| Dosha | Code | Common Name | Latin Name |
|---|---|---|---|
| Vataja | 203 | Ashwagandha | Withania somnifera |
| | 206 | Guduchi | Tinospora cordifolia |
| | 211 | Shatavari | Asparagus racemosus |
| | 301 | Amalaki | Emblica officinalis |
| | | Bibhitaki | Terminalia belerica |
| | | Haritaki | Terminalia chebula |
| Pittaja | 201 | Amalaki | Emblica officinalis |
| | 206 | Guduchi | Tinospora cordifolia |
| | 211 | Shatavari | Asparagus racemosus |
| | 301 | Amalaki | Emblica officinalis |
| | | Bibhitaki | Terminalia belerica |
| | | Haritaki | Terminalia chebula |
| Kaphaja | 206 | Guduchi | Tinospora cordifolia |
| | 209 | Punarnava | Boerhaavia diffusa |
| | 212 | Pau d'arco | Tabebuia impetiginosa |
| | 301 | Amalaki | Emblica officinalis |
| | | Bibhitaki | Terminalia belerica |
| | | Haritaki | Terminalia chebula |

| Dosha | Low Dose | High Dose |
|---|---|---|
| Vata | 1 of each X2 per day before meals | 2 of each X2 per day before meals |
| Pitta | 1 of each X2 per day with meals | 2 of each X2 per day with meals |
| Kapha | 2 of each X2 per day after meals | 3 of each X2 per day after meals |

## Description:

These are Rasayana blends for each Prakriti type. Use a blend as per the Prakriti of the person, or if there is a strong Vikriti with no Ama follow that until the person is stable; then follow the Prakriti. These blends can be used after any serious illness to help the patient recover their health and immunity.

Use the Vataja herbs if Vata is predominant in the Prakriti with a Vata Prakriti diet / lifestyle.

Use the Pittaja herbs if Pitta is predominant in the Prakriti with a Pitta Prakriti diet / lifestyle.

Use the Kaphaja herbs if Kapha is predominant in the Prakriti with a Kapha Prakriti diet / lifestyle.

## Convulsions

| Dosha | Code | Common Name | Latin Name |
|-------|------|-------------|------------|
| Vataja | 204 | Bramhi | Bacopa monnieri |
|  | 210 | Shankhpushpi | Convolvulus pluricaulis |
|  | 401 | Cumin | Cumimum cyminum |
|  |  | Fennel | Foeniculum vulgare |
|  |  | Cardamom | Elettaria cardamomum |
| Pittaja | 204 | Bramhi | Bacopa monnieri |
|  | 210 | Shankhpushpi | Convolvulus pluricaulis |
|  | 402 | Coriander | Coriandrum sativum |
|  |  | Cumin | Cumimum cyminum |
|  |  | Fennel | Foeniculum vulgare |
| Kaphaja | 204 | Bramhi | Bacopa monnieri |
|  | 210 | Shankhpushpi | Convolvulus pluricaulis |
|  | 403 | Ginger | Zingiber officinale |
|  |  | Cumin | Cumimum cyminum |
|  |  | Fenugreek | Trigonella foenum-graecum |

| Dosha | Low Dose | High Dose |
|-------|----------|-----------|
| Vata | 1 of each X2 per day before meals | 2 of each X2 per day before meals |
| Pitta | 1 of each X2 per day with meals | 2 of each X2 per day with meals |
| Kapha | 2 of each X2 per day after meals | 3 of each X2 per day after meals |

### Description:

Convulsions are when a person has uncontrollable shaking that is rapid and rhythmic, in which the muscles contract and relax repeatedly. There are many different types of seizures. Some have mild symptoms without shaking. Convulsions of all types are caused by disorganized and sudden electrical activity in the brain. There are many causes, some of which are very serious need to be correctly diagnosed and treated. This advice is mainly for idiopathic seizures.

Ayurveda views this as Vataja by function and Kaphaja by structure (Majja Dhatu). It is classified as a Vata Roga problem. Lifestyle therapies are very important and Nadishodhana pranayama should be done daily. Lifestyle needs to be very regular with stress reducing therapies. External therapies of oil and heat (Snehana and Svedhana) need to be given to the patient at least three times per week; daily treatments would be best. If this is not possible then Abhyanga should be done by the patient. Treatment should follow Vikriti; Ama can be a primary cause in idiopathic convulsions.

NOTE: There are possible interaction with psychoactive medicines or antidepressants, large doses may cause dizziness and disorientation.

- Use the Vataja herbs if Vata is predominant in the Vikriti (imbalance) with a Vata Vikriti diet / lifestyle.
- Use the Pittaja herbs if Pitta is predominant in the Vikriti (imbalance) with a Pitta Vikriti diet / lifestyle.
- Use the Kaphaja herbs if Kapha is predominant in the Vikriti (imbalance) with a Kapha Vikriti diet / lifestyle.

## Coronary artery disorders

| Dosha | Code | Common Name | Latin Name |
|-------|------|-------------|------------|
| **Vataja** | 202 | Arjuna | Terminalia arjuna |
| | 301 | Amalaki | Emblica officinalis |
| | | Bibhitaki | Terminalia belerica |
| | | Haritaki | Terminalia chebula |
| | 404 | Angelica | Angelica archangelica |
| | | Wild yam | Dioscorea villosa |
| | | Valerian | Valeriana officinalis |
| **Pittaja** | 202 | Arjuna | Terminalia arjuna |
| | 301 | Amalaki | Emblica officinalis |
| | | Bibhitaki | Terminalia belerica |
| | | Haritaki | Terminalia chebula |
| | 405 | Burdock | Arctium lappa |
| | | Yellow dock | Rumex crispus |
| | | Milk Thistle | Silybum marianum |
| | 407 | Turmeric | Curcuma longa |
| | | Barberry | Berberis vulgaris |
| | | Dandelion | Taraxacum officinale |
| **Kaphaja** | 202 | Arjuna | Terminalia arjuna |
| | 209 | Punarnava | Boerhaavia diffusa |
| | 301 | Amalaki | Emblica officinalis |
| | | Bibhitaki | Terminalia belerica |
| | | Haritaki | Terminalia chebula |
| | 407 | Turmeric | Curcuma longa |
| | | Barberry | Berberis vulgaris |
| | | Dandelion | Taraxacum officinale |

| Dosha | Low Dose | High Dose |
|-------|----------|-----------|
| **Vata** | 1 of each X2 per day before meals | 2 of each X2 per day before meals |
| **Pitta** | 1 of each X2 per day with meals | 2 of each X2 per day with meals |
| **Kapha** | 2 of each X2 per day after meals | 3 of each X2 per day after meals |

## Description:
See Cardiovascular Disease.

Use the Vataja herbs if Vata is predominant in the Vikriti (imbalance) with a Vata Vikriti diet / lifestyle.

Use the Pittaja herbs if Pitta is predominant in the Vikriti (imbalance) with a Pitta Vikriti diet / lifestyle.

Use the Kaphaja herbs if Kapha is predominant in the Vikriti (imbalance) with a Kapha Vikriti diet / lifestyle.

# Cough

| Dosha | Code | Common Name | Latin Name |
|-------|------|-------------|------------|
| Vataja | 403 | Ginger | Zingiber officinale |
| | | Cumin | Cumimum cyminum |
| | | Fenugreek | Trigonella foenum-graecum |
| | 406 | Myrrh | Commiphora myrrha |
| | | Elecampane | Inula helenium |
| | | Yellow dock | Rumex crispus |
| | 407 | Turmeric | Curcuma longa |
| | | Barberry | Berberis vulgaris |
| | | Dandelion | Taraxacum officinale |
| | 409 | Marshmallow | Althaea officinalis |
| | | Gotu kola | Centella asiatica |
| | | Stinging nettles | Urtica dioica |
| Pittaja | 402 | Coriander | Coriandrum sativum |
| | | Cumin | Cumimum cyminum |
| | | Fennel | Foeniculum vulgare |
| | 403 | Ginger | Zingiber officinale |
| | | Cumin | Cumimum cyminum |
| | | Fenugreek | Trigonella foenum-graecum |
| | 406 | Myrrh | Commiphora myrrha |
| | | Elecampane | Inula helenium |
| | | Yellow dock | Rumex crispus |
| | 407 | Turmeric | Curcuma longa |
| | | Barberry | Berberis vulgaris |
| | | Dandelion | Taraxacum officinale |
| Kaphaja | 209 | Punarnava | Boerhaavia diffusa |
| | 403 | Ginger | Zingiber officinale |
| | | Cumin | Cumimum cyminum |
| | | Fenugreek | Trigonella foenum-graecum |
| | 406 | Myrrh | Commiphora myrrha |
| | | Elecampane | Inula helenium |
| | | Yellow dock | Rumex crispus |
| | 407 | Turmeric | Curcuma longa |
| | | Barberry | Berberis vulgaris |
| | | Dandelion | Taraxacum officinale |

| Dosha | Low Dose | High Dose |
|-------|----------|-----------|
| Vata | 1 of each X2 per day before meals | 2 of each X2 per day before meals |
| Pitta | 1 of each X2 per day with meals | 2 of each X2 per day with meals |
| Kapha | 2 of each X2 per day after meals | 3 of each X2 per day after meals |

## Description:

These blends are best used for chronic coughs or coughs that persist longer than three days. Immediate relief from cough can be had from sucking on a slice of raw ginger root (pealed). If fresh ginger is a problem a tablespoon of honey and lemon is a classic remedy.

Coughs are a problem of Kapha structure (Rasa Dhatu) and weaken the lungs, throat and sinuses. Functionally coughs can be caused by Vataja, Pittaja, or Kaphaja so it is important to correctly identify which Dosha is causing the problem. General guidelines are:

- **Vataja**: dry cough, worse in early morning and afternoon
- **Pittaja**: inflammation, yellow / green mucus coughing up, worse in midday and around midnight
- **Kaphaja**: congested with lots of white or clear mucus, worse in morning and early evening

It is very important to stop coughs as soon as possible as they weaken the lungs and can cause degenerative respiratory problems later in life. These blends will clear and clean the respiratory system and strengthen it if the herbal blends are taken for several weeks after the cough stops.

Use the Vataja herbs if Vata is predominant in the Vikriti (imbalance) with a Vata Vikriti diet / lifestyle.

Use the Pittaja herbs if Pitta is predominant in the Vikriti (imbalance) with a Pitta Vikriti diet / lifestyle.

Use the Kaphaja herbs if Kapha is predominant in the Vikriti (imbalance) with a Kapha Vikriti diet / lifestyle.

## Cramps

| Dosha | Code | Common Name | Latin Name |
|---|---|---|---|
| **Vataja** | 210 | Shankhpushpi | Convolvulus pluricaulis |
| | 403 | Ginger | Zingiber officinale |
| | | Cumin | Cumimum cyminum |
| | | Fenugreek | Trigonella foenum-graecum |
| | 408 | Vitex | Vitex agnus-castus |
| | | Black cohosh | Cimicifuga racemosa |
| | | Cramp bark | Viburnum opulus |
| **Pittaja** | 210 | Shankhpushpi | Convolvulus pluricaulis |
| | 402 | Coriander | Coriandrum sativum |
| | | Cumin | Cumimum cyminum |
| | | Fennel | Foeniculum vulgare |
| | 408 | Vitex | Vitex agnus-castus |
| | | Black cohosh | Cimicifuga racemosa |
| | | Cramp bark | Viburnum opulus |
| **Kaphaja** | 210 | Shankhpushpi | Convolvulus pluricaulis |
| | 403 | Ginger | Zingiber officinale |
| | | Cumin | Cumimum cyminum |
| | | Fenugreek | Trigonella foenum-graecum |
| | 408 | Vitex | Vitex agnus-castus |
| | | Black cohosh | Cimicifuga racemosa |
| | | Cramp bark | Viburnum opulus |

| Dosha | Low Dose | High Dose |
|---|---|---|
| **Vata** | 1 of each X2 per day before meals | 2 of each X2 per day before meals |
| **Pitta** | 1 of each X2 per day with meals | 2 of each X2 per day with meals |
| **Kapha** | 2 of each X2 per day after meals | 3 of each X2 per day after meals |

## Description:

These blends are mainly for premenstrual cramps, but can be used for any muscle cramping if needed. Use as per Vikriti Dosha. This is a Vataja problem functionally.

Use the Vataja herbs if Vata is predominant in the Vikriti (imbalance) with a Vata Vikriti diet / lifestyle.

Use the Pittaja herbs if Pitta is predominant in the Vikriti (imbalance) with a Pitta Vikriti diet / lifestyle.

Use the Kaphaja herbs if Kapha is predominant in the Vikriti (imbalance) with a Kapha Vikriti diet / lifestyle.

## Cystitis

| Dosha | Code | Common Name | Latin Name |
|---|---|---|---|
| **Vataja** | 205 | Gokshura | Tribulus terrestris |
| | 402 | Coriander | Coriandrum sativum |
| | | Cumin | Cumimum cyminum |
| | | Fennel | Foeniculum vulgare |
| | 405 | Burdock | Arctium lappa |
| | | Yellow dock | Rumex crispus |
| | | Milk Thistle | Silybum marianum |
| | 409 | Marshmallow | Althaea officinalis |
| | | Gotu kola | Centella asiatica |
| | | Stinging nettles | Urtica dioica |
| **Pittaja** | 205 | Gokshura | Tribulus terrestris |
| | 402 | Coriander | Coriandrum sativum |
| | | Cumin | Cumimum cyminum |
| | | Fennel | Foeniculum vulgare |
| | 405 | Burdock | Arctium lappa |
| | | Yellow dock | Rumex crispus |
| | | Milk Thistle | Silybum marianum |
| | 409 | Marshmallow | Althaea officinalis |
| | | Gotu kola | Centella asiatica |
| | | Stinging nettles | Urtica dioica |
| **Kaphaja** | 205 | Gokshura | Tribulus terrestris |
| | 209 | Punarnava | Boerhaavia diffusa |
| | 402 | Coriander | Coriandrum sativum |
| | | Cumin | Cumimum cyminum |
| | | Fennel | Foeniculum vulgare |
| | 405 | Burdock | Arctium lappa |
| | | Yellow dock | Rumex crispus |
| | | Milk Thistle | Silybum marianum |

| Dosha | Low Dose | High Dose |
|---|---|---|
| **Vata** | 1 of each X2 per day before meals | 2 of each X2 per day before meals |
| **Pitta** | 1 of each X2 per day with meals | 2 of each X2 per day with meals |
| **Kapha** | 2 of each X2 per day after meals | 3 of each X2 per day after meals |

## Description:

Cystitis is inflammation of the urinary bladder. The condition more often affects women, but can affect either sex and all age groups. Very often cystitis is caused from an imbalance in the colon or an excessive amount of Ama in the colon. Either condition will create a bacterial imbalance in the intestinal flora that will affect the bladder by proximity. Other causes of cystitis are poor hygiene, excessive sex, not drinking enough liquids, drinking too much coffee or alcohol. For women, vaginal flora should also be monitored. This is a classic Pitta problem that often plagues Pitta Prakriti people. These herbal blends can be used as an anti-inflammatory for the whole urinary system including urethra, bladder and kidneys if needed.

The bladder and kidneys are part of Meda Dhatu so under the control of Kapha Dosha structurally. Functionally, the bladder is used by Vata Dosha (Apana Vayu) to remove urine. Any Dosha can be the cause of this disorder. Pitta is always implicated to some extent as it is behind inflammatory conditions.

If there is no clear pathology or symptomology for the patient then use these formulas according to Vikriti. A Pitta reducing diet is very important for the treatment of all urinary infections.

NOTE: use of these blends should be limited to one month in most cases; minimum period of treatment should be two weeks and maximum five weeks. FOR ACUTE cystitis use this formula and a tincture of *Hydrastis canadensis* (Golden Seal) at a dose of 25 drops X4 per day for 10 days. After ten days stop using the Golden Seal and continue with the blends as per the Vikriti.

Use the Vataja herbs if Vata is predominant in the Vikriti (imbalance) with a Pitta Vikriti diet / lifestyle.

Use the Pittaja herbs if Pitta is predominant in the Vikriti (imbalance) with a Pitta Vikriti diet / lifestyle.

Use the Kaphaja herbs if Kapha is predominant in the Vikriti (imbalance) with a Pitta Vikriti diet / lifestyle.

## Cysts

| Dosha | Code | Common Name | Latin Name |
|---|---|---|---|
| **Vataja** | 401 | Cumin | Cumimum cyminum |
| | | Fennel | Foeniculum vulgare |
| | | Cardamom | Elettaria cardamomum |
| | 406 | Myrrh | Commiphora myrrha |
| | | Elecampane | Inula helenium |
| | | Yellow dock | Rumex crispus |
| | 407 | Turmeric | Curcuma longa |
| | | Barberry | Berberis vulgaris |
| | | Dandelion | Taraxacum officinale |
| | 408 | Vitex | Vitex agnus-castus |
| | | Black cohosh | Cimicifuga racemosa |
| | | Cramp bark | Viburnum opulus |
| **Pittaja** | 402 | Coriander | Coriandrum sativum |
| | | Cumin | Cumimum cyminum |
| | | Fennel | Foeniculum vulgare |
| | 405 | Burdock | Arctium lappa |
| | | Yellow dock | Rumex crispus |
| | | Milk Thistle | Silybum marianum |
| | 407 | Turmeric | Curcuma longa |
| | | Barberry | Berberis vulgaris |
| | | Dandelion | Taraxacum officinale |
| | 408 | Vitex | Vitex agnus-castus |
| | | Black cohosh | Cimicifuga racemosa |
| | | Cramp bark | Viburnum opulus |
| **Kaphaja** | 403 | Ginger | Zingiber officinale |
| | | Cumin | Cumimum cyminum |
| | | Fenugreek | Trigonella foenum-graecum |
| | 406 | Myrrh | Commiphora myrrha |
| | | Elecampane | Inula helenium |
| | | Yellow dock | Rumex crispus |
| | 407 | Turmeric | Curcuma longa |
| | | Barberry | Berberis vulgaris |
| | | Dandelion | Taraxacum officinale |
| | 408 | Vitex | Vitex agnus-castus |
| | | Black cohosh | Cimicifuga racemosa |
| | | Cramp bark | Viburnum opulus |

| Dosha | Low Dose | High Dose |
|-------|----------|-----------|
| Vata | 1 of each X2 per day before meals | 2 of each X2 per day before meals |
| Pitta | 1 of each X2 per day with meals | 2 of each X2 per day with meals |
| Kapha | 2 of each X2 per day after meals | 3 of each X2 per day after meals |

## Description:

A cyst is a closed sac having a distinct membrane and division on the nearby tissue. It may contain air, fluids, or semi-solid material. Once formed, the cyst could go away by itself or may have to be removed using surgery. There are many different types of cysts, both functional and dysfunctional. Cystic fibrosis is another type of problem and is not actually a cyst.

This formula can be used for any growths in the body that are hormone dependent (functional). For dysfunctional cysts (not dependent on hormones) see the indications for Tumors. The purpose of this formula is to stop the endocrine imbalance that is responsible for the cyst. Once this is done the formula then reduces the size of the growth until the cyst is decreased and evacuated from the body through normal evacuation channels. These formulas will work very well from Rasa to Mamsa Dhatus, but can be used on all Dhatus. Cysts or tumors are Kaphaja by function and the location is by Dhatu (tissue, gland, or organ). Both men and women can benefit from these blends. Use the herbal blend for six to eighteen months for the best effects. If the cyst is just beginning then four to six months of treatment could resolve the problem. Plan on one year of treatment with the patient.

If there is no clear pathology or symptomology for the patient then use this formula according to Vikriti. A Kapha reducing diet is helpful for the treatment of all cysts as a Vegan diet. Lifestyle therapies are extremely important. Ayurvedic therapies such as Pranayama, yoga, exercise and relaxation are indicated.

Use the Vataja herbs if Vata is predominant in the Vikriti (imbalance) with a Kapha Vikriti diet / lifestyle.

Use the Pittaja herbs if Pitta is predominant in the Vikriti (imbalance) with a Kapha Vikriti diet / lifestyle.

Use the Kaphaja herbs if Kapha is predominant in the Vikriti (imbalance) with a Kapha Vikriti diet / lifestyle.

## Debility

| Dosha | Code | Common Name | Latin Name |
|-------|------|-------------|------------|
| Vataja | 203 | Ashwagandha | Withania somnifera |
| | 206 | Guduchi | Tinospora cordifolia |
| | 212 | Pau d'arco | Tabebuia impetiginosa |
| | 301 | Amalaki | Emblica officinalis |
| | | Bibhitaki | Terminalia belerica |
| | | Haritaki | Terminalia chebula |
| Pittaja | 201 | Amalaki | Emblica officinalis |
| | 206 | Guduchi | Tinospora cordifolia |
| | 212 | Pau d'arco | Tabebuia impetiginosa |
| | 301 | Amalaki | Emblica officinalis |
| | | Bibhitaki | Terminalia belerica |
| | | Haritaki | Terminalia chebula |
| Kaphaja | 206 | Guduchi | Tinospora cordifolia |
| | 209 | Punarnava | Boerhaavia diffusa |
| | 212 | Pau d'arco | Tabebuia impetiginosa |
| | 301 | Amalaki | Emblica officinalis |
| | | Bibhitaki | Terminalia belerica |
| | | Haritaki | Terminalia chebula |

| Dosha | Low Dose | High Dose |
|-------|----------|-----------|
| Vata | 1 of each X2 per day before meals | 2 of each X2 per day before meals |
| Pitta | 1 of each X2 per day with meals | 2 of each X2 per day with meals |
| Kapha | 2 of each X2 per day after meals | 3 of each X2 per day after meals |

## Description:

These blends are made to support and rejuvenate each Prakriti type. Debility is any condition in which the person feels tired and run down, but not suffering from a specific disorder. The blends should be used as per Vikriti. Once the Vikriti is lower and the patient wishes to continue rejuvenation use the 'Deficiency diseases' formula blends that increase Ojas and Shukra Dhatus as per Prakriti.

Use the Vataja herbs if Vata is predominant in the Vikriti (imbalance) with a Vata Vikriti diet / lifestyle.

Use the Pittaja herbs if Pitta is predominant in the Vikriti (imbalance) with a Pitta Vikriti diet / lifestyle.

Use the Kaphaja herbs if Kapha is predominant in the Vikriti (imbalance) with a Kapha Vikriti diet / lifestyle.

## Deficiency diseases (wasting diseases)

| Dosha | Code | Common Name | Latin Name |
|---|---|---|---|
| Vataja | 203 | Ashwagandha | Withania somnifera |
| | 206 | Guduchi | Tinospora cordifolia |
| | 211 | Shatavari | Asparagus racemosus |
| | 301 | Amalaki | Emblica officinalis |
| | | Bibhitaki | Terminalia belerica |
| | | Haritaki | Terminalia chebula |
| Pittaja | 201 | Amalaki | Emblica officinalis |
| | 206 | Guduchi | Tinospora cordifolia |
| | 211 | Shatavari | Asparagus racemosus |
| | 301 | Amalaki | Emblica officinalis |
| | | Bibhitaki | Terminalia belerica |
| | | Haritaki | Terminalia chebula |
| Kaphaja | 203 | Ashwagandha | Withania somnifera |
| | 206 | Guduchi | Tinospora cordifolia |
| | 209 | Punarnava | Boerhaavia diffusa |
| | 301 | Amalaki | Emblica officinalis |
| | | Bibhitaki | Terminalia belerica |
| | | Haritaki | Terminalia chebula |

| Dosha | Low Dose | High Dose |
|---|---|---|
| Vata | 1 of each X2 per day before meals | 2 of each X2 per day before meals |
| Pitta | 1 of each X2 per day with meals | 2 of each X2 per day with meals |
| Kapha | 2 of each X2 per day after meals | 3 of each X2 per day after meals |

## Description:

Deficiency diseases or 'wasting diseases' require Rasayana (rejuvenation) therapies as per Prakriti. The best approach would be to first understand and stop the cause of the disorder, then give these herbal blends to support and rejuvenate Ojas and Majja and Shukra Dhatus. If there is Ama in the system it is better to try and remove it first by using the diet, lifestyle and herbal blends for 'Ama'.

Use the Vataja herbs if Vata is predominant in the Prakriti with a Vata Prakriti diet / lifestyle.

Use the Pittaja herbs if Pitta is predominant in the Prakriti with a Pitta Prakriti diet / lifestyle.

Use the Kaphaja herbs if Kapha is predominant in the Prakriti with a Kapha Prakriti diet / lifestyle.

## Dehydration

| Dosha | Code | Common Name | Latin Name |
|---|---|---|---|
| Vataja | 211 | Shatavari | Asparagus racemosus |
| | 401 | Cumin | Cumimum cyminum |
| | | Fennel | Foeniculum vulgare |
| | | Cardamom | Elettaria cardamomum |
| | 409 | Marshmallow | Althaea officinalis |
| | | Gotu kola | Centella asiatica |
| | | Stinging nettles | Urtica dioica |
| Pittaja | 211 | Shatavari | Asparagus racemosus |
| | 402 | Coriander | Coriandrum sativum |
| | | Cumin | Cumimum cyminum |
| | | Fennel | Foeniculum vulgare |
| | 409 | Marshmallow | Althaea officinalis |
| | | Gotu kola | Centella asiatica |
| | | Stinging nettles | Urtica dioica |
| Kaphaja | 211 | Shatavari | Asparagus racemosus |
| | 403 | Ginger | Zingiber officinale |
| | | Cumin | Cumimum cyminum |
| | | Fenugreek | Trigonella foenum-graecum |
| | 409 | Marshmallow | Althaea officinalis |
| | | Gotu kola | Centella asiatica |
| | | Stinging nettles | Urtica dioica |

| Dosha | Low Dose | High Dose |
|---|---|---|
| Vata | 1 of each X2 per day before meals | 2 of each X2 per day before meals |
| Pitta | 1 of each X2 per day with meals | 2 of each X2 per day with meals |
| Kapha | 2 of each X2 per day after meals | 3 of each X2 per day after meals |

## Description:

Dehydration is a condition due to Vata Vriddhi (high Vata) that dries out the tissues of the body. It can be associated with a number of other disorders as a secondary condition. Treatment follows Vikriti.

Use the Vataja herbs if Vata is predominant in the Vikriti (imbalance) with a Vata Vikriti diet / lifestyle.

Use the Pittaja herbs if Pitta is predominant in the Vikriti (imbalance) with a Pitta Vikriti diet / lifestyle.

Use the Kaphaja herbs if Kapha is predominant in the Vikriti (imbalance) with a Kapha Vikriti diet / lifestyle.

## Delayed menstruation

| Dosha | Code | Common Name | Latin Name |
|---|---|---|---|
| Vataja | 211 | Shatavari | Asparagus racemosus |
| | 403 | Ginger | Zingiber officinale |
| | | Cumin | Cumimum cyminum |
| | | Fenugreek | Trigonella foenum-graecum |
| | 408 | Vitex | Vitex agnus-castus |
| | | Black cohosh | Cimicifuga racemosa |
| | | Cramp bark | Viburnum opulus |
| Pittaja | 211 | Shatavari | Asparagus racemosus |
| | 402 | Coriander | Coriandrum sativum |
| | | Cumin | Cumimum cyminum |
| | | Fennel | Foeniculum vulgare |
| | 407 | Turmeric | Curcuma longa |
| | | Barberry | Berberis vulgaris |
| | | Dandelion | Taraxacum officinale |
| | 408 | Vitex | Vitex agnus-castus |
| | | Black cohosh | Cimicifuga racemosa |
| | | Cramp bark | Viburnum opulus |
| Kaphaja | 208 | Manjishta | Rubia cordifolia |
| | 403 | Ginger | Zingiber officinale |
| | | Cumin | Cumimum cyminum |
| | | Fenugreek | Trigonella foenum-graecum |
| | 407 | Turmeric | Curcuma longa |
| | | Barberry | Berberis vulgaris |
| | | Dandelion | Taraxacum officinale |
| | 408 | Vitex | Vitex agnus-castus |
| | | Black cohosh | Cimicifuga racemosa |
| | | Cramp bark | Viburnum opulus |

| Dosha | Low Dose | High Dose |
|---|---|---|
| Vata | 1 of each X2 per day before meals | 2 of each X2 per day before meals |
| Pitta | 1 of each X2 per day with meals | 2 of each X2 per day with meals |
| Kapha | 2 of each X2 per day after meals | 3 of each X2 per day after meals |

## Description:

Delayed menstruation can be due to number of reasons such as a major weight loss, excessive exercise, poor diet low in nutrients, or high stress. It can also indicate more serious disorders such as thyroid problems, PCOS or different forms of PID. Of course, any kind of ongoing hormonal imbalance can also cause this kind of issue.

Menstruation is the Upadhatu of Rasa Dhatu and thus controlled by Kapha Dosha. The first place to look is at Rasa Dhatu and see if there is an insufficiency of Rasa (plasma, etc.). This happens when sudden weight loss or excessive exercise can reduce or stop menstruation. Functionally, all three Doshas have a role in menstruation, so it is important to understand the role of each Dosha. Remember the following points about menstruation (*Artava* or *Raja*):

- Kapha controls the fluid through Rasa Dhatu (Upadhatu)
- Kapha controls the growth hormones through Shukra Dhatu
- Pitta controls the uterus and gives color to the fluid through Rakta Dhatu
- Pitta controls hormone levels in the blood through liver & Rakta Dhatu
- Vata controls all cycles in time & endocrine function
- Vata controls the release of menstrual fluid through Apana Vayu
- Vata controls non-growth hormones in general
- Vata controls both Kapha and Pitta

All three Doshas need to be evaluated to understand the cause of the problem. The cause will be indicated by the Vikriti so this is what should be followed for treatment. Also, be aware that stopping the Pill can disrupt menstruation for several months. These blends can also be used to establish a normal cycle.

Use the Vataja herbs if Vata is predominant in the Vikriti (imbalance) with a Vata Vikriti diet / lifestyle.

Use the Pittaja herbs if Pitta is predominant in the Vikriti (imbalance) with a Pitta Vikriti diet / lifestyle.

Use the Kaphaja herbs if Kapha is predominant in the Vikriti (imbalance) with a Kapha Vikriti diet / lifestyle.

NOTE: a full discussion on women's health can be found in the textbook: *Ayurvedic Medicine for Westerners, Vol. 5; Application of Ayurvedic Treatments Throughout Life*, 2016

# Depression

| Dosha | Code | Common Name | Latin Name |
|-------|------|-------------|------------|
| **Vataja** | 204 | Bramhi | Bacopa monnieri |
| | 210 | Shankhpushpi | Convolvulus pluricaulis |
| | 401 | Cumin | Cumimum cyminum |
| | | Fennel | Foeniculum vulgare |
| | | Cardamom | Elettaria cardamomum |
| | 404 | Angelica | Angelica archangelica |
| | | Wild yam | Dioscorea villosa |
| | | Valerian | Valeriana officinalis |
| **Pittaja** | 204 | Bramhi | Bacopa monnieri |
| | 210 | Shankhpushpi | Convolvulus pluricaulis |
| | 402 | Coriander | Coriandrum sativum |
| | | Cumin | Cumimum cyminum |
| | | Fennel | Foeniculum vulgare |
| | 410 | Passion flower | Passiflora incarnata |
| | | Skullcap | Scutellaria lateriflora |
| | | Gotu kola | Centella asiatica |
| **Kaphaja** | 204 | Bramhi | Bacopa monnieri |
| | 403 | Ginger | Zingiber officinale |
| | | Cumin | Cumimum cyminum |
| | | Fenugreek | Trigonella foenum-graecum |
| | 406 | Myrrh | Commiphora myrrha |
| | | Elecampane | Inula helenium |
| | | Yellow dock | Rumex crispus |
| | 410 | Passion flower | Passiflora incarnata |
| | | Skullcap | Scutellaria lateriflora |
| | | Gotu kola | Centella asiatica |

| Dosha | Low Dose | High Dose |
|-------|----------|-----------|
| **Vata** | 1 of each X2 per day before meals | 2 of each X2 per day before meals |
| **Pitta** | 1 of each X2 per day with meals | 2 of each X2 per day with meals |
| **Kapha** | 2 of each X2 per day after meals | 3 of each X2 per day after meals |

## Description:

Depression is one of the most common problems today. It can be caused by any Dosha. These formulas can be used for all forms of depression *except* clinical depression, which may need additional special treatment, or counseling. These herbal blends are slightly stimulating to remove blockage in Manovahasrota. They also work on the mind and nerves by sedative and nervine action. The blends are also effective for cyclic, or hormonal forms of depression as there is a mildly balancing action on the endocrine system. These blends work best with mantra therapy, pranayama, or other methods to reduce mental stagnation or Tamas Guna in the mind. The overall action of the blends is Sattvic. The herbs should be used for at least three months and not more than twelve months.

If there is no clear pathology or symptomology for the patient then use this formula according to Vikriti. Mantra and pranayama are highly recommended to accelerate results. The type of mantra and pranayama used depends on which Dosha is causing the depression.

Diet is very important in the treatment of depression. Junk food, fast food and processed foods need to be stopped. A whole food diet will stop many forms of depression as some of the chemicals used in the food industry have been linked to behavioral modification. Ayurveda suggests a vegetarian or vegan diet for best results. Avoid all stimulants such as sugar, coffee, etc.

NOTE: There are possible interaction with psychoactive medicines or antidepressants, large doses may cause dizziness and disorientation.

Use the Vataja herbs if Vata is predominant in the Vikriti (imbalance) with a Vata Vikriti diet / lifestyle.

Use the Pittaja herbs if Pitta is predominant in the Vikriti (imbalance) with a Pitta Vikriti diet / lifestyle.

Use the Kaphaja herbs if Kapha is predominant in the Vikriti (imbalance) with a Kapha Vikriti diet / lifestyle.

## Diabetes, type II

| Dosha | Code | Common Name | Latin Name |
|---|---|---|---|
| Vataja | 205 | Gokshura | Tribulus terrestris |
| | 208 | Manjishta | Rubia cordifolia |
| | 401 | Cumin | Cumimum cyminum |
| | | Fennel | Foeniculum vulgare |
| | | Cardamom | Elettaria cardamomum |
| | 407 | Turmeric | Curcuma longa |
| | | Barberry | Berberis vulgaris |
| | | Dandelion | Taraxacum officinale |
| Pittaja | 205 | Gokshura | Tribulus terrestris |
| | 208 | Manjishta | Rubia cordifolia |
| | 402 | Coriander | Coriandrum sativum |
| | | Cumin | Cumimum cyminum |
| | | Fennel | Foeniculum vulgare |
| | 407 | Turmeric | Curcuma longa |
| | | Barberry | Berberis vulgaris |
| | | Dandelion | Taraxacum officinale |
| Kaphaja | 205 | Gokshura | Tribulus terrestris |
| | 208 | Manjishta | Rubia cordifolia |
| | 403 | Ginger | Zingiber officinale |
| | | Cumin | Cumimum cyminum |
| | | Fenugreek | Trigonella foenum-graecum |
| | 407 | Turmeric | Curcuma longa |
| | | Barberry | Berberis vulgaris |
| | | Dandelion | Taraxacum officinale |

| Dosha | Low Dose | High Dose |
|---|---|---|
| Vata | 1 of each X2 per day before meals | 2 of each X2 per day before meals |
| Pitta | 1 of each X2 per day with meals | 2 of each X2 per day with meals |
| Kapha | 2 of each X2 per day after meals | 3 of each X2 per day after meals |

### Description:
Choose the blend as per Vikriti dominance.

Use the Vataja herbs if Vata is predominant in the Vikriti (imbalance) with a Vata Vikriti diet / lifestyle.

Use the Pittaja herbs if Pitta is predominant in the Vikriti (imbalance) with a Pitta Vikriti diet / lifestyle.

Use the Kaphaja herbs if Kapha is predominant in the Vikriti (imbalance) with a Kapha Vikriti diet / lifestyle.

## Diarrhea

| Dosha | Code | Common Name | Latin Name |
|-------|------|-------------|------------|
| Vataja | 401 | Cumin | Cumimum cyminum |
| | | Fennel | Foeniculum vulgare |
| | | Cardamom | Elettaria cardamomum |
| | 407 | Turmeric | Curcuma longa |
| | | Barberry | Berberis vulgaris |
| | | Dandelion | Taraxacum officinale |
| | 409 | Marshmallow | Althaea officinalis |
| | | Gotu kola | Centella asiatica |
| | | Stinging nettles | Urtica dioica |
| Pittaja | 402 | Coriander | Coriandrum sativum |
| | | Cumin | Cumimum cyminum |
| | | Fennel | Foeniculum vulgare |
| | 407 | Turmeric | Curcuma longa |
| | | Barberry | Berberis vulgaris |
| | | Dandelion | Taraxacum officinale |
| | 409 | Marshmallow | Althaea officinalis |
| | | Gotu kola | Centella asiatica |
| | | Stinging nettles | Urtica dioica |
| Kaphaja | 403 | Ginger | Zingiber officinale |
| | | Cumin | Cumimum cyminum |
| | | Fenugreek | Trigonella foenum-graecum |
| | 407 | Turmeric | Curcuma longa |
| | | Barberry | Berberis vulgaris |
| | | Dandelion | Taraxacum officinale |
| | 409 | Marshmallow | Althaea officinalis |
| | | Gotu kola | Centella asiatica |
| | | Stinging nettles | Urtica dioica |

| Dosha | Low Dose | High Dose |
|-------|----------|-----------|
| Vata | 1 of each X2 per day before meals | 2 of each X2 per day before meals |
| Pitta | 1 of each X2 per day with meals | 2 of each X2 per day with meals |
| Kapha | 2 of each X2 per day after meals | 3 of each X2 per day after meals |

## Description:

Diarrhea is a dangerous condition, especially for children and the elderly, as it causes dehydration in the body. In extreme cases this can cause death. Hence, diarrhea should be treated quickly and not allowed to develop or create deeper more complex problems. In Ayurveda, this is a Pitta Roga condition.

There are a number causes for Diarrhea such as dysentery, bacterial infections, poor diet, bad food (old or rotten), toxic cooking oils (often found in fast food), flu, fever, or Pitta Vriddhi (high Pitta) conditions. Understanding the cause is very important as the Diarrhea could be the indication of a deeper cause.

This is a problem of Pachaka Pitta in most cases. Pachaka can be increased by the above factors or by emotions. High Vata conditions (e.g., stress) can also cause an increase in Pachaka. If the cause seems to be from virus or bacterial infections use the blends for Dysentery.

Use the Vataja herbs if Vata is predominant in the Vikriti (imbalance) with a Vata Vikriti diet / lifestyle.

Use the Pittaja herbs if Pitta is predominant in the Vikriti (imbalance) with a Pitta Vikriti diet / lifestyle.

Use the Kaphaja herbs if Kapha is predominant in the Vikriti (imbalance) with a Kapha Vikriti diet / lifestyle.

## Digestive problems

| Dosha | Code | Common Name | Latin Name |
|---|---|---|---|
| Vataja | 301 | Amalaki | Emblica officinalis |
| | | Bibhitaki | Terminalia belerica |
| | | Haritaki | Terminalia chebula |
| | 401 | Cumin | Cumimum cyminum |
| | | Fennel | Foeniculum vulgare |
| | | Cardamom | Elettaria cardamomum |
| | 407 | Turmeric | Curcuma longa |
| | | Barberry | Berberis vulgaris |
| | | Dandelion | Taraxacum officinale |
| Pittaja | 402 | Coriander | Coriandrum sativum |
| | | Cumin | Cumimum cyminum |
| | | Fennel | Foeniculum vulgare |
| | 407 | Turmeric | Curcuma longa |
| | | Barberry | Berberis vulgaris |
| | | Dandelion | Taraxacum officinale |
| Kaphaja | 403 | Ginger | Zingiber officinale |
| | | Cumin | Cumimum cyminum |
| | | Fenugreek | Trigonella foenum-graecum |
| | 407 | Turmeric | Curcuma longa |
| | | Barberry | Berberis vulgaris |
| | | Dandelion | Taraxacum officinale |

| Dosha | Low Dose | High Dose |
|---|---|---|
| Vata | 1 of each X2 per day before meals | 2 of each X2 per day before meals |
| Pitta | 1 of each X2 per day with meals | 2 of each X2 per day with meals |
| Kapha | 2 of each X2 per day after meals | 3 of each X2 per day after meals |

## Description:
These blends correct digestive issues as per Vikriti. Of course, it is important during treatment to avoid food that causes problems.

Use the Vataja herbs if Vata is predominant in the Vikriti (imbalance) with a Vata Vikriti diet / lifestyle.

Use the Pittaja herbs if Pitta is predominant in the Vikriti (imbalance) with a Pitta Vikriti diet / lifestyle.

Use the Kaphaja herbs if Kapha is predominant in the Vikriti (imbalance) with a Kapha Vikriti diet / lifestyle.

## Digestive stimulant

| Dosha | Code | Common Name | Latin Name |
|---|---|---|---|
| Vataja | 401 | Cumin | Cumimum cyminum |
| | | Fennel | Foeniculum vulgare |
| | | Cardamom | Elettaria cardamomum |
| | 404 | Angelica | Angelica archangelica |
| | | Wild yam | Dioscorea villosa |
| | | Valerian | Valeriana officinalis |
| Pittaja | 402 | Coriander | Coriandrum sativum |
| | | Cumin | Cumimum cyminum |
| | | Fennel | Foeniculum vulgare |
| | 405 | Burdock | Arctium lappa |
| | | Yellow dock | Rumex crispus |
| | | Milk Thistle | Silybum marianum |
| Kaphaja | 403 | Ginger | Zingiber officinale |
| | | Cumin | Cumimum cyminum |
| | | Fenugreek | Trigonella foenum-graecum |
| | 406 | Myrrh | Commiphora myrrha |
| | | Elecampane | Inula helenium |
| | | Yellow dock | Rumex crispus |

| Dosha | Low Dose | High Dose |
|---|---|---|
| Vata | 1 of each X2 per day before meals | 2 of each X2 per day before meals |
| Pitta | 1 of each X2 per day with meals | 2 of each X2 per day with meals |
| Kapha | 2 of each X2 per day after meals | 3 of each X2 per day after meals |

## Description:

These blends correct and stimulate digestion in a balanced manner by correcting Dosha function. As the Doshas control Agni and Agni is the main factor in digestion, these blends balance and support correct Agni function. Use the blend as per Vikriti.

Use the Vataja herbs if Vata is predominant in the Vikriti (imbalance) with a Vata Vikriti diet / lifestyle.

Use the Pittaja herbs if Pitta is predominant in the Vikriti (imbalance) with a Pitta Vikriti diet / lifestyle.

Use the Kaphaja herbs if Kapha is predominant in the Vikriti (imbalance) with a Kapha Vikriti diet / lifestyle.

## Diverticulitis

| Dosha | Code | Common Name | Latin Name |
|---|---|---|---|
| **Vataja** | 401 | Cumin | Cumimum cyminum |
| | | Fennel | Foeniculum vulgare |
| | | Cardamom | Elettaria cardamomum |
| | 404 | Angelica | Angelica archangelica |
| | | Wild yam | Dioscorea villosa |
| | | Valerian | Valeriana officinalis |
| | 407 | Turmeric | Curcuma longa |
| | | Barberry | Berberis vulgaris |
| | | Dandelion | Taraxacum officinale |
| | 409 | Marshmallow | Althaea officinalis |
| | | Gotu kola | Centella asiatica |
| | | Stinging nettles | Urtica dioica |
| **Pittaja** | 402 | Coriander | Coriandrum sativum |
| | | Cumin | Cumimum cyminum |
| | | Fennel | Foeniculum vulgare |
| | 404 | Angelica | Angelica archangelica |
| | | Wild yam | Dioscorea villosa |
| | | Valerian | Valeriana officinalis |
| | 407 | Turmeric | Curcuma longa |
| | | Barberry | Berberis vulgaris |
| | | Dandelion | Taraxacum officinale |
| | 409 | Marshmallow | Althaea officinalis |
| | | Gotu kola | Centella asiatica |
| | | Stinging nettles | Urtica dioica |
| **Kaphaja** | 403 | Ginger | Zingiber officinale |
| | | Cumin | Cumimum cyminum |
| | | Fenugreek | Trigonella foenum-graecum |
| | 404 | Angelica | Angelica archangelica |
| | | Wild yam | Dioscorea villosa |
| | | Valerian | Valeriana officinalis |
| | 407 | Turmeric | Curcuma longa |
| | | Barberry | Berberis vulgaris |
| | | Dandelion | Taraxacum officinale |

| Dosha | Low Dose | High Dose |
|---|---|---|
| **Vata** | 1 of each X2 per day before meals | 2 of each X2 per day before meals |
| **Pitta** | 1 of each X2 per day with meals | 2 of each X2 per day with meals |
| **Kapha** | 2 of each X2 per day after meals | 3 of each X2 per day after meals |

**Description:**

These herbal blends can be used to remove Ama from the G.I. tract and to heal the damaged walls of the intestines. These blends are anti-inflammatory and will heal any wounds in the mucus membrane. According to Ayurveda, diverticulitis, colitis, IBS (Irritable Bowel Syndrome) and other painful problems that have lesions or infections in the mucus membranes of the digestive tube are caused by Ama. When Ama accumulates on the intestine walls the membranes underneath the Ama become damaged. These formulas remove Ama, reduce infection, and stops pain and inflammation. It is advised to use these blends for at least three months for the best effect. Normally it takes six to twelve months to cure a chronic disorder of the GI tract like diverticulitis. These blends will give the patient fairly fast relief – in about five to seven days they should experience a reduction in symptoms in most cases.

The mucus membranes in the GI tract are under the control of Rasa Dhatu and Kapha Dosha; so structurally this is a problem of Kapha. Functionally, all three Doshas can be implicated and equally any of the Doshas can be the cause of the disorder.

Use these formulas according to Vikriti. The diet should be changed to an anti-Ama diet appropriate for the Vikriti of the person. If possible coffee, carbonated drinks, alcohol, sugar and red meat should be removed from the diet. A vegetarian, or vegan diet would be best.

Use the Vataja herbs if Vata is predominant in the Vikriti (imbalance) with a Vata Vikriti diet / lifestyle.

Use the Pittaja herbs if Pitta is predominant in the Vikriti (imbalance) with a Pitta Vikriti diet / lifestyle.

Use the Kaphaja herbs if Kapha is predominant in the Vikriti (imbalance) with a Kapha Vikriti diet / lifestyle.

## Duodenal ulcers

| Dosha | Code | Common Name | Latin Name |
|-------|------|-------------|------------|
| **Vataja** | 201 | Amalaki | Emblica officinalis |
| | 211 | Shatavari | Asparagus racemosus |
| | 401 | Cumin | Cumimum cyminum |
| | | Fennel | Foeniculum vulgare |
| | | Cardamom | Elettaria cardamomum |
| | 404 | Angelica | Angelica archangelica |
| | | Wild yam | Dioscorea villosa |
| | | Valerian | Valeriana officinalis |
| **Pittaja** | 201 | Amalaki | Emblica officinalis |
| | 211 | Shatavari | Asparagus racemosus |
| | 402 | Coriander | Coriandrum sativum |
| | | Cumin | Cumimum cyminum |
| | | Fennel | Foeniculum vulgare |
| | 405 | Burdock | Arctium lappa |
| | | Yellow dock | Rumex crispus |
| | | Milk Thistle | Silybum marianum |
| **Kaphaja** | 201 | Amalaki | Emblica officinalis |
| | 211 | Shatavari | Asparagus racemosus |
| | 402 | Coriander | Coriandrum sativum |
| | | Cumin | Cumimum cyminum |
| | | Fennel | Foeniculum vulgare |
| | 404 | Angelica | Angelica archangelica |
| | | Wild yam | Dioscorea villosa |
| | | Valerian | Valeriana officinalis |

| Dosha | Low Dose | High Dose |
|-------|----------|-----------|
| **Vata** | 1 of each X2 per day before meals | 2 of each X2 per day before meals |
| **Pitta** | 1 of each X2 per day with meals | 2 of each X2 per day with meals |
| **Kapha** | 2 of each X2 per day after meals | 3 of each X2 per day after meals |

## Description:
Ulcers are a Pitta Roga problem. Use the blend as per Vikriti.

Use the Vataja herbs if Vata is predominant in the Vikriti (imbalance) with a Vata Vikriti diet / lifestyle.

Use the Pittaja herbs if Pitta is predominant in the Vikriti (imbalance) with a Pitta Vikriti diet / lifestyle.

Use the Kaphaja herbs if Kapha is predominant in the Vikriti (imbalance) with a Kapha Vikriti diet / lifestyle.

## Dysentery

| Dosha | Code | Common Name | Latin Name |
|-------|------|-------------|------------|
| **Vataja** | 207 | Haritaki | Terminalia chebula |
| | 212 | Pau d'arco | Tabebuia impetiginosa |
| | 401 | Cumin | Cumimum cyminum |
| | | Fennel | Foeniculum vulgare |
| | | Cardamom | Elettaria cardamomum |
| | 407 | Turmeric | Curcuma longa |
| | | Barberry | Berberis vulgaris |
| | | Dandelion | Taraxacum officinale |
| **Pittaja** | 207 | Haritaki | Terminalia chebula |
| | 212 | Pau d'arco | Tabebuia impetiginosa |
| | 402 | Coriander | Coriandrum sativum |
| | | Cumin | Cumimum cyminum |
| | | Fennel | Foeniculum vulgare |
| | 407 | Turmeric | Curcuma longa |
| | | Barberry | Berberis vulgaris |
| | | Dandelion | Taraxacum officinale |
| **Kaphaja** | 207 | Haritaki | Terminalia chebula |
| | 212 | Pau d'arco | Tabebuia impetiginosa |
| | 403 | Ginger | Zingiber officinale |
| | | Cumin | Cumimum cyminum |
| | | Fenugreek | Trigonella foenum-graecum |
| | 407 | Turmeric | Curcuma longa |
| | | Barberry | Berberis vulgaris |
| | | Dandelion | Taraxacum officinale |

| Dosha | Low Dose | High Dose |
|-------|----------|-----------|
| **Vata** | 1 of each X2 per day before meals | 2 of each X2 per day before meals |
| **Pitta** | 1 of each X2 per day with meals | 2 of each X2 per day with meals |
| **Kapha** | 2 of each X2 per day after meals | 3 of each X2 per day after meals |

## Description:

See the information under "Diarrhea"; use as per Vikriti.

Use the Vataja herbs if Vata is predominant in the Vikriti (imbalance) with a Vata Vikriti diet / lifestyle.

Use the Pittaja herbs if Pitta is predominant in the Vikriti (imbalance) with a Pitta Vikriti diet / lifestyle.

Use the Kaphaja herbs if Kapha is predominant in the Vikriti (imbalance) with a Kapha Vikriti diet / lifestyle.

# Dysmenorrhea (painful menstruation)

| Dosha | Code | Common Name | Latin Name |
|---|---|---|---|
| **Vataja** | 208 | Manjishta | Rubia cordifolia |
| | 401 | Cumin | Cumimum cyminum |
| | | Fennel | Foeniculum vulgare |
| | | Cardamom | Elettaria cardamomum |
| | 404 | Angelica | Angelica archangelica |
| | | Wild yam | Dioscorea villosa |
| | | Valerian | Valeriana officinalis |
| | 408 | Vitex | Vitex agnus-castus |
| | | Black cohosh | Cimicifuga racemosa |
| | | Cramp bark | Viburnum opulus |
| **Pittaja** | 208 | Manjishta | Rubia cordifolia |
| | 402 | Coriander | Coriandrum sativum |
| | | Cumin | Cumimum cyminum |
| | | Fennel | Foeniculum vulgare |
| | 405 | Burdock | Arctium lappa |
| | | Yellow dock | Rumex crispus |
| | | Milk Thistle | Silybum marianum |
| | 408 | Vitex | Vitex agnus-castus |
| | | Black cohosh | Cimicifuga racemosa |
| | | Cramp bark | Viburnum opulus |
| **Kaphaja** | 208 | Manjishta | Rubia cordifolia |
| | 403 | Ginger | Zingiber officinale |
| | | Cumin | Cumimum cyminum |
| | | Fenugreek | Trigonella foenum-graecum |
| | 406 | Myrrh | Commiphora myrrha |
| | | Elecampane | Inula helenium |
| | | Yellow dock | Rumex crispus |
| | 408 | Vitex | Vitex agnus-castus |
| | | Black cohosh | Cimicifuga racemosa |
| | | Cramp bark | Viburnum opulus |

| Dosha | Low Dose | High Dose |
|---|---|---|
| **Vata** | 1 of each X2 per day before meals | 2 of each X2 per day before meals |
| **Pitta** | 1 of each X2 per day with meals | 2 of each X2 per day with meals |
| **Kapha** | 2 of each X2 per day after meals | 3 of each X2 per day after meals |

## Description:

Dysmenorrhea is primarily a Vata Roga disorder and so all three herbal blends address Apana Vayu to some extent and return it from the uterus back into the colon where it belongs.

Typically, Apana Vayu is affecting the menstruation channel (Artavavaha Srota). A chronic imbalance of Vata may exist. High Vata can cause a drying or constriction of Rasavaha Srota which will deplete Rasa Dhatu. Deplete Rasa Dhatu will affect Pitta, Rakta Dhatu, Raktavaha Srota and Artavavaha Srota. Treatment aims to clear the movement of Apana Vayu. There should also be signs of Vata Vriddhi in the body and menstruation.

This can also be a Pittaja problem due to an excess of Pitta in Rakta Dhatu, which includes the uterus / vagina. Once Pitta increases beyond the point that the body can regulate it, Pitta will be forced out through menstruation. When this happens, the tissues become inflamed and irritated, causing Dysmenorrhea. There should also be signs of Pitta Vriddhi in the body and menstruation.

There exists a Kaphaja type of Dysmenorrhea in which Kapha accumulates in Artavavaha Srota and causes Apana Vayu to become blocked. This is experienced as pain or cramping. There should also be signs of Kapha Vriddhi in the body and menstruation.

The information for premenstrual disorders is also relevant here and can be applied. Here are some formulas that differ somewhat in that they address the constitution more than the ones for just cramps.

Use the Vataja herbs if Vata is predominant in the Vikriti (imbalance) with a Vata Vikriti diet / lifestyle.

Use the Pittaja herbs if Pitta is predominant in the Vikriti (imbalance) with a Pitta Vikriti diet / lifestyle.

Use the Kaphaja herbs if Kapha is predominant in the Vikriti (imbalance) with a Kapha Vikriti diet / lifestyle.

Note: for more information on Women's health see the textbook: *Ayurvedic Medicine for Westerners, Vol. 5; Application of Ayurvedic Treatments Throughout Life*, 2016

# Dyspepsia (indigestion)

| Dosha | Code | Common Name | Latin Name |
|---|---|---|---|
| Vataja | 207 | Haritaki | Terminalia chebula |
| | 401 | Cumin | Cumimum cyminum |
| | | Fennel | Foeniculum vulgare |
| | | Cardamom | Elettaria cardamomum |
| | 404 | Angelica | Angelica archangelica |
| | | Wild yam | Dioscorea villosa |
| | | Valerian | Valeriana officinalis |
| Pittaja | 201 | Amalaki | Emblica officinalis |
| | 402 | Coriander | Coriandrum sativum |
| | | Cumin | Cumimum cyminum |
| | | Fennel | Foeniculum vulgare |
| | 407 | Turmeric | Curcuma longa |
| | | Barberry | Berberis vulgaris |
| | | Dandelion | Taraxacum officinale |
| Kaphaja | 207 | Haritaki | Terminalia chebula |
| | 403 | Ginger | Zingiber officinale |
| | | Cumin | Cumimum cyminum |
| | | Fenugreek | Trigonella foenum-graecum |
| | 407 | Turmeric | Curcuma longa |
| | | Barberry | Berberis vulgaris |
| | | Dandelion | Taraxacum officinale |

| Dosha | Low Dose | High Dose |
|---|---|---|
| Vata | 1 of each X2 per day before meals | 2 of each X2 per day before meals |
| Pitta | 1 of each X2 per day with meals | 2 of each X2 per day with meals |
| Kapha | 2 of each X2 per day after meals | 3 of each X2 per day after meals |

## Description:

Dyspepsia can be defined as painful, difficult, or disturbed digestion, which may be accompanied by symptoms such as gas, nausea, vomiting, heartburn, bloating, and general discomfort. Any Dosha can cause this disorder, use the blends as per Vikriti.

Use the Vataja herbs if Vata is predominant in the Vikriti (imbalance) with a Vata Vikriti diet / lifestyle.

Use the Pittaja herbs if Pitta is predominant in the Vikriti (imbalance) with a Pitta Vikriti diet / lifestyle.

Use the Kaphaja herbs if Kapha is predominant in the Vikriti (imbalance) with a Kapha Vikriti diet / lifestyle.

# Eczema

| Dosha | Code | Common Name | Latin Name |
|-------|------|-------------|------------|
| **Vataja** | 401 | Cumin | Cumimum cyminum |
| | | Fennel | Foeniculum vulgare |
| | | Cardamom | Elettaria cardamomum |
| | 404 | Angelica | Angelica archangelica |
| | | Wild yam | Dioscorea villosa |
| | | Valerian | Valeriana officinalis |
| | 407 | Turmeric | Curcuma longa |
| | | Barberry | Berberis vulgaris |
| | | Dandelion | Taraxacum officinale |
| | 410 | Passion flower | Passiflora incarnata |
| | | Skullcap | Scutellaria lateriflora |
| | | Gotu kola | Centella asiatica |
| **Pittaja** | 402 | Coriander | Coriandrum sativum |
| | | Cumin | Cumimum cyminum |
| | | Fennel | Foeniculum vulgare |
| | 405 | Burdock | Arctium lappa |
| | | Yellow dock | Rumex crispus |
| | | Milk Thistle | Silybum marianum |
| | 407 | Turmeric | Curcuma longa |
| | | Barberry | Berberis vulgaris |
| | | Dandelion | Taraxacum officinale |
| | 410 | Passion flower | Passiflora incarnata |
| | | Skullcap | Scutellaria lateriflora |
| | | Gotu kola | Centella asiatica |
| **Kaphaja** | 403 | Ginger | Zingiber officinale |
| | | Cumin | Cumimum cyminum |
| | | Fenugreek | Trigonella foenum-graecum |
| | 405 | Burdock | Arctium lappa |
| | | Yellow dock | Rumex crispus |
| | | Milk Thistle | Silybum marianum |
| | 407 | Turmeric | Curcuma longa |
| | | Barberry | Berberis vulgaris |
| | | Dandelion | Taraxacum officinale |
| | 410 | Passion flower | Passiflora incarnata |
| | | Skullcap | Scutellaria lateriflora |
| | | Gotu kola | Centella asiatica |

| Dosha | Low Dose | High Dose |
|-------|----------|-----------|
| Vata | 1 of each X2 per day before meals | 2 of each X2 per day before meals |
| Pitta | 1 of each X2 per day with meals | 2 of each X2 per day with meals |
| Kapha | 2 of each X2 per day after meals | 3 of each X2 per day after meals |

## Description:

Eczema is a form of dermatitis, or inflammation of the epidermis. The term eczema is broadly applied to a range of persistent skin conditions. These include dryness and recurring skin rashes which are characterized by one or more of these symptoms: redness, skin edema (swelling), itching and dryness, crusting, flaking, blistering, cracking, oozing, or bleeding. Areas of temporary skin discoloration may appear and are sometimes due to healed lesions, although scarring is rare. In contrast to psoriasis, eczema is often likely to be found on the flexor (interior) aspect of joints. There are a number of psychosomatic varieties of Eczema (Vataja).

From an Ayurvedic point of view the group of disorders that we call eczema are mostly related to Rasadhatu and liver digestion of nutrients. Any Dosha can cause eczema, correct identification of the cause is very important for success in treatment.

- **Vataja** – variable symptoms, skin dryness, nervousness, high stress levels, Samavata
- **Pittaja** – regular & burning symptoms, skin inflammation, toxic blood, Samapitta
- **Kaphaja** – regular symptoms, skin edema, congestion, depression, Samakapha

Treatment begins by removing all agrochemicals from the diet, by the use of organic foods, and by removing all animal products if possible. Some organic dairy products can be allowed if needed, however, dairy products are often linked to skin disorders and are best removed. Agni needs to be balanced and Ama removed from the body – especially in the digestive system.

Use the Vataja herbs if Vata is predominant in the Vikriti (imbalance) with a Vata Vikriti diet / lifestyle.

Use the Pittaja herbs if Pitta is predominant in the Vikriti (imbalance) with a Pitta Vikriti diet / lifestyle.

Use the Kaphaja herbs if Kapha is predominant in the Vikriti (imbalance) with a Kapha Vikriti diet / lifestyle.

## Edema

| Dosha | Code | Common Name | Latin Name |
|---|---|---|---|
| Vataja | 205 | Gokshura | Tribulus terrestris |
| | 209 | Punarnava | Boerhaavia diffusa |
| | 401 | Cumin | Cumimum cyminum |
| | | Fennel | Foeniculum vulgare |
| | | Cardamom | Elettaria cardamomum |
| | 409 | Marshmallow | Althaea officinalis |
| | | Gotu kola | Centella asiatica |
| | | Stinging nettles | Urtica dioica |
| Pittaja | 205 | Gokshura | Tribulus terrestris |
| | 209 | Punarnava | Boerhaavia diffusa |
| | 402 | Coriander | Coriandrum sativum |
| | | Cumin | Cumimum cyminum |
| | | Fennel | Foeniculum vulgare |
| | 409 | Marshmallow | Althaea officinalis |
| | | Gotu kola | Centella asiatica |
| | | Stinging nettles | Urtica dioica |
| Kaphaja | 209 | Punarnava | Boerhaavia diffusa |
| | 403 | Ginger | Zingiber officinale |
| | | Cumin | Cumimum cyminum |
| | | Fenugreek | Trigonella foenum-graecum |
| | 406 | Myrrh | Commiphora myrrha |
| | | Elecampane | Inula helenium |
| | | Yellow dock | Rumex crispus |

| Dosha | Low Dose | High Dose |
|---|---|---|
| Vata | 1 of each X2 per day before meals | 2 of each X2 per day before meals |
| Pitta | 1 of each X2 per day with meals | 2 of each X2 per day with meals |
| Kapha | 2 of each X2 per day after meals | 3 of each X2 per day after meals |

## Description:

Kapha Roga can be caused by any Dosha. Follow treatment as per Vikriti.

Use the Vataja herbs if Vata is predominant in the Vikriti (imbalance) with a Vata Vikriti diet / lifestyle.

Use the Pittaja herbs if Pitta is predominant in the Vikriti (imbalance) with a Pitta Vikriti diet / lifestyle.

Use the Kaphaja herbs if Kapha is predominant in the Vikriti (imbalance) with a Kapha Vikriti diet / lifestyle.

## Emaciation

| Dosha | Code | Common Name | Latin Name |
|---|---|---|---|
| **Vataja** | 203 | Ashwagandha | Withania somnifera |
| | 211 | Shatavari | Asparagus racemosus |
| | 301 | Amalaki | Emblica officinalis |
| | | Bibhitaki | Terminalia belerica |
| | | Haritaki | Terminalia chebula |
| **Pittaja** | 203 | Ashwagandha | Withania somnifera |
| | 211 | Shatavari | Asparagus racemosus |
| | 301 | Amalaki | Emblica officinalis |
| | | Bibhitaki | Terminalia belerica |
| | | Haritaki | Terminalia chebula |
| **Kaphaja** | 203 | Ashwagandha | Withania somnifera |
| | 211 | Shatavari | Asparagus racemosus |
| | 301 | Amalaki | Emblica officinalis |
| | | Bibhitaki | Terminalia belerica |
| | | Haritaki | Terminalia chebula |

| Dosha | Low Dose | High Dose |
|---|---|---|
| **Vata** | 1 of each X2 per day before meals | 2 of each X2 per day before meals |
| **Pitta** | 1 of each X2 per day with meals | 2 of each X2 per day with meals |
| **Kapha** | 2 of each X2 per day after meals | 3 of each X2 per day after meals |

## Description:

This is a symptomatic treatment to increase tissue; a Rasayana diet and lifestyle are needed as per Prakriti. Effort should be made to find out why the patient is losing structure.

Use the Vataja herbs if Vata is predominant in the Prakriti (imbalance) with a Vata Prakriti diet / lifestyle.

Use the Pittaja herbs if Pitta is predominant in the Prakriti (imbalance) with a Pitta Prakriti diet / lifestyle.

Use the Kaphaja herbs if Kapha is predominant in the Prakriti (imbalance) with a Kapha Prakriti diet / lifestyle.

## Endometriosis

| Dosha | Code | Common Name | Latin Name |
|---|---|---|---|
| Vataja | 206 | Guduchi | Tinospora cordifolia |
| | 401 | Cumin | Cumimum cyminum |
| | | Fennel | Foeniculum vulgare |
| | | Cardamom | Elettaria cardamomum |
| | 406 | Myrrh | Commiphora myrrha |
| | | Elecampane | Inula helenium |
| | | Yellow dock | Rumex crispus |
| | 407 | Turmeric | Curcuma longa |
| | | Barberry | Berberis vulgaris |
| | | Dandelion | Taraxacum officinale |
| | 408 | Vitex | Vitex agnus-castus |
| | | Black cohosh | Cimicifuga racemosa |
| | | Cramp bark | Viburnum opulus |
| Pittaja | 206 | Guduchi | Tinospora cordifolia |
| | 402 | Coriander | Coriandrum sativum |
| | | Cumin | Cumimum cyminum |
| | | Fennel | Foeniculum vulgare |
| | 405 | Burdock | Arctium lappa |
| | | Yellow dock | Rumex crispus |
| | | Milk Thistle | Silybum marianum |
| | 407 | Turmeric | Curcuma longa |
| | | Barberry | Berberis vulgaris |
| | | Dandelion | Taraxacum officinale |
| | 408 | Vitex | Vitex agnus-castus |
| | | Black cohosh | Cimicifuga racemosa |
| | | Cramp bark | Viburnum opulus |
| Kaphaja | 206 | Guduchi | Tinospora cordifolia |
| | 403 | Ginger | Zingiber officinale |
| | | Cumin | Cumimum cyminum |
| | | Fenugreek | Trigonella foenum-graecum |
| | 406 | Myrrh | Commiphora myrrha |
| | | Elecampane | Inula helenium |
| | | Yellow dock | Rumex crispus |
| | 407 | Turmeric | Curcuma longa |
| | | Barberry | Berberis vulgaris |
| | | Dandelion | Taraxacum officinale |
| | 408 | Vitex | Vitex agnus-castus |
| | | Black cohosh | Cimicifuga racemosa |
| | | Cramp bark | Viburnum opulus |

| Dosha | Low Dose | High Dose |
|-------|----------|-----------|
| Vata | 1 of each X2 per day before meals | 2 of each X2 per day before meals |
| Pitta | 1 of each X2 per day with meals | 2 of each X2 per day with meals |
| Kapha | 2 of each X2 per day after meals | 3 of each X2 per day after meals |

## Description:

This disorder is generally considered incurable by modern medicine. Patient compliance to follow dietary, herbal and lifestyle treatments is the most critical factor for success. Endometriosis can be classified as Kapha Roga by function and Pitta Roga by location. This is due to the fact that Kapha Dosha is controlling the function of the endometrial tissue growth in the uterus. As Pitta is the controller of the uterus and Raktadhatu of which the uterus belongs it can also be classified as a Pitta disorder by location. I personally classify it by function - in other words as Kapha Roga.

This disorder has its root in Pitta (uterus) that deranges the function (Kapha). Kapha provides lubrication and tissue renewal in the uterus. In this pathology Kapha over produces endometrial cells and allows them outside of the uterus; Apana Vayu provides the movement out of the uterus. This causes problems in both the uterus and the vagina. These endometrial cells can migrate to many different places in the pelvic area. Other areas outside of the pelvis can also be affected. The growth of endometrial cells depends on hormone cycles that are controlled by Vata and secondarily Kapha.

Sometimes this disorder is classified as an autoimmune disorder; this is a trend that is becoming more accepted in modern medicine over the last twenty years. According to Ayurveda the Doshas lose their capacity to function normally. This abnormal function indicates a failure of Vata Dosha to coordinate the other two Doshas, in other words Vata Dosha can be a causal factor in this disease. Another possible causal factor can be a fundamental problem with low Ojas that is reduced due to bad habits (e.g., drug abuse, etc.) and poor diet.

Use the Vataja herbs if Vata is predominant in the Vikriti (imbalance) with a Vata Vikriti diet / lifestyle.

Use the Pittaja herbs if Pitta is predominant in the Vikriti (imbalance) with a Pitta Vikriti diet / lifestyle.

Use the Kaphaja herbs if Kapha is predominant in the Vikriti (imbalance) with a Kapha Vikriti diet / lifestyle.

## Enlarged liver

| Dosha | Code | Common Name | Latin Name |
|---|---|---|---|
| **Vataja** | 205 | Gokshura | Tribulus terrestris |
| | 206 | Guduchi | Tinospora cordifolia |
| | 208 | Manjishta | Rubia cordifolia |
| | 401 | Cumin | Cumimum cyminum |
| | | Fennel | Foeniculum vulgare |
| | | Cardamom | Elettaria cardamomum |
| **Pittaja** | 205 | Gokshura | Tribulus terrestris |
| | 206 | Guduchi | Tinospora cordifolia |
| | 208 | Manjishta | Rubia cordifolia |
| | 402 | Coriander | Coriandrum sativum |
| | | Cumin | Cumimum cyminum |
| | | Fennel | Foeniculum vulgare |
| **Kaphaja** | 205 | Gokshura | Tribulus terrestris |
| | 206 | Guduchi | Tinospora cordifolia |
| | 208 | Manjishta | Rubia cordifolia |
| | 403 | Ginger | Zingiber officinale |
| | | Cumin | Cumimum cyminum |
| | | Fenugreek | Trigonella foenum-graecum |

| Dosha | Low Dose | High Dose |
|---|---|---|
| **Vata** | 1 of each X2 per day before meals | 2 of each X2 per day before meals |
| **Pitta** | 1 of each X2 per day with meals | 2 of each X2 per day with meals |
| **Kapha** | 2 of each X2 per day after meals | 3 of each X2 per day after meals |

## Description:

An enlarged liver may be a sign of other diseases. Although diseases of the liver itself often cause an enlarged liver, there are many other possible causes, including: bacteria, viruses, parasites, certain heart conditions, genetic diseases, some types of leukemia and lymphoma. It is very unusual to have an enlarged liver without other symptoms that point to an underlying disease. It is a Pitta Roga disorder.

Use the Vataja herbs if Vata is predominant in the Vikriti (imbalance) with a Vata Vikriti diet / lifestyle.

Use the Pittaja herbs if Pitta is predominant in the Vikriti (imbalance) with a Pitta Vikriti diet / lifestyle.

Use the Kaphaja herbs if Kapha is predominant in the Vikriti (imbalance) with a Kapha Vikriti diet / lifestyle.

## Enlarged spleen (splenomegaly)

| Dosha | Code | Common Name | Latin Name |
|---|---|---|---|
| Vataja | 205 | Gokshura | Tribulus terrestris |
| | 206 | Guduchi | Tinospora cordifolia |
| | 208 | Manjishta | Rubia cordifolia |
| | 401 | Cumin | Cumimum cyminum |
| | | Fennel | Foeniculum vulgare |
| | | Cardamom | Elettaria cardamomum |
| Pittaja | 205 | Gokshura | Tribulus terrestris |
| | 206 | Guduchi | Tinospora cordifolia |
| | 208 | Manjishta | Rubia cordifolia |
| | 402 | Coriander | Coriandrum sativum |
| | | Cumin | Cumimum cyminum |
| | | Fennel | Foeniculum vulgare |
| Kaphaja | 205 | Gokshura | Tribulus terrestris |
| | 206 | Guduchi | Tinospora cordifolia |
| | 208 | Manjishta | Rubia cordifolia |
| | 403 | Ginger | Zingiber officinale |
| | | Cumin | Cumimum cyminum |
| | | Fenugreek | Trigonella foenum-graecum |

| Dosha | Low Dose | High Dose |
|---|---|---|
| Vata | 1 of each X2 per day before meals | 2 of each X2 per day before meals |
| Pitta | 1 of each X2 per day with meals | 2 of each X2 per day with meals |
| Kapha | 2 of each X2 per day after meals | 3 of each X2 per day after meals |

## Description:

Many conditions can cause an enlarged spleen, including: infections, liver disease and some cancers. An enlarged spleen usually doesn't cause symptoms. It is a Pitta Roga problem and can be treated like the liver as both are part of Rakta Dhatu.

Use the Vataja herbs if Vata is predominant in the Vikriti (imbalance) with a Vata Vikriti diet / lifestyle.
Use the Pittaja herbs if Pitta is predominant in the Vikriti (imbalance) with a Pitta Vikriti diet / lifestyle.
Use the Kaphaja herbs if Kapha is predominant in the Vikriti (imbalance) with a Kapha Vikriti diet / lifestyle.

# Epilepsy

| Dosha | Code | Common Name | Latin Name |
|---|---|---|---|
| **Vataja** | 204 | Bramhi | Bacopa monnieri |
| | 210 | Shankhpushpi | Convolvulus pluricaulis |
| | 401 | Cumin | Cumimum cyminum |
| | | Fennel | Foeniculum vulgare |
| | | Cardamom | Elettaria cardamomum |
| | 410 | Passion flower | Passiflora incarnata |
| | | Skullcap | Scutellaria lateriflora |
| | | Gotu kola | Centella asiatica |
| **Pittaja** | 204 | Bramhi | Bacopa monnieri |
| | 210 | Shankhpushpi | Convolvulus pluricaulis |
| | 402 | Coriander | Coriandrum sativum |
| | | Cumin | Cumimum cyminum |
| | | Fennel | Foeniculum vulgare |
| | 410 | Passion flower | Passiflora incarnata |
| | | Skullcap | Scutellaria lateriflora |
| | | Gotu kola | Centella asiatica |
| **Kaphaja** | 204 | Bramhi | Bacopa monnieri |
| | 210 | Shankhpushpi | Convolvulus pluricaulis |
| | 403 | Ginger | Zingiber officinale |
| | | Cumin | Cumimum cyminum |
| | | Fenugreek | Trigonella foenum-graecum |
| | 410 | Passion flower | Passiflora incarnata |
| | | Skullcap | Scutellaria lateriflora |
| | | Gotu kola | Centella asiatica |

| Dosha | Low Dose | High Dose |
|---|---|---|
| **Vata** | 1 of each X2 per day before meals | 2 of each X2 per day before meals |
| **Pitta** | 1 of each X2 per day with meals | 2 of each X2 per day with meals |
| **Kapha** | 2 of each X2 per day after meals | 3 of each X2 per day after meals |

## Description:

Epilepsy is a group of neurological disorders characterized by epileptic seizures. Epileptic seizures are episodes that can vary from brief and nearly undetectable to long periods of vigorous shaking. In epilepsy, seizures tend to recur, and have no immediate underlying cause while seizures that occur due to a specific cause are not deemed to represent epilepsy.

Ayurvedic treatment focuses on the individual rather than just on their symptoms. Ayurvedic medicine seeks to treat epilepsy by unblocking the channels (Srotamsi) that may be clogged by the excess of Doshas, Mala or Ama. This opening of the Srotamsi is usually done through the Pancha Karma clinical procedures. Pancha Karma is the best and most effective group of therapies to use for treating Epilepsy and can cure this disorder in early stages (see Chapter Eight, Langhana Chikitsa - Pancha Karma in *Ayurvedic Medicine for Westerners: Vol. 2, Pathology & Diagnosis in Ayurveda*).

External oil applications, massages, and baths are a major part of the treatment. Internal treatments focus mainly on removing Ama and Dosha from the Srotamsi and reducing Vata. Treatment modalities that include strong elimination purgatives are used to alleviate the symptoms, depending upon specific requirements, are useful for epilepsy patients.

In Ayurveda, the modes of administration of herbs for epilepsy include external application, internal use, and application in the nose. This is considered to be a Vata Roga problem by function and Kapha Roga by structure. Pitta can be implicated when there is chronic infection or inflammation. Any Dosha can cause this disorder with Kaphaja, then Vataja, and then Pittaja in order of dominance. If Pancha Karma therapies are not possible, then an Ayurvedic massage therapist is needed to teach the patient and family how to give daily massage treatments with oil. A strict diet is very important and a regular lifestyle is needed to cure this problem in early stages.

These herbal blends are very useful to manage epilepsy, but like all the herbal treatments, give the best results when a strict diet and lifestyle are followed. If this is not possible the herbs should still be taken as they will slow the pathology and improve the quality of life of the patient. For more information see *Ayurvedic Medicine for Westerners, Vol. 5; Application of Ayurvedic Treatments Throughout Life*, chapter 16. NOTE: There are possible interaction with psychoactive medicines or antidepressants

Use the Vataja herbs if Vata is predominant in the Vikriti (imbalance) with a Vata Vikriti diet / lifestyle.
Use the Pittaja herbs if Pitta is predominant in the Vikriti (imbalance) with a Pitta Vikriti diet / lifestyle.
Use the Kaphaja herbs if Kapha is predominant in the Vikriti (imbalance) with a Kapha Vikriti diet / lifestyle.

## Epstein bar

| Dosha | Code | Common Name | Latin Name |
|-------|------|-------------|------------|
| **Vataja** | 206 | Guduchi | Tinospora cordifolia |
| | 212 | Pau d'arco | Tabebuia impetiginosa |
| | 401 | Cumin | Cumimum cyminum |
| | | Fennel | Foeniculum vulgare |
| | | Cardamom | Elettaria cardamomum |
| | 404 | Angelica | Angelica archangelica |
| | | Wild yam | Dioscorea villosa |
| | | Valerian | Valeriana officinalis |
| **Pittaja** | 206 | Guduchi | Tinospora cordifolia |
| | 212 | Pau d'arco | Tabebuia impetiginosa |
| | 402 | Coriander | Coriandrum sativum |
| | | Cumin | Cumimum cyminum |
| | | Fennel | Foeniculum vulgare |
| | 407 | Turmeric | Curcuma longa |
| | | Barberry | Berberis vulgaris |
| | | Dandelion | Taraxacum officinale |
| **Kaphaja** | 206 | Guduchi | Tinospora cordifolia |
| | 212 | Pau d'arco | Tabebuia impetiginosa |
| | 403 | Ginger | Zingiber officinale |
| | | Cumin | Cumimum cyminum |
| | | Fenugreek | Trigonella foenum-graecum |
| | 407 | Turmeric | Curcuma longa |
| | | Barberry | Berberis vulgaris |
| | | Dandelion | Taraxacum officinale |

| Dosha | Low Dose | High Dose |
|-------|----------|-----------|
| **Vata** | 1 of each X2 per day before meals | 2 of each X2 per day before meals |
| **Pitta** | 1 of each X2 per day with meals | 2 of each X2 per day with meals |
| **Kapha** | 2 of each X2 per day after meals | 3 of each X2 per day after meals |

## Description:

Epstein-Barr virus (EBV) is a ubiquitous virus that infects at least 95% of the population. Most persons are infected during infancy or early childhood and are asymptomatic or have nonspecific symptoms. Infection of adolescents and young adults with EBV often results in infectious mononucleosis that manifests as fever, lymphadenopathy, sore throat, and splenomegaly. Additional signs and symptoms of Epstein-Barr virus can include fatigue, headache, hepatomegaly, and rash. EBV is also associated with a number of malignancies including Hodgkin's disease, B cell lymphomas, and nasopharyngeal carcinoma.

In Ayurveda Epstein-Barr virus symptoms show weak immunity, which is often linked to low Ojas and Dosha Vriddhi. Most virus proliferate when there is Ama in the system. As any Dosha can cause Ama through derangement of the Agni any Dosha can cause the EBV to grow and take hold of the body.

Treat the patient according to the Vikriti dominance. An anti-Ama diet is useful and can accelerate therapeutic results. In most cases of infectious mononucleosis, the patient should be isolated and quarantined from others. Rest is very important. These herbal blends help to strengthen immunity so the body can fight off the virus.

Use the Vataja herbs if Vata is predominant in the Vikriti (imbalance) with a Vata Vikriti diet / lifestyle.

Use the Pittaja herbs if Pitta is predominant in the Vikriti (imbalance) with a Pitta Vikriti diet / lifestyle.

Use the Kaphaja herbs if Kapha is predominant in the Vikriti (imbalance) with a Kapha Vikriti diet / lifestyle.

## Eye disorders

| Dosha | Code | Common Name | Latin Name |
|---|---|---|---|
| **Vataja** | 301 | Amalaki | Emblica officinalis |
| | | Bibhitaki | Terminalia belerica |
| | | Haritaki | Terminalia chebula |
| **Pittaja** | 301 | Amalaki | Emblica officinalis |
| | | Bibhitaki | Terminalia belerica |
| | | Haritaki | Terminalia chebula |
| **Kaphaja** | 301 | Amalaki | Emblica officinalis |
| | | Bibhitaki | Terminalia belerica |
| | | Haritaki | Terminalia chebula |

| Dosha | Low Dose | High Dose |
|---|---|---|
| **Vata** | 1 of each X2 per day before meals | 2 of each X2 per day before meals |
| **Pitta** | 1 of each X2 per day with meals | 2 of each X2 per day with meals |
| **Kapha** | 2 of each X2 per day after meals | 3 of each X2 per day after meals |

## Description:

The main treatment for the eyes is external for which instructions are given below. Internally Triphala is considered to be one of the best Rasayana for the eyes. The eyes are controlled by Alochaka Pitta and so eye disorders are Pitta Roga. Functionally any Dosha can cause eye problems. Internal treatment with Triphala should be accompanied by the diet and lifestyle as per Vikriti and the external treatment.

Note for this external treatment the patient needs to buy Triphala in a powder form from an herbal supplier or therapist. This treatment is used for the following eye problems and may be used for other disorders not listed here:

- Chorioretinal inflammation
- Corneal dystrophies
- Glaucoma
- Disorders of conjunctiva
- Varies inflammations of eye parts
- Loss of vision
- Weakening of the eye due to old age

Take one half of a level teaspoon of Triphala powder (1 gram) and place it in a teacup. Add 1/2 cup (120 ml) of hot water that has just boiled. Let the Triphala infuse until it is the same temperature as your body.

Once the infusion has cooled to body temperature DO NOT STIR IT. Take a sterile round cotton pad that is used for make-up or for medical reasons. Dip the cotton pad into the infusion and remove it. Squeeze it so that some liquid remains, but that it is not dripping wet.

Place a towel on your pillow, under your head. Lay down on your bed. Place the cotton pad over one of your eyes. Blink. Repeat this for the second eye. Leave for at least fifteen minutes. Twenty minutes is an optimal time for this treatment and thirty minutes is the maximum time.

There should be enough liquid that some runs into your eye. The first few times that you do the treatment it may cause a burning sensation. This will pass after two or three days in most cases. If it burns it means you need this treatment. If the burning persists more than a week it is not normal - see your doctor.

For loss of vision due to age or life style do this ONE time per day, evening is best before bed so your eyes can rest after the treatment. Do not read or look at a screen after treatment.

For all other disorders do the treatment TWO times per day. Make sure to rest the eyes for thirty to sixty minutes before using the computer or other screens. For very serious disorders do the treatment THREE times per day.

Triphala is primarily astringent in nature and is a rejuvenator of tissue. The longer you use this treatment the better results it gives. Minimum time of treatment should be one month. Maximum treatment should be not more than twelve months unless told to do so by your Ayurvedic practitioner.

Use the Vataja herbs if Vata is predominant in the Vikriti (imbalance) with a Vata Vikriti diet / lifestyle.

Use the Pittaja herbs if Pitta is predominant in the Vikriti (imbalance) with a Pitta Vikriti diet / lifestyle.

Use the Kaphaja herbs if Kapha is predominant in the Vikriti (imbalance) with a Kapha Vikriti diet / lifestyle.

## Fatigue

| Dosha | Code | Common Name | Latin Name |
|-------|------|-------------|------------|
| **Vataja** | 203 | Ashwagandha | Withania somnifera |
| | 211 | Shatavari | Asparagus racemosus |
| | 401 | Cumin | Cumimum cyminum |
| | | Fennel | Foeniculum vulgare |
| | | Cardamom | Elettaria cardamomum |
| | 407 | Turmeric | Curcuma longa |
| | | Barberry | Berberis vulgaris |
| | | Dandelion | Taraxacum officinale |
| **Pittaja** | 203 | Ashwagandha | Withania somnifera |
| | 211 | Shatavari | Asparagus racemosus |
| | 402 | Coriander | Coriandrum sativum |
| | | Cumin | Cumimum cyminum |
| | | Fennel | Foeniculum vulgare |
| | 407 | Turmeric | Curcuma longa |
| | | Barberry | Berberis vulgaris |
| | | Dandelion | Taraxacum officinale |
| **Kaphaja** | 203 | Ashwagandha | Withania somnifera |
| | 211 | Shatavari | Asparagus racemosus |
| | 403 | Ginger | Zingiber officinale |
| | | Cumin | Cumimum cyminum |
| | | Fenugreek | Trigonella foenum-graecum |
| | 407 | Turmeric | Curcuma longa |
| | | Barberry | Berberis vulgaris |
| | | Dandelion | Taraxacum officinale |

| Dosha | Low Dose | High Dose |
|-------|----------|-----------|
| **Vata** | 1 of each X2 per day before meals | 2 of each X2 per day before meals |
| **Pitta** | 1 of each X2 per day with meals | 2 of each X2 per day with meals |
| **Kapha** | 2 of each X2 per day after meals | 3 of each X2 per day after meals |

## Description:
A tonic blend to use as per Vikriti.

Use the Vataja herbs if Vata is predominant in the Vikriti (imbalance) with a Vata Vikriti diet / lifestyle.

Use the Pittaja herbs if Pitta is predominant in the Vikriti (imbalance) with a Pitta Vikriti diet / lifestyle.

Use the Kaphaja herbs if Kapha is predominant in the Vikriti (imbalance) with a Kapha Vikriti diet / lifestyle.

## Fever

| Dosha | Code | Common Name | Latin Name |
|-------|------|-------------|------------|
| **Vataja** | 206 | Guduchi | Tinospora cordifolia |
| | 207 | Haritaki | Terminalia chebula |
| | 212 | Pau d'arco | Tabebuia impetiginosa |
| | 401 | Cumin | Cumimum cyminum |
| | | Fennel | Foeniculum vulgare |
| | | Cardamom | Elettaria cardamomum |
| | 407 | Turmeric | Curcuma longa |
| | | Barberry | Berberis vulgaris |
| | | Dandelion | Taraxacum officinale |
| **Pittaja** | 206 | Guduchi | Tinospora cordifolia |
| | 212 | Pau d'arco | Tabebuia impetiginosa |
| | 402 | Coriander | Coriandrum sativum |
| | | Cumin | Cumimum cyminum |
| | | Fennel | Foeniculum vulgare |
| | 405 | Burdock | Arctium lappa |
| | | Yellow dock | Rumex crispus |
| | | Milk Thistle | Silybum marianum |
| | 407 | Turmeric | Curcuma longa |
| | | Barberry | Berberis vulgaris |
| | | Dandelion | Taraxacum officinale |
| **Kaphaja** | 206 | Guduchi | Tinospora cordifolia |
| | 212 | Pau d'arco | Tabebuia impetiginosa |
| | 403 | Ginger | Zingiber officinale |
| | | Cumin | Cumimum cyminum |
| | | Fenugreek | Trigonella foenum-graecum |
| | 405 | Burdock | Arctium lappa |
| | | Yellow dock | Rumex crispus |
| | | Milk Thistle | Silybum marianum |
| | 407 | Turmeric | Curcuma longa |
| | | Barberry | Berberis vulgaris |
| | | Dandelion | Taraxacum officinale |

| Dosha | Low Dose | High Dose |
|-------|----------|-----------|
| **Vata** | 1 of each X2 per day before meals | 2 of each X2 per day before meals |
| **Pitta** | 1 of each X2 per day with meals | 2 of each X2 per day with meals |
| **Kapha** | 2 of each X2 per day after meals | 3 of each X2 per day after meals |

## Description:

Fever is a normal immune response to kill pathogens in the body. Virus are especially susceptible to high body heat which kills them very effectively. Fever can be deadly. In the olden times fever was one of the most common causes of death. If the body is not able to kill off the pathogens quickly the body can continue to increase the heat, become dehydrated and dry out. If this happens the internal organs begin to slow down and eventually stop. It is said the brain stops functioning after 107.6° F (42° C) and higher temperatures may cause brain damage. A high fever is not harmful to the body itself until it goes over these levels. In general, it's not the fever that is lethal as much as it is the pathogen that causes the fever. Note for children the safe level is considered to be 100.4° F (38° C), at this level or above chemical medication should be given, or an ice bath, to bring the temperature down to safe levels.

In Ayurveda fever is often associated with Ama conditions which allow pathogens to grow and flourish in the body. A fever is used by the body to remove Ama as well as pathogens. Thus, low grade, chronic fevers are usually due to the presence of Ama in the body. Any Dosha can cause the increase of Ama, and thus pathogens, in the body.

Keep the body hydrated with a lot of liquids – fresh ginger root tea is the best – to prevent dehydration. It is better not to eat, or eat very little to assist the immune system in ridding the body of the pathogens. Use the above herbal blends as per Vikriti. These blends can be used in the treatment of both chronic low grade fevers as well as acute fever. Use cold baths, or ice baths to control the body temperature in conjunction with herbal and dietary treatments.

Use the Vataja herbs if Vata is predominant in the Vikriti (imbalance) with a Vata Vikriti diet / lifestyle.

Use the Pittaja herbs if Pitta is predominant in the Vikriti (imbalance) with a Pitta Vikriti diet / lifestyle.

Use the Kaphaja herbs if Kapha is predominant in the Vikriti (imbalance) with a Kapha Vikriti diet / lifestyle.

## Fertility Male

| Dosha | Code | Common Name | Latin Name |
|---|---|---|---|
| **Vataja** | 203 | Ashwagandha | Withania somnifera |
| | 205 | Gokshura | Tribulus terrestris |
| | 211 | Shatavari | Asparagus racemosus |
| | 401 | Cumin | Cumimum cyminum |
| | | Fennel | Foeniculum vulgare |
| | | Cardamom | Elettaria cardamomum |
| **Pittaja** | 203 | Ashwagandha | Withania somnifera |
| | 205 | Gokshura | Tribulus terrestris |
| | 211 | Shatavari | Asparagus racemosus |
| | 402 | Coriander | Coriandrum sativum |
| | | Cumin | Cumimum cyminum |
| | | Fennel | Foeniculum vulgare |
| **Kaphaja** | 203 | Ashwagandha | Withania somnifera |
| | 205 | Gokshura | Tribulus terrestris |
| | 211 | Shatavari | Asparagus racemosus |
| | 403 | Ginger | Zingiber officinale |
| | | Cumin | Cumimum cyminum |
| | | Fenugreek | Trigonella foenum-graecum |

| Dosha | Low Dose | High Dose |
|---|---|---|
| **Vata** | 1 of each X2 per day before meals | 2 of each X2 per day before meals |
| **Pitta** | 1 of each X2 per day with meals | 2 of each X2 per day with meals |
| **Kapha** | 2 of each X2 per day after meals | 3 of each X2 per day after meals |

## Description:

These herbal blends can be used to treat unexplained infertility. The herbs will tend to increase sperm counts and fluids. Use as per Vikriti, if there is one, or Prakriti if no pathology is apparent.

Use the Vataja herbs if Vata is predominant in the Vikriti (imbalance) with a Vata Vikriti diet / lifestyle.

Use the Pittaja herbs if Pitta is predominant in the Vikriti (imbalance) with a Pitta Vikriti diet / lifestyle.

Use the Kaphaja herbs if Kapha is predominant in the Vikriti (imbalance) with a Kapha Vikriti diet / lifestyle.

# Fertility Female

| Dosha | Code | Common Name | Latin Name |
|---|---|---|---|
| **Vataja** | 203 | Ashwagandha | Withania somnifera |
| | 211 | Shatavari | Asparagus racemosus |
| | 301 | Amalaki | Emblica officinalis |
| | | Bibhitaki | Terminalia belerica |
| | | Haritaki | Terminalia chebula |
| | 401 | Cumin | Cumimum cyminum |
| | | Fennel | Foeniculum vulgare |
| | | Cardamom | Elettaria cardamomum |
| | 408 | Vitex | Vitex agnus-castus |
| | | Black cohosh | Cimicifuga racemosa |
| | | Cramp bark | Viburnum opulus |
| **Pittaja** | 201 | Amalaki | Emblica officinalis |
| | 203 | Ashwagandha | Withania somnifera |
| | 211 | Shatavari | Asparagus racemosus |
| | 402 | Coriander | Coriandrum sativum |
| | | Cumin | Cumimum cyminum |
| | | Fennel | Foeniculum vulgare |
| | 408 | Vitex | Vitex agnus-castus |
| | | Black cohosh | Cimicifuga racemosa |
| | | Cramp bark | Viburnum opulus |
| **Kaphaja** | 203 | Ashwagandha | Withania somnifera |
| | 211 | Shatavari | Asparagus racemosus |
| | 301 | Amalaki | Emblica officinalis |
| | | Bibhitaki | Terminalia belerica |
| | | Haritaki | Terminalia chebula |
| | 403 | Ginger | Zingiber officinale |
| | | Cumin | Cumimum cyminum |
| | | Fenugreek | Trigonella foenum-graecum |
| | 408 | Vitex | Vitex agnus-castus |
| | | Black cohosh | Cimicifuga racemosa |
| | | Cramp bark | Viburnum opulus |

| Dosha | Low Dose | High Dose |
|---|---|---|
| **Vata** | 1 of each X2 per day before meals | 2 of each X2 per day before meals |
| **Pitta** | 1 of each X2 per day with meals | 2 of each X2 per day with meals |
| **Kapha** | 2 of each X2 per day after meals | 3 of each X2 per day after meals |

## Description:

These herbal blends can be used to treat unexplained infertility. Use as per Vikriti, if there is one, or Prakriti if no pathology is apparent.

According to Ayurveda any existing disorder in the body should be treated before trying to give Vajikarana medicines or fertility therapies. If there is no apparent cause of infertility, then it can be classified as Unexplained Infertility which affects twenty to twenty-five percent of couples that are having difficulty to conceive. I always treat both women and men when a couple is having difficulty to conceive. There are two primary problems that I see in clinical practice, those due to Ama and those due to an excess of Pitta or Kapha in the uterus.

The vast majority of infertility problems that I see are due to Ama congesting Shukra Dhatu and the Srotas that permit correct function of all the reproductive system. This usually means one or several of the Srotas are congested by Ama and prevent the normal movement of the ovum or sperm. Protocol is simple; remove Ama before giving Vajikarana medicines to the patients. This usually means a minimum of three or a maximum of twelve months of mild Shodhana therapies to remove Ama, balance Doshas and Agni. See the advice for Ama in this section.

Another issue that is common and that I see as a major cause of Unexplained Infertility is the condition of the uterus. The ovum and sperm need a very specific environment to live in the body, if the environment is too acidic or too alkaline they die. As the uterus is part of Rakta Dhatu and under the control of Pitta it tends to be more acidic than alkaline to kill off pathogens and to protect the health of the woman. If it becomes too acidic then it also kills off the sperm and ovum. On the other hand, if the Kapha aspect – Rasa Dhatu – begins to dominate then the uterus can begin to become too alkaline and this will also create the same destructive environment to the sperm and ovum.

Use the Vataja herbs if Vata is predominant in the Vikriti (imbalance) with a Vata Vikriti diet / lifestyle.

Use the Pittaja herbs if Pitta is predominant in the Vikriti (imbalance) with a Pitta Vikriti diet / lifestyle.

Use the Kaphaja herbs if Kapha is predominant in the Vikriti (imbalance) with a Kapha Vikriti diet / lifestyle.

## Fibroids

| Dosha | Code | Common Name | Latin Name |
|---|---|---|---|
| **Vataja** | 207 | Haritaki | Terminalia chebula |
| | 404 | Angelica | Angelica archangelica |
| | | Wild yam | Dioscorea villosa |
| | | Valerian | Valeriana officinalis |
| | 406 | Myrrh | Commiphora myrrha |
| | | Elecampane | Inula helenium |
| | | Yellow dock | Rumex crispus |
| | 407 | Turmeric | Curcuma longa |
| | | Barberry | Berberis vulgaris |
| | | Dandelion | Taraxacum officinale |
| | 408 | Vitex | Vitex agnus-castus |
| | | Black cohosh | Cimicifuga racemosa |
| | | Cramp bark | Viburnum opulus |
| **Pittaja** | 201 | Amalaki | Emblica officinalis |
| | 405 | Burdock | Arctium lappa |
| | | Yellow dock | Rumex crispus |
| | | Milk Thistle | Silybum marianum |
| | 406 | Myrrh | Commiphora myrrha |
| | | Elecampane | Inula helenium |
| | | Yellow dock | Rumex crispus |
| | 407 | Turmeric | Curcuma longa |
| | | Barberry | Berberis vulgaris |
| | | Dandelion | Taraxacum officinale |
| | 408 | Vitex | Vitex agnus-castus |
| | | Black cohosh | Cimicifuga racemosa |
| | | Cramp bark | Viburnum opulus |
| **Kaphaja** | 207 | Haritaki | Terminalia chebula |
| | 406 | Myrrh | Commiphora myrrha |
| | | Elecampane | Inula helenium |
| | | Yellow dock | Rumex crispus |
| | 407 | Turmeric | Curcuma longa |
| | | Barberry | Berberis vulgaris |
| | | Dandelion | Taraxacum officinale |
| | 408 | Vitex | Vitex agnus-castus |
| | | Black cohosh | Cimicifuga racemosa |
| | | Cramp bark | Viburnum opulus |

| Dosha | Low Dose | High Dose |
|-------|----------|-----------|
| Vata | 1 of each X2 per day before meals | 2 of each X2 per day before meals |
| Pitta | 1 of each X2 per day with meals | 2 of each X2 per day with meals |
| Kapha | 2 of each X2 per day after meals | 3 of each X2 per day after meals |

## Description:

Fibroids are muscular tumors that grow in or outside the uterus (womb). Another medical term for fibroids is *leiomyoma* or just *myoma*. Fibroids are almost always benign (non-cancerous). Fibroids can grow as a single tumor, or there can be many of them in the uterus. They can be as small as an apple seed or as big as a grapefruit.

The leading cause of having a hysterectomy in the United States is due to fibroids. One out of three hysterectomies are performed because of fibroids in the United States (2014). Fibroids are known to grow with increased estrogen and decrease with an increase of progesterone and are therefore called 'functional'. There is an obvious relation to endocrine function and external factors such as estrogenic chemicals in the food chain.

There are four classifications of fibroids in modern medicine. Nevertheless, all four types can be treated through the same Ayurvedic formulas and therapies. Each of these four can cause different problems and some pain when in a chronic state, very large or pushing against another organ.

Fibroids are mainly classified as Pitta Roga because Pitta controls the uterus as part of Rakta Dhatu. Fibroids are usually associated with Vata Vriddhi, specifically Apana Vayu which causes the accumulation of Pitta or Kapha in the uterus. There is always a Kapha aspect to fibroids because of the increased growth due to estrogen. Functionally it is possible to say that fibroids are Kapha Roga because Kapha controls growth. For more information see *Ayurvedic Medicine for Westerners, Vol. 5 Application of Ayurvedic Treatments Throughout Life*, chapter 9.

Use the Vataja herbs if Vata is predominant in the Vikriti (imbalance) with a Vata Vikriti diet / lifestyle.

Use the Pittaja herbs if Pitta is predominant in the Vikriti (imbalance) with a Pitta Vikriti diet / lifestyle.

Use the Kaphaja herbs if Kapha is predominant in the Vikriti (imbalance) with a Kapha Vikriti diet / lifestyle.

## Flatulence

| Dosha | Code | Common Name | Latin Name |
|---|---|---|---|
| **Vataja** | 207 | Haritaki | Terminalia chebula |
| | 401 | Cumin | Cumimum cyminum |
| | | Fennel | Foeniculum vulgare |
| | | Cardamom | Elettaria cardamomum |
| | 404 | Angelica | Angelica archangelica |
| | | Wild yam | Dioscorea villosa |
| | | Valerian | Valeriana officinalis |
| **Pittaja** | 201 | Amalaki | Emblica officinalis |
| | 402 | Coriander | Coriandrum sativum |
| | | Cumin | Cumimum cyminum |
| | | Fennel | Foeniculum vulgare |
| | 407 | Turmeric | Curcuma longa |
| | | Barberry | Berberis vulgaris |
| | | Dandelion | Taraxacum officinale |
| **Kaphaja** | 207 | Haritaki | Terminalia chebula |
| | 403 | Ginger | Zingiber officinale |
| | | Cumin | Cumimum cyminum |
| | | Fenugreek | Trigonella foenum-graecum |
| | 407 | Turmeric | Curcuma longa |
| | | Barberry | Berberis vulgaris |
| | | Dandelion | Taraxacum officinale |

| Dosha | Low Dose | High Dose |
|---|---|---|
| **Vata** | 1 of each X2 per day before meals | 2 of each X2 per day before meals |
| **Pitta** | 1 of each X2 per day with meals | 2 of each X2 per day with meals |
| **Kapha** | 2 of each X2 per day after meals | 3 of each X2 per day after meals |

## Description:

Use as per Vikriti to stop or control intestinal gas.

Use the Vataja herbs if Vata is predominant in the Vikriti (imbalance) with a Vata Vikriti diet / lifestyle.

Use the Pittaja herbs if Pitta is predominant in the Vikriti (imbalance) with a Pitta Vikriti diet / lifestyle.

Use the Kaphaja herbs if Kapha is predominant in the Vikriti (imbalance) with a Kapha Vikriti diet / lifestyle.

# Flu

| Dosha | Code | Common Name | Latin Name |
|-------|------|-------------|------------|
| Vataja | 206 | Guduchi | Tinospora cordifolia |
| | 212 | Pau d'arco | Tabebuia impetiginosa |
| | 403 | Ginger | Zingiber officinale |
| | | Cumin | Cumimum cyminum |
| | | Fenugreek | Trigonella foenum-graecum |
| Pittaja | 206 | Guduchi | Tinospora cordifolia |
| | 212 | Pau d'arco | Tabebuia impetiginosa |
| | 403 | Ginger | Zingiber officinale |
| | | Cumin | Cumimum cyminum |
| | | Fenugreek | Trigonella foenum-graecum |
| Kaphaja | 206 | Guduchi | Tinospora cordifolia |
| | 212 | Pau d'arco | Tabebuia impetiginosa |
| | 403 | Ginger | Zingiber officinale |
| | | Cumin | Cumimum cyminum |
| | | Fenugreek | Trigonella foenum-graecum |

| Dosha | Low Dose | High Dose |
|-------|----------|-----------|
| Vata | 1 of each X2 per day before meals | 2 of each X2 per day before meals |
| Pitta | 1 of each X2 per day with meals | 2 of each X2 per day with meals |
| Kapha | 2 of each X2 per day after meals | 3 of each X2 per day after meals |

## Description:

This is a symptomatic treatment for the influenza virus. The same blend is used for all types as these herbs help to remove Ama and support Agni. In Ayurveda, a flu is showing low immunity and disrupted Agni. This usually allows Ama to accumulate in the body which further lowers immunity and allows for virus to grow and become strong enough to make the person sick.

The diet and lifestyle should normally follow the Vikriti of the person. Note that an anti-Ama diet is very useful. See the discussion under fever for more information.

Use the Vataja herbs if Vata is predominant in the Vikriti (imbalance) with a Vata Vikriti diet / lifestyle.

Use the Pittaja herbs if Pitta is predominant in the Vikriti (imbalance) with a Pitta Vikriti diet / lifestyle.

Use the Kaphaja herbs if Kapha is predominant in the Vikriti (imbalance) with a Kapha Vikriti diet / lifestyle.

# Food allergies

| Dosha | Code | Common Name | Latin Name |
|---|---|---|---|
| **Vataja** | 207 | Haritaki | Terminalia chebula |
| | 401 | Cumin | Cumimum cyminum |
| | | Fennel | Foeniculum vulgare |
| | | Cardamom | Elettaria cardamomum |
| | 404 | Angelica | Angelica archangelica |
| | | Wild yam | Dioscorea villosa |
| | | Valerian | Valeriana officinalis |
| | 407 | Turmeric | Curcuma longa |
| | | Barberry | Berberis vulgaris |
| | | Dandelion | Taraxacum officinale |
| | 409 | Marshmallow | Althaea officinalis |
| | | Gotu kola | Centella asiatica |
| | | Stinging nettles | Urtica dioica |
| **Pittaja** | 402 | Coriander | Coriandrum sativum |
| | | Cumin | Cumimum cyminum |
| | | Fennel | Foeniculum vulgare |
| | 405 | Burdock | Arctium lappa |
| | | Yellow dock | Rumex crispus |
| | | Milk Thistle | Silybum marianum |
| | 407 | Turmeric | Curcuma longa |
| | | Barberry | Berberis vulgaris |
| | | Dandelion | Taraxacum officinale |
| **Kaphaja** | 207 | Haritaki | Terminalia chebula |
| | 403 | Ginger | Zingiber officinale |
| | | Cumin | Cumimum cyminum |
| | | Fenugreek | Trigonella foenum-graecum |
| | 404 | Angelica | Angelica archangelica |
| | | Wild yam | Dioscorea villosa |
| | | Valerian | Valeriana officinalis |
| | 407 | Turmeric | Curcuma longa |
| | | Barberry | Berberis vulgaris |
| | | Dandelion | Taraxacum officinale |

| Dosha | Low Dose | High Dose |
|---|---|---|
| **Vata** | 1 of each X2 per day before meals | 2 of each X2 per day before meals |
| **Pitta** | 1 of each X2 per day with meals | 2 of each X2 per day with meals |
| **Kapha** | 2 of each X2 per day after meals | 3 of each X2 per day after meals |

## Description:

Food sensitivities and allergies are an indication of deeper problems. The immunity is beginning to fail and is making mistakes to identify food as an allergen. If these problems are not corrected, then the next step of pathology would some kind of autoimmune disorder. Allergies need to be treated as soon as possible by correcting the underlying problem. According to Ayurveda the main cause of food sensitivities and allergies is Ama.

Ama is the result of poor Agni function, which is the result of poor Dosha function. Hence, any Dosha can cause Ama to form in the body. When there is Vishama Agni use the Vataja blend; when there is Tikshna Agni use the Pittaja blend; and when there is Munda Agni use the Kaphaja blend of herbs. This will target the correct sub-Dosha and balance Agni. These blends will also remove the Ama that has accumulated in the digestive system. Modifying diet and reducing heavy foods during treatment is needed to achieve good results. The patient should use the herbal blend, diet and lifestyle as per Vikriti.

During the course of treatment, it is advised to avoid any food that is causing problems. Once the Ama is removed and the Agni is stable then foods can slowly be reintroduced. Avoid reintroducing problematic foods too quickly; avoid binging on foods. Sugar, dairy, refined flour, refined food, and fast food should all be avoided during treatment. The problem with gluten and lactose allergies is rooted in overly refined food that is indigestible and causes Ama. Once Ama is formed the body confuses the rotting food (Ama) with the food source; e. g., refined wheat and pasteurized dairy products. A diet based on whole food is critical for success in reeducating the digestive system and immunity.

Use the Vataja herbs if Vata is predominant in the Vikriti (imbalance) with a Vata Vikriti diet / lifestyle.

Use the Pittaja herbs if Pitta is predominant in the Vikriti (imbalance) with a Pitta Vikriti diet / lifestyle.

Use the Kaphaja herbs if Kapha is predominant in the Vikriti (imbalance) with a Kapha Vikriti diet / lifestyle.

## Frequent urination

| Dosha | Code | Common Name | Latin Name |
|---|---|---|---|
| Vataja | 401 | Cumin | Cumimum cyminum |
| | | Fennel | Foeniculum vulgare |
| | | Cardamom | Elettaria cardamomum |
| | 409 | Marshmallow | Althaea officinalis |
| | | Gotu kola | Centella asiatica |
| | | Stinging nettles | Urtica dioica |
| Pittaja | 402 | Coriander | Coriandrum sativum |
| | | Cumin | Cumimum cyminum |
| | | Fennel | Foeniculum vulgare |
| | 409 | Marshmallow | Althaea officinalis |
| | | Gotu kola | Centella asiatica |
| | | Stinging nettles | Urtica dioica |
| Kaphaja | 403 | Ginger | Zingiber officinale |
| | | Cumin | Cumimum cyminum |
| | | Fenugreek | Trigonella foenum-graecum |
| | 409 | Marshmallow | Althaea officinalis |
| | | Gotu kola | Centella asiatica |
| | | Stinging nettles | Urtica dioica |

| Dosha | Low Dose | High Dose |
|---|---|---|
| Vata | 1 of each X2 per day before meals | 2 of each X2 per day before meals |
| Pitta | 1 of each X2 per day with meals | 2 of each X2 per day with meals |
| Kapha | 2 of each X2 per day after meals | 3 of each X2 per day after meals |

## Description:

These blends can be used to strengthen Mutravaha Srota and the kidneys (Meda Dhatu). This problem is Kaphaja by structure (Meda Dhatu) and Vataja by function (Apana Vayu). The blend and diet should follow Vikriti in most cases. Avoid all alcoholic beverages, sodas and carbonated beverages of any kind.

Use the Vataja herbs if Vata is predominant in the Vikriti (imbalance) with a Vata Vikriti diet / lifestyle.
Use the Pittaja herbs if Pitta is predominant in the Vikriti (imbalance) with a Pitta Vikriti diet / lifestyle.
Use the Kaphaja herbs if Kapha is predominant in the Vikriti (imbalance) with a Kapha Vikriti diet / lifestyle.

# Frigidity

| Dosha | Code | Common Name | Latin Name |
|-------|------|-------------|------------|
| **Vataja** | 203 | Ashwagandha | Withania somnifera |
| | 211 | Shatavari | Asparagus racemosus |
| | 401 | Cumin | Cumimum cyminum |
| | | Fennel | Foeniculum vulgare |
| | | Cardamom | Elettaria cardamomum |
| | 408 | Vitex | Vitex agnus-castus |
| | | Black cohosh | Cimicifuga racemosa |
| | | Cramp bark | Viburnum opulus |
| **Pittaja** | 201 | Amalaki | Emblica officinalis |
| | 203 | Ashwagandha | Withania somnifera |
| | 211 | Shatavari | Asparagus racemosus |
| | 402 | Coriander | Coriandrum sativum |
| | | Cumin | Cumimum cyminum |
| | | Fennel | Foeniculum vulgare |
| | 408 | Vitex | Vitex agnus-castus |
| | | Black cohosh | Cimicifuga racemosa |
| | | Cramp bark | Viburnum opulus |
| **Kaphaja** | 203 | Ashwagandha | Withania somnifera |
| | 207 | Haritaki | Terminalia chebula |
| | 211 | Shatavari | Asparagus racemosus |
| | 403 | Ginger | Zingiber officinale |
| | | Cumin | Cumimum cyminum |
| | | Fenugreek | Trigonella foenum-graecum |
| | 408 | Vitex | Vitex agnus-castus |
| | | Black cohosh | Cimicifuga racemosa |
| | | Cramp bark | Viburnum opulus |

| Dosha | Low Dose | High Dose |
|-------|----------|-----------|
| **Vata** | 1 of each X2 per day before meals | 2 of each X2 per day before meals |
| **Pitta** | 1 of each X2 per day with meals | 2 of each X2 per day with meals |
| **Kapha** | 2 of each X2 per day after meals | 3 of each X2 per day after meals |

## Description:

The Encyclopedia Britannica tells us that frigidity is the inability of a woman to attain orgasm during sexual intercourse. In popular usage, the word has been used to describe a variety of behaviors, ranging from general coldness of manner, or lack of interest in physical affection, to aversion to the act of sexual intercourse. The lay term frigidity encompasses three distinct problems recognized by sex therapists: inability to experience a sexual response of any kind; ability to achieve sexual arousal only with great difficulty (hyposexuality); and the inability to achieve orgasm (anorgasmia).

Ayurveda recognizes a wide variety of causes from physical to psychological with varying degrees of complexity. All three Doshas have roles in sexual function, so any of the Doshas can cause physical imbalances in the body. Use the advice as per Vikriti in most cases.

These blends are primarily working on the physical aspect of frigidity and support a balanced health of the female reproductive system. Diet is very important in reproductive health. There are studies that show a higher rate of reproductive disorders in low-income households which tend to eat unhealthy diets. A whole food diet, a balanced lifestyle and herbal blends offer a physical support that in turn supports the psychology.

For psychological aspects of this issue the patient should consult with a woman psychologist to understand possible issues.

Use the Vataja herbs if Vata is predominant in the Vikriti (imbalance) with a Vata Vikriti diet / lifestyle.

Use the Pittaja herbs if Pitta is predominant in the Vikriti (imbalance) with a Pitta Vikriti diet / lifestyle.

Use the Kaphaja herbs if Kapha is predominant in the Vikriti (imbalance) with a Kapha Vikriti diet / lifestyle.

## Fungal infections

| Dosha | Code | Common Name | Latin Name |
|-------|------|-------------|------------|
| **Vataja** | 207 | Haritaki | Terminalia chebula |
| | 212 | Pau d'arco | Tabebuia impetiginosa |
| | 401 | Cumin | Cumimum cyminum |
| | | Fennel | Foeniculum vulgare |
| | | Cardamom | Elettaria cardamomum |
| | 404 | Angelica | Angelica archangelica |
| | | Wild yam | Dioscorea villosa |
| | | Valerian | Valeriana officinalis |
| **Pittaja** | 212 | Pau d'arco | Tabebuia impetiginosa |
| | 402 | Coriander | Coriandrum sativum |
| | | Cumin | Cumimum cyminum |
| | | Fennel | Foeniculum vulgare |
| **Kaphaja** | 207 | Haritaki | Terminalia chebula |
| | 212 | Pau d'arco | Tabebuia impetiginosa |
| | 403 | Ginger | Zingiber officinale |
| | | Cumin | Cumimum cyminum |
| | | Fenugreek | Trigonella foenum-graecum |

| Dosha | Low Dose | High Dose |
|-------|----------|-----------|
| **Vata** | 1 of each X2 per day before meals | 2 of each X2 per day before meals |
| **Pitta** | 1 of each X2 per day with meals | 2 of each X2 per day with meals |
| **Kapha** | 2 of each X2 per day after meals | 3 of each X2 per day after meals |

## Description:

Ayurveda views fungal infections much like viral or bacterial infections in that they are all associated with Ama conditions. This means that any Dosha can cause an environment favorable for fungal infections in the body by disrupting the function of Agni. Treatment follows the Vikriti and an anti-Ama diet will accelerate results.

Use the Vataja herbs if Vata is predominant in the Vikriti (imbalance) with a Vata Vikriti diet / lifestyle.

Use the Pittaja herbs if Pitta is predominant in the Vikriti (imbalance) with a Pitta Vikriti diet / lifestyle.

Use the Kaphaja herbs if Kapha is predominant in the Vikriti (imbalance) with a Kapha Vikriti diet / lifestyle.

## Gallbladder stones

| Dosha | Code | Common Name | Latin Name |
|---|---|---|---|
| **Vataja** | 208 | Manjishta | Rubia cordifolia |
| | 401 | Cumin | Cumimum cyminum |
| | | Fennel | Foeniculum vulgare |
| | | Cardamom | Elettaria cardamomum |
| | 404 | Angelica | Angelica archangelica |
| | | Wild yam | Dioscorea villosa |
| | | Valerian | Valeriana officinalis |
| | 405 | Burdock | Arctium lappa |
| | | Yellow dock | Rumex crispus |
| | | Milk Thistle | Silybum marianum |
| **Pittaja** | 208 | Manjishta | Rubia cordifolia |
| | 402 | Coriander | Coriandrum sativum |
| | | Cumin | Cumimum cyminum |
| | | Fennel | Foeniculum vulgare |
| | 405 | Burdock | Arctium lappa |
| | | Yellow dock | Rumex crispus |
| | | Milk Thistle | Silybum marianum |
| | 407 | Turmeric | Curcuma longa |
| | | Barberry | Berberis vulgaris |
| | | Dandelion | Taraxacum officinale |
| **Kaphaja** | 208 | Manjishta | Rubia cordifolia |
| | 403 | Ginger | Zingiber officinale |
| | | Cumin | Cumimum cyminum |
| | | Fenugreek | Trigonella foenum-graecum |
| | 405 | Burdock | Arctium lappa |
| | | Yellow dock | Rumex crispus |
| | | Milk Thistle | Silybum marianum |
| | 407 | Turmeric | Curcuma longa |
| | | Barberry | Berberis vulgaris |
| | | Dandelion | Taraxacum officinale |

| Dosha | Low Dose | High Dose |
|---|---|---|
| **Vata** | 1 of each X2 per day before meals | 2 of each X2 per day before meals |
| **Pitta** | 1 of each X2 per day with meals | 2 of each X2 per day with meals |
| **Kapha** | 2 of each X2 per day after meals | 3 of each X2 per day after meals |

## Description:

There are many different causes of Gallbladder disorders. In Ayurveda, the gallbladder is part of the liver, which in itself is the

Mulasthana of Rakta Dhatu. Thus, structurally all gallbladder problems are Pitta Roga. Functionally, any Dosha can cause problems in the liver and gallbladder. Kapha causes problems by congesting the bile flow, Vata though drying out the bile, and Pitta through causing excess bile production and inflammation (cholecystitis). The gallbladder's main function is to store the bile produced by the liver and secrete it into the small intestine. This liver bile helps to digest food in the small intestine.

In most cases gallstones are Vataja because they are 'stones' that are actually dried out bile that accumulate in the ducts and gall bladder itself. These stones are sandy, hard and small – all indications of Vataja pathology. If the congestion in the gallbladder is general and shows cysts, fatty tissues or polyps then these generally indicate Kaphaja pathologies. Of course, Pittaja problems are associated with various forms of inflammation. Gallstones can cause inflammatory issues in the ducts, in these cases it can be Vataja / Pittaja problems. Treatment should target the casual Dosha and then secondary Rakta Dhatu and Pitta Dosha. A Pitta reducing diet is very important in early stages of treatment.

Note that gallstones are very slow to dissolve. Diet and herbs will not dissolve the stones in emergency situations, they require from six to twelve months to remove the stones slowly and without pain or trauma. Hence, it is better to start treatment before crisis of pain develop. Radical methods of removing the stones can damage the bile ducts and generally better to avoid. Junk food diets and rich, fatty diets are a main cause of gallstone formation.

Use the Vataja herbs if Vata is predominant in the Vikriti (imbalance) with a Pitta Vikriti diet and Vata lifestyle.

Use the Pittaja herbs if Pitta is predominant in the Vikriti (imbalance) with a Pitta Vikriti diet / lifestyle.

Use the Kaphaja herbs if Kapha is predominant in the Vikriti (imbalance) with a Pitta Vikriti diet and Kapha lifestyle.

## Gas

| Dosha | Code | Common Name | Latin Name |
|-------|------|-------------|------------|
| Vataja | 207 | Haritaki | Terminalia chebula |
|  | 401 | Cumin | Cumimum cyminum |
|  |  | Fennel | Foeniculum vulgare |
|  |  | Cardamom | Elettaria cardamomum |
|  | 404 | Angelica | Angelica archangelica |
|  |  | Wild yam | Dioscorea villosa |
|  |  | Valerian | Valeriana officinalis |
| Pittaja | 201 | Amalaki | Emblica officinalis |
|  | 402 | Coriander | Coriandrum sativum |
|  |  | Cumin | Cumimum cyminum |
|  |  | Fennel | Foeniculum vulgare |
|  | 407 | Turmeric | Curcuma longa |
|  |  | Barberry | Berberis vulgaris |
|  |  | Dandelion | Taraxacum officinale |
| Kaphaja | 207 | Haritaki | Terminalia chebula |
|  | 403 | Ginger | Zingiber officinale |
|  |  | Cumin | Cumimum cyminum |
|  |  | Fenugreek | Trigonella foenum-graecum |
|  | 407 | Turmeric | Curcuma longa |
|  |  | Barberry | Berberis vulgaris |
|  |  | Dandelion | Taraxacum officinale |

| Dosha | Low Dose | High Dose |
|-------|----------|-----------|
| Vata | 1 of each X2 per day before meals | 2 of each X2 per day before meals |
| Pitta | 1 of each X2 per day with meals | 2 of each X2 per day with meals |
| Kapha | 2 of each X2 per day after meals | 3 of each X2 per day after meals |

## Description:
See "flatulence" for the description.

Use the Vataja herbs if Vata is predominant in the Vikriti (imbalance) with a Vata Vikriti diet / lifestyle.

Use the Pittaja herbs if Pitta is predominant in the Vikriti (imbalance) with a Pitta Vikriti diet / lifestyle.

Use the Kaphaja herbs if Kapha is predominant in the Vikriti (imbalance) with a Kapha Vikriti diet / lifestyle.

## Gastric ulcers

| Dosha | Code | Common Name | Latin Name |
|---|---|---|---|
| **Vataja** | 201 | Amalaki | Emblica officinalis |
| | 211 | Shatavari | Asparagus racemosus |
| | 401 | Cumin | Cumimum cyminum |
| | | Fennel | Foeniculum vulgare |
| | | Cardamom | Elettaria cardamomum |
| | 404 | Angelica | Angelica archangelica |
| | | Wild yam | Dioscorea villosa |
| | | Valerian | Valeriana officinalis |
| **Pittaja** | 201 | Amalaki | Emblica officinalis |
| | 211 | Shatavari | Asparagus racemosus |
| | 402 | Coriander | Coriandrum sativum |
| | | Cumin | Cumimum cyminum |
| | | Fennel | Foeniculum vulgare |
| | 405 | Burdock | Arctium lappa |
| | | Yellow dock | Rumex crispus |
| | | Milk Thistle | Silybum marianum |
| **Kaphaja** | 201 | Amalaki | Emblica officinalis |
| | 211 | Shatavari | Asparagus racemosus |
| | 402 | Coriander | Coriandrum sativum |
| | | Cumin | Cumimum cyminum |
| | | Fennel | Foeniculum vulgare |
| | 404 | Angelica | Angelica archangelica |
| | | Wild yam | Dioscorea villosa |
| | | Valerian | Valeriana officinalis |

| Dosha | Low Dose | High Dose |
|---|---|---|
| **Vata** | 1 of each X2 per day before meals | 2 of each X2 per day before meals |
| **Pitta** | 1 of each X2 per day with meals | 2 of each X2 per day with meals |
| **Kapha** | 2 of each X2 per day after meals | 3 of each X2 per day after meals |

## Description:
Gastric ulcers are Pitta Roga due to Tikshna Agni. It is rare that Kapha will cause this disorder, usually it is a Pittaja or Vataja disorder.

Use the Vataja herbs if Vata is predominant in the Vikriti (imbalance) with a Vata Vikriti diet / lifestyle.

Use the Pittaja herbs if Pitta is predominant in the Vikriti (imbalance) with a Pitta Vikriti diet / lifestyle.

Use the Kaphaja herbs if Kapha is predominant in the Vikriti (imbalance) with a Kapha Vikriti diet / lifestyle.

# Gastritis

| Dosha | Code | Common Name | Latin Name |
|---|---|---|---|
| **Vataja** | 401 | Cumin | Cumimum cyminum |
| | | Fennel | Foeniculum vulgare |
| | | Cardamom | Elettaria cardamomum |
| | 404 | Angelica | Angelica archangelica |
| | | Wild yam | Dioscorea villosa |
| | | Valerian | Valeriana officinalis |
| | 407 | Turmeric | Curcuma longa |
| | | Barberry | Berberis vulgaris |
| | | Dandelion | Taraxacum officinale |
| | 409 | Passion flower | Passiflora incarnata |
| | | Skullcap | Scutellaria lateriflora |
| | | Gotu kola | Centella asiatica |
| **Pittaja** | 402 | Coriander | Coriandrum sativum |
| | | Cumin | Cumimum cyminum |
| | | Fennel | Foeniculum vulgare |
| | 405 | Burdock | Arctium lappa |
| | | Yellow dock | Rumex crispus |
| | | Milk Thistle | Silybum marianum |
| | 407 | Turmeric | Curcuma longa |
| | | Barberry | Berberis vulgaris |
| | | Dandelion | Taraxacum officinale |
| | 409 | Passion flower | Passiflora incarnata |
| | | Skullcap | Scutellaria lateriflora |
| | | Gotu kola | Centella asiatica |
| **Kaphaja** | 403 | Ginger | Zingiber officinale |
| | | Cumin | Cumimum cyminum |
| | | Fenugreek | Trigonella foenum-graecum |
| | 404 | Angelica | Angelica archangelica |
| | | Wild yam | Dioscorea villosa |
| | | Valerian | Valeriana officinalis |
| | 407 | Turmeric | Curcuma longa |
| | | Barberry | Berberis vulgaris |
| | | Dandelion | Taraxacum officinale |

| Dosha | Low Dose | High Dose |
|---|---|---|
| **Vata** | 1 of each X2 per day before meals | 2 of each X2 per day before meals |
| **Pitta** | 1 of each X2 per day with meals | 2 of each X2 per day with meals |
| **Kapha** | 2 of each X2 per day after meals | 3 of each X2 per day after meals |

## Description:

Gastritis describes a group of conditions with one thing in common: inflammation of the lining of the stomach. The inflammation aspect of gastritis is most often the result of infection of some kind and is usually termed acute or chronic. Common causes include bacterial infection, the use of NSAIDs, excessive alcohol consumption, smoking, cocaine, some autoimmune problems, radiation therapy and Crohn's disease, among others. It is thought that up to half of the worlds populations suffers from some form of gastritis.

This is a Pitta Roga condition in Ayurveda. Causes can be due to any Dosha that disrupts Agni function and allows an imbalance in the bacterial levels of the digestive system. Food and beverages further disrupt Agni and can also contribute. An anti-Pitta diet is recommended that avoids fermented, acid and pungent food. The herbal blend and lifestyle should follow the dominant Vikriti.

These herbal blends will heal the intestinal walls and cure the problem if diet and lifestyle are followed.

Use the Vataja herbs if Vata is predominant in the Vikriti (imbalance) with a Pitta Vikriti diet and Vata lifestyle.

Use the Pittaja herbs if Pitta is predominant in the Vikriti (imbalance) with a Pitta Vikriti diet / lifestyle.

Use the Kaphaja herbs if Kapha is predominant in the Vikriti (imbalance) with a Pitta Vikriti diet and Kapha lifestyle.

## General debility

| Dosha | Code | Common Name | Latin Name |
|---|---|---|---|
| **Vataja** | 203 | Ashwagandha | Withania somnifera |
| | 206 | Guduchi | Tinospora cordifolia |
| | 211 | Shatavari | Asparagus racemosus |
| | 301 | Amalaki | Emblica officinalis |
| | | Bibhitaki | Terminalia belerica |
| | | Haritaki | Terminalia chebula |
| **Pittaja** | 201 | Amalaki | Emblica officinalis |
| | 206 | Guduchi | Tinospora cordifolia |
| | 211 | Shatavari | Asparagus racemosus |
| | 301 | Amalaki | Emblica officinalis |
| | | Bibhitaki | Terminalia belerica |
| | | Haritaki | Terminalia chebula |
| **Kaphaja** | 206 | Guduchi | Tinospora cordifolia |
| | 209 | Punarnava | Boerhaavia diffusa |
| | 212 | Pau d'arco | Tabebuia impetiginosa |
| | 301 | Amalaki | Emblica officinalis |
| | | Bibhitaki | Terminalia belerica |
| | | Haritaki | Terminalia chebula |

| Dosha | Low Dose | High Dose |
|---|---|---|
| **Vata** | 1 of each X2 per day before meals | 2 of each X2 per day before meals |
| **Pitta** | 1 of each X2 per day with meals | 2 of each X2 per day with meals |
| **Kapha** | 2 of each X2 per day after meals | 3 of each X2 per day after meals |

### Description:

These are herbal blends that help the body and mind recover from illness, burnout and any situation that causes weakness in the body. These blends should be used as per Prakriti with Prakriti diets and lifestyles. If there is a notable amount of Ama on the tongue it is best to avoid using these blends until the Ama has been reduced.

Use the Vataja herbs if Vata is predominant in the Prakriti (imbalance) with a Vata Prakriti diet / lifestyle.

Use the Pittaja herbs if Pitta is predominant in the Prakriti (imbalance) with a Pitta Prakriti diet / lifestyle.

Use the Kaphaja herbs if Kapha is predominant in the Prakriti (imbalance) with a Kapha Prakriti diet / lifestyle.

# Genital herpes

| Dosha | Code | Common Name | Latin Name |
|---|---|---|---|
| Vataja | 207 | Haritaki | Terminalia chebula |
| | 208 | Manjishta | Rubia cordifolia |
| | 212 | Pau d'arco | Tabebuia impetiginosa |
| | 401 | Cumin | Cumimum cyminum |
| | | Fennel | Foeniculum vulgare |
| | | Cardamom | Elettaria cardamomum |
| Pittaja | 207 | Haritaki | Terminalia chebula |
| | 208 | Manjishta | Rubia cordifolia |
| | 212 | Pau d'arco | Tabebuia impetiginosa |
| | 402 | Coriander | Coriandrum sativum |
| | | Cumin | Cumimum cyminum |
| | | Fennel | Foeniculum vulgare |
| Kaphaja | 207 | Haritaki | Terminalia chebula |
| | 208 | Manjishta | Rubia cordifolia |
| | 212 | Pau d'arco | Tabebuia impetiginosa |
| | 403 | Ginger | Zingiber officinale |
| | | Cumin | Cumimum cyminum |
| | | Fenugreek | Trigonella foenum-graecum |

| Dosha | Low Dose | High Dose |
|---|---|---|
| Vata | 1 of each X2 per day before meals | 2 of each X2 per day before meals |
| Pitta | 1 of each X2 per day with meals | 2 of each X2 per day with meals |
| Kapha | 2 of each X2 per day after meals | 3 of each X2 per day after meals |

## Description:

This is a symptomatic treatment of the Herpes virus as per Prakriti. This is a Pitta Roga problem reflecting low immunity. These problems should be treated after the virus is eliminated. It may not be possible to remove the virus completely if Pitta is unstable and the immune system is not working correctly, or if there is low immunity.

Use the Vataja herbs if Vata is predominant in the Prakriti with a Vata Prakriti diet / lifestyle.

Use the Pittaja herbs if Pitta is predominant in the Prakriti with a Pitta Prakriti diet / lifestyle.

Use the Kaphaja herbs if Kapha is predominant in the Prakriti with a Kapha Prakriti diet / lifestyle.

## Glaucoma

| Dosha | Code | Common Name | Latin Name |
|-------|------|-------------|------------|
| Vataja | 301 | Amalaki | Emblica officinalis |
| | | Bibhitaki | Terminalia belerica |
| | | Haritaki | Terminalia chebula |
| | 404 | Angelica | Angelica archangelica |
| | | Wild yam | Dioscorea villosa |
| | | Valerian | Valeriana officinalis |
| Pittaja | 301 | Amalaki | Emblica officinalis |
| | | Bibhitaki | Terminalia belerica |
| | | Haritaki | Terminalia chebula |
| | 405 | Burdock | Arctium lappa |
| | | Yellow dock | Rumex crispus |
| | | Milk Thistle | Silybum marianum |
| Kaphaja | 301 | Amalaki | Emblica officinalis |
| | | Bibhitaki | Terminalia belerica |
| | | Haritaki | Terminalia chebula |
| | 406 | Myrrh | Commiphora myrrha |
| | | Elecampane | Inula helenium |
| | | Yellow dock | Rumex crispus |

| Dosha | Low Dose | High Dose |
|-------|----------|-----------|
| Vata | 1 of each X2 per day before meals | 2 of each X2 per day before meals |
| Pitta | 1 of each X2 per day with meals | 2 of each X2 per day with meals |
| Kapha | 2 of each X2 per day after meals | 3 of each X2 per day after meals |

## Description:

The eyes are under the control of Pitta (Alochaka Pitta) and have support from both Kapha in structure and Vata in function. Hence, any Dosha can cause eye diseases according to location and function. As the structure is under the control of Kapha and Majja Dhatu Kapha is implicated in glaucoma. Pitta is controlling the function of "seeing" and Vata controls both Kapha and Pitta and coordinates images received in the brain and their interpretation.

Generally, the cause of glaucoma is a failure of the eye to maintain an appropriate balance between the amount of internal (intraocular) fluid produced and the amount that drains away; this is a Vata function of coordination. When something affects the ability of internal eye structures to regulate Intraocular Pressure (IOP), eye pressure can rise to dangerously high levels — causing glaucoma.

Glaucoma can also occur when internal eye pressure is normal (normal-tension glaucoma). People with this condition have highly pressure-sensitive optic nerves that are susceptible to irreversible damage from what ordinarily would be considered 'normal' IOP. Some studies also indicate that poor blood flow within the eye is associated with blind spots (scotomas) that develop within the visual field, similar to those that occur in glaucoma. When glaucoma progresses, injury to neurons ultimately leads to eye damage in the form of peripheral vision loss. However, eye damage appears to begin first in the brain as connectivity is lost.

Vata type weak nerves, dryness, poor blood circulation
Pitta type inflammation, IOP is hypertension
Kapha type, poor blood circulation, IOP is hypotension

Internal treatment should follow the Vikriti with the above blends of herbs. External treatment of the eyes is explained under the 'Eye disorders' description. Follow the instructions for Triphala tea to use on the eyes externally for best results.

Use the Vataja herbs if Vata is predominant in the Vikriti (imbalance) with a Vata Vikriti diet / lifestyle.

Use the Pittaja herbs if Pitta is predominant in the Vikriti (imbalance) with a Pitta Vikriti diet / lifestyle.

Use the Kaphaja herbs if Kapha is predominant in the Vikriti (imbalance) with a Kapha Vikriti diet / lifestyle.

## Goiter

| Dosha | Code | Common Name | Latin Name |
|---|---|---|---|
| **Vataja** | 203 | Ashwagandha | Withania somnifera |
| | 206 | Guduchi | Tinospora cordifolia |
| | 401 | Cumin | Cumimum cyminum |
| | | Fennel | Foeniculum vulgare |
| | | Cardamom | Elettaria cardamomum |
| | 404 | Angelica | Angelica archangelica |
| | | Wild yam | Dioscorea villosa |
| | | Valerian | Valeriana officinalis |
| **Pittaja** | 203 | Ashwagandha | Withania somnifera |
| | 206 | Guduchi | Tinospora cordifolia |
| | 402 | Coriander | Coriandrum sativum |
| | | Cumin | Cumimum cyminum |
| | | Fennel | Foeniculum vulgare |
| | 405 | Burdock | Arctium lappa |
| | | Yellow dock | Rumex crispus |
| | | Milk Thistle | Silybum marianum |
| **Kaphaja** | 203 | Ashwagandha | Withania somnifera |
| | 206 | Guduchi | Tinospora cordifolia |
| | 403 | Ginger | Zingiber officinale |
| | | Cumin | Cumimum cyminum |
| | | Fenugreek | Trigonella foenum-graecum |
| | 406 | Myrrh | Commiphora myrrha |
| | | Elecampane | Inula helenium |
| | | Yellow dock | Rumex crispus |

| Dosha | Low Dose | High Dose |
|---|---|---|
| **Vata** | 1 of each X2 per day before meals | 2 of each X2 per day before meals |
| **Pitta** | 1 of each X2 per day with meals | 2 of each X2 per day with meals |
| **Kapha** | 2 of each X2 per day after meals | 3 of each X2 per day after meals |

### Description:

Goiter is an abnormal enlargement of the thyroid gland. The thyroid gland is part of Majja Dhatu and controlled by Kapha Dosha structurally. Pitta is using the thyroid to regulate the metabolism, so most functional problems are related to Pitta. Vata coordinates both Kapha and Pitta in the thyroid gland.

Goiter can be related to either a hypo or hyper function of the thyroid gland. Hypothyroid is due to a Munda Dhatu Agni in Majja,

Hyperthyroid is due to a Tikshna Dhatu Agni in Majja Dhatu. Autoimmune disorders of the thyroid – such as Hashimoto's – often fluctuate between hypo or hyper functions of the thyroid and indicate a Vishama Dhatu Agni disruption in Majja Dhatu. In all of these conditions Goiter is a possible result of Dhatu Agni disruption.

Causes of thyroid disruption are many, ranging from radiation, chemical, pollution, to stress, shock or dietary. Correct diagnosis is helpful to cure these problems. Treatment of Majja is difficult and takes months to modify; treatments should last at least nine to twelve months. Diet and lifestyle are critical for a cure. Thyroid conditions that are older than five years are not curable in most cases according to my clinical experience, but are able to be managed.

These herbal blends can be mixed with thyroid medications because they work on the structure / function and not the endocrine aspect of the thyroid gland; therefore, there is little or no drug / herb interactions.

Use the Vataja herbs if Vata is predominant in the Vikriti (imbalance) with a Vata Vikriti diet / lifestyle.

Use the Pittaja herbs if Pitta is predominant in the Vikriti (imbalance) with a Pitta Vikriti diet / lifestyle.

Use the Kaphaja herbs if Kapha is predominant in the Vikriti (imbalance) with a Kapha Vikriti diet / lifestyle.

## Gout

| Dosha | Code | Common Name | Latin Name |
|-------|------|-------------|------------|
| **Vataja** | 207 | Haritaki | Terminalia chebula |
| | 208 | Manjishta | Rubia cordifolia |
| | 401 | Cumin | Cumimum cyminum |
| | | Fennel | Foeniculum vulgare |
| | | Cardamom | Elettaria cardamomum |
| | 404 | Angelica | Angelica archangelica |
| | | Wild yam | Dioscorea villosa |
| | | Valerian | Valeriana officinalis |
| **Pittaja** | 201 | Amalaki | Emblica officinalis |
| | 208 | Manjishta | Rubia cordifolia |
| | 402 | Coriander | Coriandrum sativum |
| | | Cumin | Cumimum cyminum |
| | | Fennel | Foeniculum vulgare |
| | 405 | Burdock | Arctium lappa |
| | | Yellow dock | Rumex crispus |
| | | Milk Thistle | Silybum marianum |
| **Kaphaja** | 207 | Haritaki | Terminalia chebula |
| | 208 | Manjishta | Rubia cordifolia |
| | 403 | Ginger | Zingiber officinale |
| | | Cumin | Cumimum cyminum |
| | | Fenugreek | Trigonella foenum-graecum |
| | 406 | Myrrh | Commiphora myrrha |
| | | Elecampane | Inula helenium |
| | | Yellow dock | Rumex crispus |

| Dosha | Low Dose | High Dose |
|-------|----------|-----------|
| **Vata** | 1 of each X2 per day before meals | 2 of each X2 per day before meals |
| **Pitta** | 1 of each X2 per day with meals | 2 of each X2 per day with meals |
| **Kapha** | 2 of each X2 per day after meals | 3 of each X2 per day after meals |

## Description:

Gout is a form of inflammatory arthritis that develops in some people who have high levels of uric acid in the blood. Gout occurs more commonly in those who eat meat, drink alcohol, or are overweight. Uric acid is a byproduct of a diet based on animal food; e.g., meat, dairy, etc.

Arthritis is a general term for over one hundred disorders affecting the joints. Pain or stiffness are common symptoms of these types of joint disorders. Gout is a specific inflammatory type of arthritis that often begins in the big toe. Ayurveda views this group of disorders differently than modern medicine in that they recognize non-inflammatory types of arthritis. In Ayurveda, these arthritic disorders are due to the accumulation of Ama in the body.

Gout is classified as Vata Roga by location and structure, Asthi Dhatu, and functionally any Dosha can cause this problem when mixed with Ama. Because gout is an inflammatory disorder Pitta is always involved, but may not be the cause of the pathology. The main treatment for gout is diet and lifestyle with herbal support. A vegan diet is best for treatment as per Vikriti. Pancha Karma treatments are very useful to cure gout.

Use the Vataja herbs if Vata is predominant in the Vikriti (imbalance) with a Vata Vikriti diet / lifestyle.

Use the Pittaja herbs if Pitta is predominant in the Vikriti (imbalance) with a Pitta Vikriti diet / lifestyle.

Use the Kaphaja herbs if Kapha is predominant in the Vikriti (imbalance) with a Kapha Vikriti diet / lifestyle.

## Hay fever

| Dosha | Code | Common Name | Latin Name |
|-------|------|-------------|------------|
| Vataja | 212 | Pau d'arco | Tabebuia impetiginosa |
| | 401 | Cumin | Cumimum cyminum |
| | | Fennel | Foeniculum vulgare |
| | | Cardamom | Elettaria cardamomum |
| | 409 | Marshmallow | Althaea officinalis |
| | | Gotu kola | Centella asiatica |
| | | Stinging nettles | Urtica dioica |
| Pittaja | 212 | Pau d'arco | Tabebuia impetiginosa |
| | 402 | Coriander | Coriandrum sativum |
| | | Cumin | Cumimum cyminum |
| | | Fennel | Foeniculum vulgare |
| | 407 | Turmeric | Curcuma longa |
| | | Barberry | Berberis vulgaris |
| | | Dandelion | Taraxacum officinale |
| Kaphaja | 209 | Punarnava | Boerhaavia diffusa |
| | 212 | Pau d'arco | Tabebuia impetiginosa |
| | 403 | Ginger | Zingiber officinale |
| | | Cumin | Cumimum cyminum |
| | | Fenugreek | Trigonella foenum-graecum |

| Dosha | Low Dose | High Dose |
|-------|----------|-----------|
| Vata | 1 of each X2 per day before meals | 2 of each X2 per day before meals |
| Pitta | 1 of each X2 per day with meals | 2 of each X2 per day with meals |
| Kapha | 2 of each X2 per day after meals | 3 of each X2 per day after meals |

## Description:

Hay Fever is due to incorrect immune function. Start treatment six months before Hay fever season for best results. These blends will increase and stabilize the immune system and generally cure Hay fever if done for six months and repeated several years. For example, start the treatment in November if Hay fever starts at the end of April.

Use the Vataja herbs if Vata is predominant in the Vikriti (imbalance) with a Vata Vikriti diet / lifestyle.

Use the Pittaja herbs if Pitta is predominant in the Vikriti (imbalance) with a Pitta Vikriti diet / lifestyle.

Use the Kaphaja herbs if Kapha is predominant in the Vikriti (imbalance) with a Kapha Vikriti diet / lifestyle.

# Headaches

| Dosha | Code | Common Name | Latin Name |
|-------|------|-------------|------------|
| Vataja | 401 | Cumin | Cumimum cyminum |
| | | Fennel | Foeniculum vulgare |
| | | Cardamom | Elettaria cardamomum |
| | 404 | Angelica | Angelica archangelica |
| | | Wild yam | Dioscorea villosa |
| | | Valerian | Valeriana officinalis |
| | 407 | Turmeric | Curcuma longa |
| | | Barberry | Berberis vulgaris |
| | | Dandelion | Taraxacum officinale |
| Pittaja | 402 | Coriander | Coriandrum sativum |
| | | Cumin | Cumimum cyminum |
| | | Fennel | Foeniculum vulgare |
| | 405 | Burdock | Arctium lappa |
| | | Yellow dock | Rumex crispus |
| | | Milk Thistle | Silybum marianum |
| | 407 | Turmeric | Curcuma longa |
| | | Barberry | Berberis vulgaris |
| | | Dandelion | Taraxacum officinale |
| Kaphaja | 403 | Ginger | Zingiber officinale |
| | | Cumin | Cumimum cyminum |
| | | Fenugreek | Trigonella foenum-graecum |
| | 406 | Myrrh | Commiphora myrrha |
| | | Elecampane | Inula helenium |
| | | Yellow dock | Rumex crispus |
| | 407 | Turmeric | Curcuma longa |
| | | Barberry | Berberis vulgaris |
| | | Dandelion | Taraxacum officinale |

| Dosha | Low Dose | High Dose |
|-------|----------|-----------|
| Vata | 1 of each X2 per day before meals | 2 of each X2 per day before meals |
| Pitta | 1 of each X2 per day with meals | 2 of each X2 per day with meals |
| Kapha | 2 of each X2 per day after meals | 3 of each X2 per day after meals |

## Description:

Headaches can be due to a number of reasons. These herbal blends cure headaches that are due to Ama and digestive disorders. For headaches linked to hormone causes see 'Hormone Related Headaches'. Any Dosha can cause headaches that are due to deranged Agni and the formation of Ama that goes into the bloodstream, causing headaches.

These types of headaches are Pitta Roga by location as the bloodstream is under the control of Rakta Dhatu. Vata moves the blood and Ama so can be implicated by function. Kapha is often the cause of headaches due to Munda Agni causing heavy, sticky Ama to form in the digestive system.

Vataja – variable or quick onset, sharp, throbbing pain, sides of the head

Pittaja – steady, progressive onset, light sensitive, burning or sharp pain, behind the eyes and forehead area

Kaphaja – slow onset, dull pain, deep in head or base of skull

Use the Vataja herbs if Vata is predominant in the Vikriti (imbalance) with a Vata Vikriti diet / lifestyle.

Use the Pittaja herbs if Pitta is predominant in the Vikriti (imbalance) with a Pitta Vikriti diet / lifestyle.

Use the Kaphaja herbs if Kapha is predominant in the Vikriti (imbalance) with a Kapha Vikriti diet / lifestyle.

# Heartburn (acidity)

| Dosha | Code | Common Name | Latin Name |
|---|---|---|---|
| Vataja | 201 | Amalaki | Emblica officinalis |
| | 210 | Shankhpushpi | Convolvulus pluricaulis |
| | 211 | Shatavari | Asparagus racemosus |
| Pittaja | 201 | Amalaki | Emblica officinalis |
| | 405 | Burdock | Arctium lappa |
| | | Yellow dock | Rumex crispus |
| | | Milk Thistle | Silybum marianum |
| Kaphaja | 201 | Amalaki | Emblica officinalis |
| | 407 | Turmeric | Curcuma longa |
| | | Barberry | Berberis vulgaris |
| | | Dandelion | Taraxacum officinale |

| Dosha | Low Dose | High Dose |
|---|---|---|
| Vata | 1 of each X2 per day before meals | 2 of each X2 per day before meals |
| Pitta | 1 of each X2 per day with meals | 2 of each X2 per day with meals |
| Kapha | 2 of each X2 per day after meals | 3 of each X2 per day after meals |

## Description:
See 'Acidity' and the description there.

Use the Vataja herbs if Vata is predominant in the Vikriti (imbalance) with a Vata Vikriti diet / lifestyle.

Use the Pittaja herbs if Pitta is predominant in the Vikriti (imbalance) with a Pitta Vikriti diet / lifestyle.

Use the Kaphaja herbs if Kapha is predominant in the Vikriti (imbalance) with a Kapha Vikriti diet / lifestyle.

## Hemorrhoids

| Dosha | Code | Common Name | Latin Name |
|---|---|---|---|
| **Vataja** | 206 | Guduchi | Tinospora cordifolia |
| | 207 | Haritaki | Terminalia chebula |
| | 403 | Ginger | Zingiber officinale |
| | | Cumin | Cumimum cyminum |
| | | Fenugreek | Trigonella foenum-graecum |
| | 404 | Angelica | Angelica archangelica |
| | | Wild yam | Dioscorea villosa |
| | | Valerian | Valeriana officinalis |
| **Pittaja** | 206 | Guduchi | Tinospora cordifolia |
| | 207 | Haritaki | Terminalia chebula |
| | 402 | Coriander | Coriandrum sativum |
| | | Cumin | Cumimum cyminum |
| | | Fennel | Foeniculum vulgare |
| | 407 | Turmeric | Curcuma longa |
| | | Barberry | Berberis vulgaris |
| | | Dandelion | Taraxacum officinale |
| **Kaphaja** | 206 | Guduchi | Tinospora cordifolia |
| | 207 | Haritaki | Terminalia chebula |
| | 403 | Ginger | Zingiber officinale |
| | | Cumin | Cumimum cyminum |
| | | Fenugreek | Trigonella foenum-graecum |
| | 407 | Turmeric | Curcuma longa |
| | | Barberry | Berberis vulgaris |
| | | Dandelion | Taraxacum officinale |

| Dosha | Low Dose | High Dose |
|---|---|---|
| **Vata** | 1 of each X2 per day before meals | 2 of each X2 per day before meals |
| **Pitta** | 1 of each X2 per day with meals | 2 of each X2 per day with meals |
| **Kapha** | 2 of each X2 per day after meals | 3 of each X2 per day after meals |

## Description:

Hemorrhoids are swollen veins located around the anus or in the lower rectum. It is estimated that about fifty percent of adults have hemorrhoids by the age of fifty. Hemorrhoids can either be internal or external. Internal hemorrhoids develop within the anus or rectum. External hemorrhoids develop outside of the anus.

Hemorrhoids are part of the colon / rectum and are thus part of both Rasa and Mamsa Dhatus. This means they are Kapha Roga by structure. Functionally they are usually Kaphaja or Vataja, although there are Pittaja type as well. Kapha type of hemorrhoids are due to Munda Agni and congestion in the GI tract. Usually the stool is soft, sticky and abundant, however slow to be removed, often taking several days between evacuations. This kind of hemorrhoids will tend to be external and filled with fluid, not necessarily blood. These types of hemorrhoids are usually associated with a Kapha (congested, sticky) type of constipation.

Vata type of hemorrhoids are due to dryness from an excess activity of Apana Vayu. The dryness results in a hard stool that does not move out of the rectum and damages the walls due to the hardness of the stool. Vataja hemorrhoids often cause bleeding as the anus gets damaged. Vata also makes internal hemorrhoids more often than Kapha or Pitta due to the same reasons already indicated. These types of hemorrhoids are usually associated with a Vata (dry) type of constipation.

Pitta type of hemorrhoids are inflamed and bleeding. Usually they are related to burning feelings and acidity in the GI tract. The colon / rectum gets irritated from the high acidity and becomes inflamed and irritated. The stool is usually loose and burns a bit on evacuation. There can be several stools per day. This is caused from a Tikshna Agni and high Pitta conditions. The hemorrhoids are usually external and bleeding; often filled with blood.

These herbal blends work on the Agni and change the Dosha that is causing the hemorrhoids. They help to reduce the inflammation in the rectum and soften the stools for Vata and Kapha to avoid damage to the walls of the rectum.

In emergencies, the patient can buy Turmeric powder and mix it with equal parts of honey to the size of pea, or Chick pea. This can be placed on the hemorrhoids. A sanitary napkin should be used to protect the underwear as Turmeric stains everything. It is strongly hemostatic and will stop bleeding and pain in a day or two.

Use the Vataja herbs if Vata is predominant in the Vikriti (imbalance) with a Vata Vikriti diet / lifestyle.

Use the Pittaja herbs if Pitta is predominant in the Vikriti (imbalance) with a Pitta Vikriti diet / lifestyle.

Use the Kaphaja herbs if Kapha is predominant in the Vikriti (imbalance) with a Kapha Vikriti diet / lifestyle.

## Hepatitis

| Dosha | Code | Common Name | Latin Name |
|---|---|---|---|
| **Vataja** | 206 | Guduchi | Tinospora cordifolia |
| | 207 | Haritaki | Terminalia chebula |
| | 401 | Cumin | Cumimum cyminum |
| | | Fennel | Foeniculum vulgare |
| | | Cardamom | Elettaria cardamomum |
| | 407 | Turmeric | Curcuma longa |
| | | Barberry | Berberis vulgaris |
| | | Dandelion | Taraxacum officinale |
| **Pittaja** | 206 | Guduchi | Tinospora cordifolia |
| | 207 | Haritaki | Terminalia chebula |
| | 402 | Coriander | Coriandrum sativum |
| | | Cumin | Cumimum cyminum |
| | | Fennel | Foeniculum vulgare |
| | 405 | Burdock | Arctium lappa |
| | | Yellow dock | Rumex crispus |
| | | Milk Thistle | Silybum marianum |
| | 407 | Turmeric | Curcuma longa |
| | | Barberry | Berberis vulgaris |
| | | Dandelion | Taraxacum officinale |
| **Kaphaja** | 206 | Guduchi | Tinospora cordifolia |
| | 207 | Haritaki | Terminalia chebula |
| | 403 | Ginger | Zingiber officinale |
| | | Cumin | Cumimum cyminum |
| | | Fenugreek | Trigonella foenum-graecum |
| | 405 | Burdock | Arctium lappa |
| | | Yellow dock | Rumex crispus |
| | | Milk Thistle | Silybum marianum |
| | 407 | Turmeric | Curcuma longa |
| | | Barberry | Berberis vulgaris |
| | | Dandelion | Taraxacum officinale |

| Dosha | Low Dose | High Dose |
|---|---|---|
| **Vata** | 1 of each X2 per day before meals | 2 of each X2 per day before meals |
| **Pitta** | 1 of each X2 per day with meals | 2 of each X2 per day with meals |
| **Kapha** | 2 of each X2 per day after meals | 3 of each X2 per day after meals |

## Description:

These herbal blends can be used for all forms of hepatitis. These herbs will work on both Sama and Nirama conditions of hepatitis.

This is a Pittaja problem by both structure and function; the blends work primarily on Rakta Dhatu. The formulas act as tonic to the liver and at the same time they remove Ama and/or the hepatitis virus, so it is both a reducing and tonic formula to the Pitta tissues. Vata Prakriti people need to limit the use of these blends to a two-month period. There is no restriction for Pitta or Kapha types on the duration of using these herbs. A typical treatment should last six months or longer to cure the problem. For chronic conditions expect at least a year of treatment. We do not suggest using the blends longer than one year.

Some people find that this virus will flare up after or during periods of stress. This is because stress reduces the body's immune response. Normally the immune system will prevent virus from manifesting, growing, or causing problems. When stress reduces the immunity, the viruses are free to express their nature.

Use the Vataja herbs if Vata is predominant in the Vikriti (imbalance) with a Vata Vikriti diet / lifestyle.

Use the Pittaja herbs if Pitta is predominant in the Vikriti (imbalance) with a Pitta Vikriti diet / lifestyle.

Use the Kaphaja herbs if Kapha is predominant in the Vikriti (imbalance) with a Kapha Vikriti diet / lifestyle.

## Herpes virus (I & II)

| Dosha | Code | Common Name | Latin Name |
|---|---|---|---|
| Vataja | 207 | Haritaki | Terminalia chebula |
| | 208 | Manjishta | Rubia cordifolia |
| | 212 | Pau d'arco | Tabebuia impetiginosa |
| | 401 | Cumin | Cumimum cyminum |
| | | Fennel | Foeniculum vulgare |
| | | Cardamom | Elettaria cardamomum |
| Pittaja | 207 | Haritaki | Terminalia chebula |
| | 208 | Manjishta | Rubia cordifolia |
| | 212 | Pau d'arco | Tabebuia impetiginosa |
| | 402 | Coriander | Coriandrum sativum |
| | | Cumin | Cumimum cyminum |
| | | Fennel | Foeniculum vulgare |
| Kaphaja | 207 | Haritaki | Terminalia chebula |
| | 208 | Manjishta | Rubia cordifolia |
| | 212 | Pau d'arco | Tabebuia impetiginosa |
| | 403 | Ginger | Zingiber officinale |
| | | Cumin | Cumimum cyminum |
| | | Fenugreek | Trigonella foenum-graecum |

| Dosha | Low Dose | High Dose |
|---|---|---|
| Vata | 1 of each X2 per day before meals | 2 of each X2 per day before meals |
| Pitta | 1 of each X2 per day with meals | 2 of each X2 per day with meals |
| Kapha | 2 of each X2 per day after meals | 3 of each X2 per day after meals |

## Description:

These herbal blends can be used for all types of herpes, oral or genital. This is a Pittaja problem by both structure and function. The formulas work mainly on reducing Pitta in Rakta Dhatu as well as having a special action on the herpes virus. By cleaning the blood most forms of herpes will be cured. This formula can be used from two to six months. Long term use over six months should be avoided.

Use the Vataja herbs if Vata is predominant in the Vikriti (imbalance) with a Vata Vikriti diet / lifestyle.

Use the Pittaja herbs if Pitta is predominant in the Vikriti (imbalance) with a Pitta Vikriti diet / lifestyle.

Use the Kaphaja herbs if Kapha is predominant in the Vikriti (imbalance) with a Kapha Vikriti diet / lifestyle.

## Hiatus hernia

| Dosha | Code | Common Name | Latin Name |
|---|---|---|---|
| Vataja | 403 | Ginger | Zingiber officinale |
| | | Cumin | Cumimum cyminum |
| | | Fenugreek | Trigonella foenum-graecum |
| | 409 | Marshmallow | Althaea officinalis |
| | | Gotu kola | Centella asiatica |
| | | Stinging nettles | Urtica dioica |
| Pittaja | 403 | Ginger | Zingiber officinale |
| | | Cumin | Cumimum cyminum |
| | | Fenugreek | Trigonella foenum-graecum |
| | 409 | Marshmallow | Althaea officinalis |
| | | Gotu kola | Centella asiatica |
| | | Stinging nettles | Urtica dioica |
| Kaphaja | 403 | Ginger | Zingiber officinale |
| | | Cumin | Cumimum cyminum |
| | | Fenugreek | Trigonella foenum-graecum |
| | 409 | Marshmallow | Althaea officinalis |
| | | Gotu kola | Centella asiatica |
| | | Stinging nettles | Urtica dioica |

| Dosha | Low Dose | High Dose |
|---|---|---|
| Vata | 1 of each X2 per day before meals | 2 of each X2 per day before meals |
| Pitta | 1 of each X2 per day with meals | 2 of each X2 per day with meals |
| Kapha | 2 of each X2 per day after meals | 3 of each X2 per day after meals |

## Description:

This is a symptomatic treatment for a hiatus hernia to repair the damaged tissue. It is Kaphaja by structure and is usually caused by some wrong use of the body; although other causes may exist.

Use the Vataja herbs if Vata is predominant in the Vikriti (imbalance) with a Vata Vikriti diet / lifestyle.

Use the Pittaja herbs if Pitta is predominant in the Vikriti (imbalance) with a Pitta Vikriti diet / lifestyle.

Use the Kaphaja herbs if Kapha is predominant in the Vikriti (imbalance) with a Kapha Vikriti diet / lifestyle.

## High blood pressure

| Dosha | Code | Common Name | Latin Name |
|---|---|---|---|
| Vataja | 202 | Arjuna | Terminalia arjuna |
| | 203 | Ashwagandha | Withania somnifera |
| | 210 | Shankhpushpi | Convolvulus pluricaulis |
| | 401 | Cumin | Cumimum cyminum |
| | | Fennel | Foeniculum vulgare |
| | | Cardamom | Elettaria cardamomum |
| Pittaja | 202 | Arjuna | Terminalia arjuna |
| | 402 | Coriander | Coriandrum sativum |
| | | Cumin | Cumimum cyminum |
| | | Fennel | Foeniculum vulgare |
| | 405 | Burdock | Arctium lappa |
| | | Yellow dock | Rumex crispus |
| | | Milk Thistle | Silybum marianum |
| Kaphaja | 202 | Arjuna | Terminalia arjuna |
| | 403 | Ginger | Zingiber officinale |
| | | Cumin | Cumimum cyminum |
| | | Fenugreek | Trigonella foenum-graecum |
| | 405 | Burdock | Arctium lappa |
| | | Yellow dock | Rumex crispus |
| | | Milk Thistle | Silybum marianum |
| | 407 | Turmeric | Curcuma longa |
| | | Barberry | Berberis vulgaris |
| | | Dandelion | Taraxacum officinale |

| Dosha | Low Dose | High Dose |
|---|---|---|
| Vata | 1 of each X2 per day before meals | 2 of each X2 per day before meals |
| Pitta | 1 of each X2 per day with meals | 2 of each X2 per day with meals |
| Kapha | 2 of each X2 per day after meals | 3 of each X2 per day after meals |

## Description:

These herbal blends can be used for high blood pressure or hypertension. It is a problem of Raktavahasrota and is generally classified as a Pittaja condition by structure, although any Dosha can cause this problem functionally. These formulas are both clearing and tonic to Raktavahasrota and Rakta Dhatu. The Vata blend has an effect on Majja Dhatu and the nervous function related to blood circulation (Vyana Vayu). There is both a stimulating and calming action of this formula. It has an effect to remove Sama conditions from Raktavahasrota. This formula should be used for at least three months and not more than twelve months as needed.

Reducing stress and eating a simple diet are very important for these herbal blends to work effectively. Taking time for relaxation is important. Breathing methods to quiet the mind and body are strongly recommended.

Use the Vataja herbs if Vata is predominant in the Vikriti (imbalance) with a Vata Vikriti diet / lifestyle.

Use the Pittaja herbs if Pitta is predominant in the Vikriti (imbalance) with a Pitta Vikriti diet / lifestyle.

Use the Kaphaja herbs if Kapha is predominant in the Vikriti (imbalance) with a Kapha Vikriti diet / lifestyle.

# High blood sugar (hyperglycemia)

| Dosha | Code | Common Name | Latin Name |
|-------|------|-------------|------------|
| **Vataja** | 205 | Gokshura | Tribulus terrestris |
| | 208 | Manjishta | Rubia cordifolia |
| | 301 | Amalaki | Emblica officinalis |
| | | Bibhitaki | Terminalia belerica |
| | | Haritaki | Terminalia chebula |
| | 401 | Cumin | Cumimum cyminum |
| | | Fennel | Foeniculum vulgare |
| | | Cardamom | Elettaria cardamomum |
| **Pittaja** | 205 | Gokshura | Tribulus terrestris |
| | 208 | Manjishta | Rubia cordifolia |
| | 402 | Coriander | Coriandrum sativum |
| | | Cumin | Cumimum cyminum |
| | | Fennel | Foeniculum vulgare |
| | 407 | Turmeric | Curcuma longa |
| | | Barberry | Berberis vulgaris |
| | | Dandelion | Taraxacum officinale |
| **Kaphaja** | 205 | Gokshura | Tribulus terrestris |
| | 208 | Manjishta | Rubia cordifolia |
| | 403 | Ginger | Zingiber officinale |
| | | Cumin | Cumimum cyminum |
| | | Fenugreek | Trigonella foenum-graecum |
| | 407 | Turmeric | Curcuma longa |
| | | Barberry | Berberis vulgaris |
| | | Dandelion | Taraxacum officinale |

| Dosha | Low Dose | High Dose |
|-------|----------|-----------|
| **Vata** | 1 of each X2 per day before meals | 2 of each X2 per day before meals |
| **Pitta** | 1 of each X2 per day with meals | 2 of each X2 per day with meals |
| **Kapha** | 2 of each X2 per day after meals | 3 of each X2 per day after meals |

## Description:

High blood sugar (hyperglycemia) is a condition in which an excessive amount of glucose circulates in the blood plasma. Diabetes mellitus is by far the most common cause of chronic hyperglycemia, although many people suffer from mild forms. Diabetes treatments aim at maintaining blood sugar (glucose) at a level as close to normal as possible, to avoid serious long-term complications. Having high blood sugar levels for long periods of time (over months or years) can result in permanent damage to parts of the body such as the eyes, nerves, kidneys and blood vessels.

In Ayurveda hyperglycemia is considered to be a Kaphaja problem by structure and mainly a Kaphaja problem by function, although less common there are forms of Pittaja and Vataja high blood sugar. All three Doshas are involved in the hemostasis and negative feedback that maintain the correct glucose levels in the blood. As it is the Kapha gland, pancreas, that is carrying much of the burden, Kapha is always implicated. Ayurveda considers this disorder to be a problem of Ambhuvahasrota, or Udakavahasrota. This is a complex system and channels that metabolize liquid in the body. This Srota includes the pancreas, liver, kidneys, Rasa Dhatu, Rakta Dhatu and Meda Dhatu. The function of maintaining blood plasma glucose levels is done in Ambhuvahasrota by Kapha and Vata.

Use the Vataja herbs if Vata is predominant in the Vikriti (imbalance) with a Vata Vikriti diet / lifestyle.

Use the Pittaja herbs if Pitta is predominant in the Vikriti (imbalance) with a Pitta Vikriti diet / lifestyle.

Use the Kaphaja herbs if Kapha is predominant in the Vikriti (imbalance) with a Kapha Vikriti diet / lifestyle.

## High Kapha

| Dosha | Code | Common Name | Latin Name |
|---|---|---|---|
| Vataja | 0 | | |
| Pittaja | 0 | | |
| Kaphaja | 209<br>403<br><br><br>406 | Punarnava<br>Ginger<br>Cumin<br>Fenugreek<br>Myrrh<br>Elecampane<br>Yellow dock | Boerhaavia diffusa<br>Zingiber officinale<br>Cumimum cyminum<br>Trigonella foenum-graecum<br>Commiphora myrrha<br>Inula helenium<br>Rumex crispus |

| Dosha | Low Dose | High Dose |
|---|---|---|
| Kapha | 2 of each X2 per day after meals | 3 of each X2 per day after meals |

## Description:

High Kapha conditions are called Kapha Vriddhi. This is when Kapha increases and fills up its home (Mulasthana) and then then moves out into the outer pathway (Bahyamarga) and causes disorders. The following stages of Kapha Vriddhi can be seen as:

- Kapha Chaya begins to accumulate in the stomach resulting in lassitude, heaviness, indigestion and laziness.
- Kapha Prakopa causes loss of appetite, indigestion, nausea, increased salivation and disgust for food in general.
- Kapha Prasara causes cough, difficult breathing or gasping for air, swollen glands, low grade fever, vomiting, indigestion, exhaustion and mucus in the stools.

Use the Kaphaja herbs if Kapha is predominant in the Vikriti (imbalance) with a Kapha Vikriti diet / lifestyle.

(Please refer to *Ayurvedic Medicine for Westerners, Vol. 2, Pathology and Diagnosis in Ayurveda* for more information on Dosha pathology.)

## High Pitta

| Dosha | Code | Common Name | Latin Name |
|---|---|---|---|
| Vataja | 0 | | |
| Pittaja | 201 | Amalaki | Emblica officinalis |
| | 402 | Coriander | Coriandrum sativum |
| | | Cumin | Cumimum cyminum |
| | | Fennel | Foeniculum vulgare |
| | 405 | Burdock | Arctium lappa |
| | | Yellow dock | Rumex crispus |
| | | Milk Thistle | Silybum marianum |
| Kaphaja | 0 | | |

| Dosha | Low Dose | High Dose |
|---|---|---|
| Pitta | 1 of each X2 per day with meals | 2 of each X2 per day with meals |

### Description:

High Pitta conditions are called Pitta Vriddhi. This is when Pitta increases and fills up its home (Mulasthana) and then moves out into the outer pathway (Bahyamarga) and causes disorders. The following stages of Pitta Vriddhi can be seen as:

- Pitta Chaya begins to accumulate in the small intestine producing burning sensation, bitter taste in the mouth, yellow coloring of the skin and irritability.
- Pitta Prakopa causes increased acidity, acid regurgitation, burning pain in the abdomen and excessive thirst.
- Pitta Prasara causes inflammatory diseases, skin disorders, conjunctivitis, gingivitis, dizziness, headache, high fever, bilious vomiting, as well as diarrhea with burning sensation.

Use the Pittaja herbs if Pitta is predominant in the Vikriti (imbalance) with a Pitta Vikriti diet / lifestyle.

(Please refer to *Ayurvedic Medicine for Westerners, Vol. 2, Pathology and Diagnosis in Ayurveda* for more information on Dosha pathology.)

## High Vata

| Dosha | Code | Common Name | Latin Name |
|---|---|---|---|
| Vataja | 207 | Haritaki | Terminalia chebula |
| | 401 | Cumin | Cumimum cyminum |
| | | Fennel | Foeniculum vulgare |
| | | Cardamom | Elettaria cardamomum |
| | 404 | Angelica | Angelica archangelica |
| | | Wild yam | Dioscorea villosa |
| | | Valerian | Valeriana officinalis |
| Pittaja | 0 | | |
| Kaphaja | 0 | | |

| Dosha | Low Dose | High Dose |
|---|---|---|
| Vata | 1 of each X2 per day before meals | 2 of each X2 per day before meals |

### Description:

High Vata conditions are called Vata Vriddhi. This is when Vata increases and fills up its home (Mulasthana) and then then moves out into the outer pathway (Bahyamarga) and causes disorders. The following stages of Vata Vriddhi can be seen as:

- Vata Chaya begins to accumulate in the colon causing distention, gas, dry stools, fatigue and general dryness.
- Vata Prakopa causes further accumulation of gas with growling or rumbling, along with upper abdominal distention. Dryness in the colon now causes constipation.
- Vata Prasara causes dry skin, pain or stiffness of the joints, lower back pain, convulsions, spasm, headache, dry cough, intermittent fever, as well as continued abdominal pain with constipation and painful bowel movements and general fatigue.

Use the Vataja herbs if Vata is predominant in the Vikriti (imbalance) with a Vata Vikriti diet / lifestyle.

(Please refer to *Ayurvedic Medicine for Westerners, Vol. 2, Pathology and Diagnosis in Ayurveda* for more information on Dosha pathology.)

## HIV

| Dosha | Code | Common Name | Latin Name |
|-------|------|-------------|------------|
| Vataja | 203 | Ashwagandha | Withania somnifera |
|  | 206 | Guduchi | Tinospora cordifolia |
|  | 212 | Pau d'arco | Tabebuia impetiginosa |
|  | 301 | Amalaki | Emblica officinalis |
|  |  | Bibhitaki | Terminalia belerica |
|  |  | Haritaki | Terminalia chebula |
| Pittaja | 201 | Amalaki | Emblica officinalis |
|  | 206 | Guduchi | Tinospora cordifolia |
|  | 212 | Pau d'arco | Tabebuia impetiginosa |
|  | 301 | Amalaki | Emblica officinalis |
|  |  | Bibhitaki | Terminalia belerica |
|  |  | Haritaki | Terminalia chebula |
| Kaphaja | 206 | Guduchi | Tinospora cordifolia |
|  | 209 | Punarnava | Boerhaavia diffusa |
|  | 212 | Pau d'arco | Tabebuia impetiginosa |
|  | 301 | Amalaki | Emblica officinalis |
|  |  | Bibhitaki | Terminalia belerica |
|  |  | Haritaki | Terminalia chebula |

| Dosha | Low Dose | High Dose |
|-------|----------|-----------|
| Vata | 1 of each X2 per day before meals | 2 of each X2 per day before meals |
| Pitta | 1 of each X2 per day with meals | 2 of each X2 per day with meals |
| Kapha | 2 of each X2 per day after meals | 3 of each X2 per day after meals |

## Description:

These herbal blends can also be used as a starting point for building immunity and increasing nutrient absorption in the intestines. They build Ojas and Shukra Dhatu as well. Care needs to be given regarding Agni and Ama when using these herbal blends as they are heavy to digest. It is best to begin with low doses and work up to the higher doses over one month. These blends can be used when there is a small amount of Ama present on the tongue as there are enough digestive herbs to help remove Ama. Usually all Doshas are implicated in this pathology so it is advised to follow the Prakriti of the patient for diet and lifestyle. This formula is safe to use for several years, the minimum time for treatment would be three months.

If there is a high level of Ama showing up it is better to begin with formula to lower or remove Ama before beginning with this formula. This herbal blend can be used for a number of wasting disorders such as: AIDS, HIV positive, low Ojas, low immunity, Cachexia, chronic lung disorders, multiple sclerosis (MS), congestive heart failure, and tuberculosis (TB).

Use the Vataja herbs if Vata is predominant in the Prakriti with a Vata Prakriti diet / lifestyle.

Use the Pittaja herbs if Pitta is predominant in the Prakriti with a Pitta Prakriti diet / lifestyle.

Use the Kaphaja herbs if Kapha is predominant in the Prakriti with a Kapha Prakriti diet / lifestyle.

## Hodgkin's disease (Hodgkin's lymphoma)

| Dosha | Code | Common Name | Latin Name |
|-------|------|-------------|------------|
| Vataja | 203 | Ashwagandha | Withania somnifera |
| | 206 | Guduchi | Tinospora cordifolia |
| | 212 | Pau d'arco | Tabebuia impetiginosa |
| | 401 | Cumin | Cumimum cyminum |
| | | Fennel | Foeniculum vulgare |
| | | Cardamom | Elettaria cardamomum |
| Pittaja | 203 | Ashwagandha | Withania somnifera |
| | 206 | Guduchi | Tinospora cordifolia |
| | 212 | Pau d'arco | Tabebuia impetiginosa |
| | 402 | Coriander | Coriandrum sativum |
| | | Cumin | Cumimum cyminum |
| | | Fennel | Foeniculum vulgare |
| Kaphaja | 203 | Ashwagandha | Withania somnifera |
| | 206 | Guduchi | Tinospora cordifolia |
| | 212 | Pau d'arco | Tabebuia impetiginosa |
| | 403 | Ginger | Zingiber officinale |
| | | Cumin | Cumimum cyminum |
| | | Fenugreek | Trigonella foenum-graecum |

| Dosha | Low Dose | High Dose |
|-------|----------|-----------|
| Vata | 1 of each X2 per day before meals | 2 of each X2 per day before meals |
| Pitta | 1 of each X2 per day with meals | 2 of each X2 per day with meals |
| Kapha | 2 of each X2 per day after meals | 3 of each X2 per day after meals |

### Description:

Hodgkin disease is a type of lymphoma. Lymphoma is a cancer of the lymphatic system, which is part of the immune system. The first sign of Hodgkin disease is often an enlarged lymph node. The disease can spread to nearby lymph nodes. As with most cancers all Doshas tend to be implicated in Hodgkin's lymphoma.

The herbal blends, diet and lifestyle indicated here are not meant to cure Hodgkin's lymphoma. According to Ayurvedic logic they will support correct Dosha function and immunity. Cancer should be treated by qualified medical personal and these suggestions should be approved by the doctors overseeing the treatment.

*Remember that it is illegal to treat cancer. Do not try to treat cancer, instead work with the primary care doctors to support the patient with diet, lifestyle and to balance Dosha and Agni.*

Use the Vataja herbs if Vata is predominant in the Vikriti (imbalance) with a Vata Vikriti diet / lifestyle.

Use the Pittaja herbs if Pitta is predominant in the Vikriti (imbalance) with a Pitta Vikriti diet / lifestyle.

Use the Kaphaja herbs if Kapha is predominant in the Vikriti (imbalance) with a Kapha Vikriti diet / lifestyle.

## Hormonal deficiency (women)

| Dosha | Code | Common Name | Latin Name |
|---|---|---|---|
| **Vataja** | 401 | Cumin | Cumimum cyminum |
| | | Fennel | Foeniculum vulgare |
| | | Cardamom | Elettaria cardamomum |
| | 404 | Angelica | Angelica archangelica |
| | | Wild yam | Dioscorea villosa |
| | | Valerian | Valeriana officinalis |
| | 407 | Turmeric | Curcuma longa |
| | | Barberry | Berberis vulgaris |
| | | Dandelion | Taraxacum officinale |
| | 408 | Vitex | Vitex agnus-castus |
| | | Black cohosh | Cimicifuga racemosa |
| | | Cramp bark | Viburnum opulus |
| | 409 | Marshmallow | Althaea officinalis |
| | | Gotu kola | Centella asiatica |
| | | Stinging nettles | Urtica dioica |
| **Pittaja** | 402 | Coriander | Coriandrum sativum |
| | | Cumin | Cumimum cyminum |
| | | Fennel | Foeniculum vulgare |
| | 407 | Turmeric | Curcuma longa |
| | | Barberry | Berberis vulgaris |
| | | Dandelion | Taraxacum officinale |
| | 408 | Vitex | Vitex agnus-castus |
| | | Black cohosh | Cimicifuga racemosa |
| | | Cramp bark | Viburnum opulus |
| | 409 | Marshmallow | Althaea officinalis |
| | | Gotu kola | Centella asiatica |
| | | Stinging nettles | Urtica dioica |
| **Kaphaja** | 403 | Ginger | Zingiber officinale |
| | | Cumin | Cumimum cyminum |
| | | Fenugreek | Trigonella foenum-graecum |
| | 407 | Turmeric | Curcuma longa |
| | | Barberry | Berberis vulgaris |
| | | Dandelion | Taraxacum officinale |
| | 408 | Vitex | Vitex agnus-castus |
| | | Black cohosh | Cimicifuga racemosa |
| | | Cramp bark | Viburnum opulus |
| | 409 | Marshmallow | Althaea officinalis |
| | | Gotu kola | Centella asiatica |
| | | Stinging nettles | Urtica dioica |

| Dosha | Low Dose | High Dose |
|-------|----------|-----------|
| Vata | 1 of each X2 per day before meals | 2 of each X2 per day before meals |
| Pitta | 1 of each X2 per day with meals | 2 of each X2 per day with meals |
| Kapha | 2 of each X2 per day after meals | 3 of each X2 per day after meals |

## Description:

These herbal blends can be used as a general support for women of all ages after menstruation begins at adolescence. It can be used when no apparent pathology is present or when the patient desires to bring balance to endocrine function (i.e., cycle). These herbal blends are tonics for Majja Dhatu and Shukra Dhatu and can be used whenever there is an imbalance in these areas. The formula is also very useful to take after, or during, the use of birth control pills, HRT, ERT or any other hormone therapy to restore balance and correct function. This is a safe formula to use for teenagers once menstruation begins. This formula is useful because it also has a mild cleansing effect on the liver and digestive system; it removes Ama from these areas of the body. These blends should be used for at least three months and not more than twelve months. NOTE: For PMS and for perimenopause (pre-menopause) use the herbal blends under these headings.

All three Doshas have a role in endocrine function. Kapha controls the fabrication of hormones, their structure and growth hormones; Pitta controls their transformative functions and metabolic functions; Vata controls the cycles in time and the other two Doshas. Correct diagnosis is needed for results.

Use the Vataja herbs if Vata is predominant in the Vikriti (imbalance) with a Vata Vikriti diet / lifestyle.

Use the Pittaja herbs if Pitta is predominant in the Vikriti (imbalance) with a Pitta Vikriti diet / lifestyle.

Use the Kaphaja herbs if Kapha is predominant in the Vikriti (imbalance) with a Kapha Vikriti diet / lifestyle.

## Hormone related headaches

| Dosha | Code | Common Name | Latin Name |
|---|---|---|---|
| Vataja | 301 | Amalaki | Emblica officinalis |
| | | Bibhitaki | Terminalia belerica |
| | | Haritaki | Terminalia chebula |
| | 404 | Angelica | Angelica archangelica |
| | | Wild yam | Dioscorea villosa |
| | | Valerian | Valeriana officinalis |
| | 408 | Vitex | Vitex agnus-castus |
| | | Black cohosh | Cimicifuga racemosa |
| | | Cramp bark | Viburnum opulus |
| Pittaja | 208 | Manjishta | Rubia cordifolia |
| | 301 | Amalaki | Emblica officinalis |
| | | Bibhitaki | Terminalia belerica |
| | | Haritaki | Terminalia chebula |
| | 408 | Vitex | Vitex agnus-castus |
| | | Black cohosh | Cimicifuga racemosa |
| | | Cramp bark | Viburnum opulus |
| Kaphaja | 301 | Amalaki | Emblica officinalis |
| | | Bibhitaki | Terminalia belerica |
| | | Haritaki | Terminalia chebula |
| | 404 | Angelica | Angelica archangelica |
| | | Wild yam | Dioscorea villosa |
| | | Valerian | Valeriana officinalis |
| | 408 | Vitex | Vitex agnus-castus |
| | | Black cohosh | Cimicifuga racemosa |
| | | Cramp bark | Viburnum opulus |

| Dosha | Low Dose | High Dose |
|---|---|---|
| Vata | 1 of each X2 per day before meals | 2 of each X2 per day before meals |
| Pitta | 1 of each X2 per day with meals | 2 of each X2 per day with meals |
| Kapha | 2 of each X2 per day after meals | 3 of each X2 per day after meals |

## Description:

This herbal approach to headaches is based on hormonal disturbance of premenstrual origin. If it is the kind of headache that comes with the menstruation cycle it is endocrine based and linked to Vata functions. Any cyclic headache will tend to be endocrine based, thus under the control of Vata Dosha and Vataja in origin. The idea is that Pitta, which controls Rakta Dhatu, has become disturbed from Vata Vriddhi. Modifications in blood circulation due to hormones will cause headaches. This treatment first tries to balance Vata and then treats Pitta secondary. Pitta is the actual physical cause of the blood vessels becoming dilated and pressing on the nerves and causing pain. Therefore, this disorder is Pittaja by structure and Vataja by function.

These herbal blends will not help normal headaches, for those kinds of headaches due to the digestion or that are functional please see the herbs under the "Headaches" heading.

Use the Vataja herbs if Vata is predominant in the Vikriti (imbalance) with a Vata Vikriti diet / lifestyle.

Use the Pittaja herbs if Pitta is predominant in the Vikriti (imbalance) with a Pitta Vikriti diet / lifestyle.

Use the Kaphaja herbs if Kapha is predominant in the Vikriti (imbalance) with a Kapha Vikriti diet / lifestyle.

## Hot flashes

| Dosha | Code | Common Name | Latin Name |
|---|---|---|---|
| **Vataja** | 211 | Shatavari | Asparagus racemosus |
| | 401 | Cumin | Cumimum cyminum |
| | | Fennel | Foeniculum vulgare |
| | | Cardamom | Elettaria cardamomum |
| | 408 | Vitex | Vitex agnus-castus |
| | | Black cohosh | Cimicifuga racemosa |
| | | Cramp bark | Viburnum opulus |
| | 409 | Marshmallow | Althaea officinalis |
| | | Gotu kola | Centella asiatica |
| | | Stinging nettles | Urtica dioica |
| **Pittaja** | 211 | Shatavari | Asparagus racemosus |
| | 402 | Coriander | Coriandrum sativum |
| | | Cumin | Cumimum cyminum |
| | | Fennel | Foeniculum vulgare |
| | 408 | Vitex | Vitex agnus-castus |
| | | Black cohosh | Cimicifuga racemosa |
| | | Cramp bark | Viburnum opulus |
| | 409 | Marshmallow | Althaea officinalis |
| | | Gotu kola | Centella asiatica |
| | | Stinging nettles | Urtica dioica |
| **Kaphaja** | 403 | Ginger | Zingiber officinale |
| | | Cumin | Cumimum cyminum |
| | | Fenugreek | Trigonella foenum-graecum |
| | 408 | Vitex | Vitex agnus-castus |
| | | Black cohosh | Cimicifuga racemosa |
| | | Cramp bark | Viburnum opulus |
| | 409 | Marshmallow | Althaea officinalis |
| | | Gotu kola | Centella asiatica |
| | | Stinging nettles | Urtica dioica |

| Dosha | Low Dose | High Dose |
|---|---|---|
| **Vata** | 1 of each X2 per day before meals | 2 of each X2 per day before meals |
| **Pitta** | 1 of each X2 per day with meals | 2 of each X2 per day with meals |
| **Kapha** | 2 of each X2 per day after meals | 3 of each X2 per day after meals |

## Description:

These herbal blends can be used for perimenopause or menopause when there are either hot flashes or night sweating. These herbal blends work on supporting Shukra Dhatu, Majja Dhatu, Vata and

Pitta Doshas. These blends can be used long term by everyone for up to two years.

The pathology of this problem comes from Vata (Udana Vayu) moving Pitta (Pachaka) upwards into the Kapha zone. It happens most often with Pitta Prakriti and secondary with Vata Prakriti women. In my experience, it happens less often to pure Kapha type women, or when it does, it does not last long. It is best to follow the Prakriti of the patient for this problem as it a reflection of changing from the Pitta period of life to the Vata period of life, so the Udana Vayu is the primary cause and the main target of the treatment, with Pitta being a secondary target.

Use the Vataja herbs if Vata is predominant in the Prakriti (imbalance) with a Vata Prakriti diet / lifestyle.

Use the Pittaja herbs if Pitta is predominant in the Prakriti (imbalance) with a Pitta Prakriti diet / lifestyle.

Use the Kaphaja herbs if Kapha is predominant in the Prakriti (imbalance) with a Kapha Prakriti diet / lifestyle.

## Hyperacidity

| Dosha | Code | Common Name | Latin Name |
|---|---|---|---|
| Vataja | 201 | Amalaki | Emblica officinalis |
| | 210 | Shankhpushpi | Convolvulus pluricaulis |
| | 211 | Shatavari | Asparagus racemosus |
| Pittaja | 201 | Amalaki | Emblica officinalis |
| | 405 | Burdock | Arctium lappa |
| | | Yellow dock | Rumex crispus |
| | | Milk Thistle | Silybum marianum |
| Kaphaja | 201 | Amalaki | Emblica officinalis |
| | 406 | Myrrh | Commiphora myrrha |
| | | Elecampane | Inula helenium |
| | | Yellow dock | Rumex crispus |

| Dosha | Low Dose | High Dose |
|---|---|---|
| Vata | 1 of each X2 per day before meals | 2 of each X2 per day before meals |
| Pitta | 1 of each X2 per day with meals | 2 of each X2 per day with meals |
| Kapha | 2 of each X2 per day after meals | 3 of each X2 per day after meals |

## Description:

These herbal blends can be used whenever there are signs of high Pitta in the digestive area. These herbal blends treat hyperacidity, ulcers, inflammation of the mucus membrane and any other Pitta Vriddhi problem in the stomach, small intestine or colon. The herbs target the small intestine, but have an effect on all of the digestive system. It is also effective as a tonic for Rakta Dhatu. These herbal blends should be used for at least one month and not more than six months.

This is Pittaja problem by function and a Kaphaja problem by structure (mucus membranes are part of Rasa Dhatu). Therefore, it is more effective to give the herbs according to the imbalance or Vikriti. These herbal blends reduce Pitta in Rakta Dhatu and at the same time they heal or build mucus membrane and tissue in the digestive system. An anti-Pitta diet should be given to help these blends; also, avoiding red meat, fermented food, acidic food and all forms of alcohol. After the herbal blends have controlled the pathology diet is usually enough to manage the problem.

Use the Vataja herbs if Vata is predominant in the Vikriti (imbalance) with a Vata Vikriti diet / lifestyle.

Use the Pittaja herbs if Pitta is predominant in the Vikriti (imbalance) with a Pitta Vikriti diet / lifestyle.

Use the Kaphaja herbs if Kapha is predominant in the Vikriti (imbalance) with a Kapha Vikriti diet / lifestyle.

## Hyperglycemia

| Dosha | Code | Common Name | Latin Name |
|---|---|---|---|
| **Vataja** | 205 | Gokshura | Tribulus terrestris |
| | 210 | Shankhpushpi | Convolvulus pluricaulis |
| | 401 | Cumin | Cumimum cyminum |
| | | Fennel | Foeniculum vulgare |
| | | Cardamom | Elettaria cardamomum |
| | 407 | Turmeric | Curcuma longa |
| | | Barberry | Berberis vulgaris |
| | | Dandelion | Taraxacum officinale |
| **Pittaja** | 205 | Gokshura | Tribulus terrestris |
| | 208 | Manjishta | Rubia cordifolia |
| | 402 | Coriander | Coriandrum sativum |
| | | Cumin | Cumimum cyminum |
| | | Fennel | Foeniculum vulgare |
| | 407 | Turmeric | Curcuma longa |
| | | Barberry | Berberis vulgaris |
| | | Dandelion | Taraxacum officinale |
| **Kaphaja** | 205 | Gokshura | Tribulus terrestris |
| | 208 | Manjishta | Rubia cordifolia |
| | 403 | Ginger | Zingiber officinale |
| | | Cumin | Cumimum cyminum |
| | | Fenugreek | Trigonella foenum-graecum |
| | 407 | Turmeric | Curcuma longa |
| | | Barberry | Berberis vulgaris |
| | | Dandelion | Taraxacum officinale |

| Dosha | Low Dose | High Dose |
|---|---|---|
| **Vata** | 1 of each X2 per day before meals | 2 of each X2 per day before meals |
| **Pitta** | 1 of each X2 per day with meals | 2 of each X2 per day with meals |
| **Kapha** | 2 of each X2 per day after meals | 3 of each X2 per day after meals |

## Description:
See 'High Blood Sugar' description.

Use the Vataja herbs if Vata is predominant in the Vikriti (imbalance) with a Vata Vikriti diet / lifestyle.

Use the Pittaja herbs if Pitta is predominant in the Vikriti (imbalance) with a Pitta Vikriti diet / lifestyle.

Use the Kaphaja herbs if Kapha is predominant in the Vikriti (imbalance) with a Kapha Vikriti diet / lifestyle.

## Hypertension

| Dosha | Code | Common Name | Latin Name |
|---|---|---|---|
| **Vataja** | 202 | Arjuna | Terminalia arjuna |
| | 203 | Ashwagandha | Withania somnifera |
| | 210 | Shankhpushpi | Convolvulus pluricaulis |
| | 401 | Cumin | Cumimum cyminum |
| | | Fennel | Foeniculum vulgare |
| | | Cardamom | Elettaria cardamomum |
| **Pittaja** | 202 | Arjuna | Terminalia arjuna |
| | 402 | Coriander | Coriandrum sativum |
| | | Cumin | Cumimum cyminum |
| | | Fennel | Foeniculum vulgare |
| | 405 | Burdock | Arctium lappa |
| | | Yellow dock | Rumex crispus |
| | | Milk Thistle | Silybum marianum |
| **Kaphaja** | 202 | Arjuna | Terminalia arjuna |
| | 403 | Ginger | Zingiber officinale |
| | | Cumin | Cumimum cyminum |
| | | Fenugreek | Trigonella foenum-graecum |
| | 405 | Burdock | Arctium lappa |
| | | Yellow dock | Rumex crispus |
| | | Milk Thistle | Silybum marianum |
| | 407 | Turmeric | Curcuma longa |
| | | Barberry | Berberis vulgaris |
| | | Dandelion | Taraxacum officinale |

| Dosha | Low Dose | High Dose |
|---|---|---|
| **Vata** | 1 of each X2 per day before meals | 2 of each X2 per day before meals |
| **Pitta** | 1 of each X2 per day with meals | 2 of each X2 per day with meals |
| **Kapha** | 2 of each X2 per day after meals | 3 of each X2 per day after meals |

## Description:

These herbal blends can be used for high blood pressure or hypertension. It is a problem of Raktavahasrota and is generally classified as a Pitta Roga condition, although any Dosha can cause this problem functionally. These herbal blends are both clearing and tonic to Raktavahasrota. They have an effect on Majja Dhatu and the nervous function related to blood circulation. There is both a stimulating and calming action of these blends. They have an effect to remove Sama conditions from Raktavahasrota. These blends should be used for at least three months and not more than twelve months as needed. Ayurvedic therapies such as Pranayama, yoga, exercise and relaxation are indicated.

Do not use these blends with modern medications for high blood pressure. If the patient is already on medication it may be possible to use *Terminalia arjuna* (Arjuna), product number 202, at the lowest dose X2 per day after meals alone without any other herbs.

Use the Vataja herbs if Vata is predominant in the Vikriti (imbalance) with a Vata Vikriti diet / lifestyle.

Use the Pittaja herbs if Pitta is predominant in the Vikriti (imbalance) with a Pitta Vikriti diet / lifestyle.

Use the Kaphaja herbs if Kapha is predominant in the Vikriti (imbalance) with a Kapha Vikriti diet / lifestyle.

## Hypoglycemia

| Dosha | Code | Common Name | Latin Name |
|-------|------|-------------|------------|
| **Vataja** | 401 | Cumin | Cumimum cyminum |
| | | Fennel | Foeniculum vulgare |
| | | Cardamom | Elettaria cardamomum |
| | 404 | Angelica | Angelica archangelica |
| | | Wild yam | Dioscorea villosa |
| | | Valerian | Valeriana officinalis |
| | 407 | Turmeric | Curcuma longa |
| | | Barberry | Berberis vulgaris |
| | | Dandelion | Taraxacum officinale |
| **Pittaja** | 402 | Coriander | Coriandrum sativum |
| | | Cumin | Cumimum cyminum |
| | | Fennel | Foeniculum vulgare |
| | 405 | Burdock | Arctium lappa |
| | | Yellow dock | Rumex crispus |
| | | Milk Thistle | Silybum marianum |
| | 407 | Turmeric | Curcuma longa |
| | | Barberry | Berberis vulgaris |
| | | Dandelion | Taraxacum officinale |
| **Kaphaja** | 403 | Ginger | Zingiber officinale |
| | | Cumin | Cumimum cyminum |
| | | Fenugreek | Trigonella foenum-graecum |
| | 405 | Burdock | Arctium lappa |
| | | Yellow dock | Rumex crispus |
| | | Milk Thistle | Silybum marianum |
| | 407 | Turmeric | Curcuma longa |
| | | Barberry | Berberis vulgaris |
| | | Dandelion | Taraxacum officinale |

| Dosha | Low Dose | High Dose |
|-------|----------|-----------|
| **Vata** | 1 of each X2 per day before meals | 2 of each X2 per day before meals |
| **Pitta** | 1 of each X2 per day with meals | 2 of each X2 per day with meals |
| **Kapha** | 2 of each X2 per day after meals | 3 of each X2 per day after meals |

## Description:

Hypoglycemia, also called low blood glucose or low blood sugar, occurs when the level of glucose in your blood drops below normal. Hypoglycemia is commonly associated with the treatment of diabetes. However, a variety of conditions can cause low blood sugar in people without diabetes. Hypoglycemia isn't a disease itself it is an indication of an underlying disorder.

Hypo conditions are usually associated with Kapha Dosha in Ayurveda; however, hypoglycemia is actually a Vataja disorder by function. Hypoglycemia is considered to be a Kaphaja problem by structure. There are forms of Pittaja and Kaphaja low blood sugar functionally. All three Doshas are involved in the hemostasis and negative feedback that maintain the correct glucose levels in the blood. As it is the Kapha gland, pancreas, that is carrying much of the burden, Kapha is always implicated by structure. Ayurveda considers this disorder to be a problem of Ambhuvahasrota (also called Udakavahasrota). This is a complex system made up of channels that metabolize liquid in the body. This Srota includes the pancreas, liver, kidneys, Rasa Dhatu, Rakta Dhatu and Meda Dhatu. The function of maintaining blood plasma glucose levels is done in Ambhuvahasrota by Kapha and Vata Doshas. Pitta has a secondary role as the manager of Rakta Dhatu. The Mulasthana of Rakta Dhatu is the liver, thus it is an important part of blood regulation.

Use the Vataja herbs if Vata is predominant in the Vikriti (imbalance) with a Vata Vikriti diet / lifestyle.
Use the Pittaja herbs if Pitta is predominant in the Vikriti (imbalance) with a Pitta Vikriti diet / lifestyle.
Use the Kaphaja herbs if Kapha is predominant in the Vikriti (imbalance) with a Kapha Vikriti diet / lifestyle.

## Hysteria

| Dosha | Code | Common Name | Latin Name |
|---|---|---|---|
| **Vataja** | 204 | Bramhi | Bacopa monnieri |
| | 210 | Shankhpushpi | Convolvulus pluricaulis |
| | 401 | Cumin | Cumimum cyminum |
| | | Fennel | Foeniculum vulgare |
| | | Cardamom | Elettaria cardamomum |
| **Pittaja** | 204 | Bramhi | Bacopa monnieri |
| | 210 | Shankhpushpi | Convolvulus pluricaulis |
| | 402 | Coriander | Coriandrum sativum |
| | | Cumin | Cumimum cyminum |
| | | Fennel | Foeniculum vulgare |
| **Kaphaja** | 204 | Bramhi | Bacopa monnieri |
| | 210 | Shankhpushpi | Convolvulus pluricaulis |
| | 403 | Ginger | Zingiber officinale |
| | | Cumin | Cumimum cyminum |
| | | Fenugreek | Trigonella foenum-graecum |

| Dosha | Low Dose | High Dose |
|---|---|---|
| **Vata** | 1 of each X2 per day before meals | 2 of each X2 per day before meals |
| **Pitta** | 1 of each X2 per day with meals | 2 of each X2 per day with meals |
| **Kapha** | 2 of each X2 per day after meals | 3 of each X2 per day after meals |

### Description:

Hysteria is any exaggerated or uncontrollable emotion or excitement expressed. Although not used much in modern times hysteria was a common medical disorder in the past (perhaps we are all hysteric now so it seems normal?).

In Ayurveda hysteria is a Vata disorder and is Vataja by function and Kaphaja by structure (Majja Dhatu). It is a typical Vata Vriddhi condition and can be treated effectively by the use of Vata reducing lifestyle therapies.

Use the Vataja herbs if Vata is predominant in the Vikriti (imbalance) with a Vata Vikriti diet / lifestyle.

Use the Pittaja herbs if Pitta is predominant in the Vikriti (imbalance) with a Pitta Vikriti diet / lifestyle.

Use the Kaphaja herbs if Kapha is predominant in the Vikriti (imbalance) with a Kapha Vikriti diet / lifestyle.

## Impotence (Erectile Dysfunction, ED)

| Dosha | Code | Common Name | Latin Name |
|---|---|---|---|
| **Vataja** | 203 | Ashwagandha | Withania somnifera |
| | 205 | Gokshura | Tribulus terrestris |
| | 211 | Shatavari | Asparagus racemosus |
| | 403 | Ginger | Zingiber officinale |
| | | Cumin | Cumimum cyminum |
| | | Fenugreek | Trigonella foenum-graecum |
| **Pittaja** | 203 | Ashwagandha | Withania somnifera |
| | 205 | Gokshura | Tribulus terrestris |
| | 211 | Shatavari | Asparagus racemosus |
| | 301 | Amalaki | Emblica officinalis |
| | | Bibhitaki | Terminalia belerica |
| | | Haritaki | Terminalia chebula |
| **Kaphaja** | 203 | Ashwagandha | Withania somnifera |
| | 205 | Gokshura | Tribulus terrestris |
| | 211 | Shatavari | Asparagus racemosus |
| | 403 | Ginger | Zingiber officinale |
| | | Cumin | Cumimum cyminum |
| | | Fenugreek | Trigonella foenum-graecum |

| Dosha | Low Dose | High Dose |
|---|---|---|
| **Vata** | 1 of each X2 per day before meals | 2 of each X2 per day before meals |
| **Pitta** | 1 of each X2 per day with meals | 2 of each X2 per day with meals |
| **Kapha** | 2 of each X2 per day after meals | 3 of each X2 per day after meals |

## Description:

Erectile dysfunction or impotence is sexual dysfunction characterized by the inability to develop or maintain an erection of the penis during sexual activity. A penile erection is the hydraulic effect of blood entering and being retained in sponge-like bodies within the penis. The process is most often initiated as a result of sexual arousal, when signals are transmitted from the brain to nerves in the penis. The most important organic causes are cardiovascular disease, diabetes, neurological problems (for example, prostate surgery), hormonal insufficiencies and drug side effects. Research indicates that erectile dysfunction is common, and it is suggested that approximately 40% of males suffer from erectile dysfunction or impotence, at least occasionally.

This is basically a Vataja problem that is rooted in the polarity of

Apana and Prana Vayus. Overwork, anxiety and stress are factors that derange Prana Vayu and can cause this problem at any age. Psychological issues that disturb the mind will, with time, disrupt the function of Apana. Likewise, the over stimulation of Apana will disrupt the function of Prana Vayu. The treatment needs to focus on this polarity and offer solutions for both forms of Vata. Kapha and Pitta are both implicated by structure. Therefore, both Kapha (Shukra Dhatu) and Pitta (Rakta Dhatu) can be a causal factor in erectile dysfunction.

The different forms of ED can be seen as per Dosha:

Vataja – stress, anxiety, variable symptoms, low Ojas

Pittaja – stress, frustration, regular symptoms, low Ojas

Kaphaja – depression, exhaustion, regular symptoms, low Ojas

The treatment needs to include lifestyle therapies that work on the mind as well as the body. Often overwork is primary cause of ED and this issue needs to be addressed. Pranayama is an extremely important therapeutic tool to balance the functions of Vata. Diet is also very important. The removal of all stimulants such as coffee, alcohol, cannabis and other drugs is very important. Note that while cannabis is a short-term stimulant, it is a long-term suppressant of sexual function and so should be discontinued as part the treatment of erectile dysfunction.

Use the Vataja herbs if Vata is predominant in the Vikriti (imbalance) with a Vata Vikriti diet / lifestyle.

Use the Pittaja herbs if Pitta is predominant in the Vikriti (imbalance) with a Pitta Vikriti diet / lifestyle.

Use the Kaphaja herbs if Kapha is predominant in the Vikriti (imbalance) with a Kapha Vikriti diet / lifestyle.

## Incontinence (Urinary)

| Dosha | Code | Common Name | Latin Name |
|---|---|---|---|
| **Vataja** | 401 | Cumin | Cumimum cyminum |
| | | Fennel | Foeniculum vulgare |
| | | Cardamom | Elettaria cardamomum |
| | 407 | Turmeric | Curcuma longa |
| | | Barberry | Berberis vulgaris |
| | | Dandelion | Taraxacum officinale |
| | 409 | Marshmallow | Althaea officinalis |
| | | Gotu kola | Centella asiatica |
| | | Stinging nettles | Urtica dioica |
| **Pittaja** | 402 | Coriander | Coriandrum sativum |
| | | Cumin | Cumimum cyminum |
| | | Fennel | Foeniculum vulgare |
| | 407 | Turmeric | Curcuma longa |
| | | Barberry | Berberis vulgaris |
| | | Dandelion | Taraxacum officinale |
| | 409 | Marshmallow | Althaea officinalis |
| | | Gotu kola | Centella asiatica |
| | | Stinging nettles | Urtica dioica |
| **Kaphaja** | 403 | Ginger | Zingiber officinale |
| | | Cumin | Cumimum cyminum |
| | | Fenugreek | Trigonella foenum-graecum |
| | 407 | Turmeric | Curcuma longa |
| | | Barberry | Berberis vulgaris |
| | | Dandelion | Taraxacum officinale |
| | 409 | Marshmallow | Althaea officinalis |
| | | Gotu kola | Centella asiatica |
| | | Stinging nettles | Urtica dioica |

| Dosha | Low Dose | High Dose |
|---|---|---|
| **Vata** | 1 of each X2 per day before meals | 2 of each X2 per day before meals |
| **Pitta** | 1 of each X2 per day with meals | 2 of each X2 per day with meals |
| **Kapha** | 2 of each X2 per day after meals | 3 of each X2 per day after meals |

## Description:
Urinary incontinence, or the loss of bladder control, is a common and often embarrassing problem. The severity ranges from occasionally leaking urine when you cough or sneeze to having an urge to urinate suddenly. This is a Vataja problem functionally and is controlled by Apana Vayu. Structurally Kapha controls the urinary

bladder and kidneys as well as Mutravaha Srota. Thus, the causal Dosha needs to be identified in order for the treatment to cure the patient. Even if these blends are mainly symptomatic an adaptation of treatment as per causal Dosha will give better results.

These herbal blends work on both the function and structure and try to support the whole urinary system, not just the bladder. The purpose is to rejuvenate the structure and secondary to control Vata Dosha. Vata can be treated better through functional choices in life. This means lifestyle and dietary therapies are critically important for the success of the treatment. All forms of alcohol should be stopped as well as coffee and black or green tea.

Use the Vataja herbs if Vata is predominant in the Vikriti (imbalance) with a Vata Vikriti diet / lifestyle.

Use the Pittaja herbs if Pitta is predominant in the Vikriti (imbalance) with a Pitta Vikriti diet / lifestyle.

Use the Kaphaja herbs if Kapha is predominant in the Vikriti (imbalance) with a Kapha Vikriti diet / lifestyle.

## Indigestion (Dyspepsia)

| Dosha | Code | Common Name | Latin Name |
|---|---|---|---|
| **Vataja** | 207 | Haritaki | Terminalia chebula |
| | 401 | Cumin | Cumimum cyminum |
| | | Fennel | Foeniculum vulgare |
| | | Cardamom | Elettaria cardamomum |
| | 404 | Angelica | Angelica archangelica |
| | | Wild yam | Dioscorea villosa |
| | | Valerian | Valeriana officinalis |
| **Pittaja** | 201 | Amalaki | Emblica officinalis |
| | 402 | Coriander | Coriandrum sativum |
| | | Cumin | Cumimum cyminum |
| | | Fennel | Foeniculum vulgare |
| | 407 | Turmeric | Curcuma longa |
| | | Barberry | Berberis vulgaris |
| | | Dandelion | Taraxacum officinale |
| **Kaphaja** | 207 | Haritaki | Terminalia chebula |
| | 403 | Ginger | Zingiber officinale |
| | | Cumin | Cumimum cyminum |
| | | Fenugreek | Trigonella foenum-graecum |
| | 407 | Turmeric | Curcuma longa |
| | | Barberry | Berberis vulgaris |
| | | Dandelion | Taraxacum officinale |

| Dosha | Low Dose | High Dose |
|---|---|---|
| **Vata** | 1 of each X2 per day before meals | 2 of each X2 per day before meals |
| **Pitta** | 1 of each X2 per day with meals | 2 of each X2 per day with meals |
| **Kapha** | 2 of each X2 per day after meals | 3 of each X2 per day after meals |

## Description:

Indigestion (dyspepsia) is a general term for pain or discomfort felt in the stomach and abdomen. Indigestion is not a disease, but rather a set of symptoms experienced. All three Doshas have a role in digestion so any Dosha can cause this problem.

Use the Vataja herbs if Vata is predominant in the Vikriti (imbalance) with a Vata Vikriti diet / lifestyle.

Use the Pittaja herbs if Pitta is predominant in the Vikriti (imbalance) with a Pitta Vikriti diet / lifestyle.

Use the Kaphaja herbs if Kapha is predominant in the Vikriti (imbalance) with a Kapha Vikriti diet / lifestyle.

## Infection of urethra

| Dosha | Code | Common Name | Latin Name |
|---|---|---|---|
| Vataja | 205 | Gokshura | Tribulus terrestris |
| | 206 | Guduchi | Tinospora cordifolia |
| | 409 | Marshmallow | Althaea officinalis |
| | | Gotu kola | Centella asiatica |
| | | Stinging nettles | Urtica dioica |
| Pittaja | 205 | Gokshura | Tribulus terrestris |
| | 206 | Guduchi | Tinospora cordifolia |
| | 409 | Marshmallow | Althaea officinalis |
| | | Gotu kola | Centella asiatica |
| | | Stinging nettles | Urtica dioica |
| Kaphaja | 205 | Gokshura | Tribulus terrestris |
| | 206 | Guduchi | Tinospora cordifolia |
| | 409 | Marshmallow | Althaea officinalis |
| | | Gotu kola | Centella asiatica |
| | | Stinging nettles | Urtica dioica |

| Dosha | Low Dose | High Dose |
|---|---|---|
| Vata | 1 of each X2 per day before meals | 2 of each X2 per day before meals |
| Pitta | 1 of each X2 per day with meals | 2 of each X2 per day with meals |
| Kapha | 2 of each X2 per day after meals | 3 of each X2 per day after meals |

## Description:

This is a symptomatic treatment for the urethra. Infections are classified as Pitta Roga in Ayurveda. These blends reduce Pitta in Mutravaha Srota and strengthen the structure. Do not use these blends for longer than three weeks – it is important to find the cause of the problem and not to treat only the symptoms.

Use the Vataja herbs if Vata is predominant in the Vikriti (imbalance) with a Vata Vikriti diet / lifestyle.

Use the Pittaja herbs if Pitta is predominant in the Vikriti (imbalance) with a Pitta Vikriti diet / lifestyle.

Use the Kaphaja herbs if Kapha is predominant in the Vikriti (imbalance) with a Kapha Vikriti diet / lifestyle.

## Infertility (male)

| Dosha | Code | Common Name | Latin Name |
|---|---|---|---|
| Vataja | 203 | Ashwagandha | Withania somnifera |
| | 205 | Gokshura | Tribulus terrestris |
| | 211 | Shatavari | Asparagus racemosus |
| | 401 | Cumin | Cumimum cyminum |
| | | Fennel | Foeniculum vulgare |
| | | Cardamom | Elettaria cardamomum |
| Pittaja | 203 | Ashwagandha | Withania somnifera |
| | 205 | Gokshura | Tribulus terrestris |
| | 211 | Shatavari | Asparagus racemosus |
| | 402 | Coriander | Coriandrum sativum |
| | | Cumin | Cumimum cyminum |
| | | Fennel | Foeniculum vulgare |
| Kaphaja | 203 | Ashwagandha | Withania somnifera |
| | 205 | Gokshura | Tribulus terrestris |
| | 211 | Shatavari | Asparagus racemosus |
| | 403 | Ginger | Zingiber officinale |
| | | Cumin | Cumimum cyminum |
| | | Fenugreek | Trigonella foenum-graecum |

| Dosha | Low Dose | High Dose |
|---|---|---|
| Vata | 1 of each X2 per day before meals | 2 of each X2 per day before meals |
| Pitta | 1 of each X2 per day with meals | 2 of each X2 per day with meals |
| Kapha | 2 of each X2 per day after meals | 3 of each X2 per day after meals |

## Description:

Infertility has come to be defined as the inability to conceive within twelve months. This means that fifteen percent of couples attempting to conceive will not be able to do so in twelve months and are therefore classified as being infertile. There are two types of infertility:

- Primary infertility – where someone who has never conceived a child in the past has difficulty conceiving
- Secondary infertility – where a person has had one or more pregnancies in the past, but is having difficulty conceiving again

It is estimated that forty percent of infertility problems are due to problems with the man. Causes of male infertility are lifestyle habits such as smoking, poor dietary intake, sedentary habits, the use of illegal drugs and steroid medications. Stress and overwork can also be a factor in male infertility.

In Ayurveda, the reproductive system is controlled by Kapha, therefore all infertility issues will implicate Kapha Dosha and Shukra Dhatu. Functionally there is a number of causes as all three Doshas have a role in male ejaculation, even if Kapha controls the sperm production, Vata and Pitta are controlling the erection and ejaculation. Hence, any Dosha can cause this problem functionally.

These herbal blends, lifestyle and dietary therapies are for the treatment of Unexplained Infertility which account for twenty to twenty-five percent of infertility issues and strengthen Shukra Dhatu and sperm quality. Lifestyle and diet should be used to target the Dosha that is functionally causing the problem.

Use the Vataja herbs if Vata is predominant in the Vikriti (imbalance) with a Vata Vikriti diet / lifestyle.

Use the Pittaja herbs if Pitta is predominant in the Vikriti (imbalance) with a Pitta Vikriti diet / lifestyle.

Use the Kaphaja herbs if Kapha is predominant in the Vikriti (imbalance) with a Kapha Vikriti diet / lifestyle.

For a full discussion on fertility issues and other treatment options please refer to the textbook: *Ayurvedic Medicine for Westerners, Vol. 5, Application of Ayurvedic Treatments Throughout Life.*

# Infertility (female)

| Dosha | Code | Common Name | Latin Name |
|-------|------|-------------|------------|
| **Vataja** | 203 | Ashwagandha | Withania somnifera |
| | 211 | Shatavari | Asparagus racemosus |
| | 301 | Amalaki | Emblica officinalis |
| | | Bibhitaki | Terminalia belerica |
| | | Haritaki | Terminalia chebula |
| | 401 | Cumin | Cumimum cyminum |
| | | Fennel | Foeniculum vulgare |
| | | Cardamom | Elettaria cardamomum |
| | 408 | Vitex | Vitex agnus-castus |
| | | Black cohosh | Cimicifuga racemosa |
| | | Cramp bark | Viburnum opulus |
| **Pittaja** | 201 | Amalaki | Emblica officinalis |
| | 203 | Ashwagandha | Withania somnifera |
| | 211 | Shatavari | Asparagus racemosus |
| | 402 | Coriander | Coriandrum sativum |
| | | Cumin | Cumimum cyminum |
| | | Fennel | Foeniculum vulgare |
| | 408 | Vitex | Vitex agnus-castus |
| | | Black cohosh | Cimicifuga racemosa |
| | | Cramp bark | Viburnum opulus |
| **Kaphaja** | 203 | Ashwagandha | Withania somnifera |
| | 211 | Shatavari | Asparagus racemosus |
| | 301 | Amalaki | Emblica officinalis |
| | | Bibhitaki | Terminalia belerica |
| | | Haritaki | Terminalia chebula |
| | 403 | Ginger | Zingiber officinale |
| | | Cumin | Cumimum cyminum |
| | | Fenugreek | Trigonella foenum-graecum |
| | 408 | Vitex | Vitex agnus-castus |
| | | Black cohosh | Cimicifuga racemosa |
| | | Cramp bark | Viburnum opulus |

| Dosha | Low Dose | High Dose |
|-------|----------|-----------|
| **Vata** | 1 of each X2 per day before meals | 2 of each X2 per day before meals |
| **Pitta** | 1 of each X2 per day with meals | 2 of each X2 per day with meals |
| **Kapha** | 2 of each X2 per day after meals | 3 of each X2 per day after meals |

## Description:

Infertility has come to be defined as the inability to conceive within twelve months. This means that fifteen percent of couples attempting to conceive will not be able to do so in twelve months and are therefore classified as being infertile. There are two types of infertility:

- Primary infertility – where someone who has never conceived a child in the past has difficulty conceiving
- Secondary infertility – where a person has had one or more pregnancies in the past, but is having difficulty conceiving again

There are a number of causes of female infertility, often from other disorders of the reproductive system. The treatment protocols for these diseases should be followed first and the causal pathology removed. Once the pathology has been stopped then it is possible to treat fertility directly, not before. Examples of these disorders are:

- Endometriosis
- Polycystic Ovarian Syndrome (PCOS)
- Pelvic inflammatory disease (PID)
- Sexually transmitted infection (STI)
- Uterine fibroids

Infertility in women is also linked to age. The biggest decrease in fertility begins during the mid-thirties. Among women who are thirty-five years old, ninety-five percent will get pregnant after three years of having regular unprotected sex. For women who are thirty-eight, only seventy-five percent will get pregnant after three years of having regular unprotected sex.

In Ayurveda, the reproductive system is controlled by Kapha, therefore all infertility issues will implicate Kapha Dosha and Shukra Dhatu. Functionally there is a number of causes as all three Doshas have a role in the female reproductive system. Kapha controls the ovum production; Pitta controls the uterus and environment that receives the ovum and sperm; and Vata controls both Kapha and Pitta through regulating endocrine functions. Hence, any Dosha can cause this problem functionally.

These herbal blends, lifestyle and dietary therapies are for the treatment of Unexplained Infertility which account for twenty to twenty-five percent of infertility issues and strengthen Shukra Dhatu and ovum quality. Lifestyle and diet should be used to target the Dosha that is functionally causing the problem.

Use the Vataja herbs if Vata is predominant in the Vikriti (imbalance) with a Vata Vikriti diet / lifestyle.

Use the Pittaja herbs if Pitta is predominant in the Vikriti (imbalance) with a Pitta Vikriti diet / lifestyle.

Use the Kaphaja herbs if Kapha is predominant in the Vikriti (imbalance) with a Kapha Vikriti diet / lifestyle.

For a full discussion on fertility issues and other treatment options please refer to the textbook: *Ayurvedic Medicine for Westerners, Vol. 5, Application of Ayurvedic Treatments Throughout Life*.

## Inflammation (intestines)

| Dosha | Code | Common Name | Latin Name |
|---|---|---|---|
| **Vataja** | 201 | Amalaki | Emblica officinalis |
| | 206 | Guduchi | Tinospora cordifolia |
| | 407 | Turmeric | Curcuma longa |
| | | Barberry | Berberis vulgaris |
| | | Dandelion | Taraxacum officinale |
| **Pittaja** | 201 | Amalaki | Emblica officinalis |
| | 206 | Guduchi | Tinospora cordifolia |
| | 407 | Turmeric | Curcuma longa |
| | | Barberry | Berberis vulgaris |
| | | Dandelion | Taraxacum officinale |
| **Kaphaja** | 201 | Amalaki | Emblica officinalis |
| | 206 | Guduchi | Tinospora cordifolia |
| | 407 | Turmeric | Curcuma longa |
| | | Barberry | Berberis vulgaris |
| | | Dandelion | Taraxacum officinale |

| Dosha | Low Dose | High Dose |
|---|---|---|
| **Vata** | 1 of each X2 per day before meals | 2 of each X2 per day before meals |
| **Pitta** | 1 of each X2 per day with meals | 2 of each X2 per day with meals |
| **Kapha** | 2 of each X2 per day after meals | 3 of each X2 per day after meals |

## Description:

This is a symptomatic treatment for inflammation in the gastrointestinal tract (GI). Inflammation are classified as Pitta Roga in Ayurveda. These blends reduce Pitta in Annavaha Srota and strengthen the structure of the GI tract. Do not use these blends for longer than three weeks – it is important to find the cause of the problem and not to treat only the symptoms.

Use the Vataja herbs if Vata is predominant in the Vikriti (imbalance) with a Vata Vikriti diet / lifestyle.

Use the Pittaja herbs if Pitta is predominant in the Vikriti (imbalance) with a Pitta Vikriti diet / lifestyle.

Use the Kaphaja herbs if Kapha is predominant in the Vikriti (imbalance) with a Kapha Vikriti diet / lifestyle.

# Inflammation (prostrate)

| Dosha | Code | Common Name | Latin Name |
|---|---|---|---|
| **Vataja** | 205 | Gokshura | Tribulus terrestris |
| | 401 | Cumin | Cumimum cyminum |
| | | Fennel | Foeniculum vulgare |
| | | Cardamom | Elettaria cardamomum |
| | 407 | Turmeric | Curcuma longa |
| | | Barberry | Berberis vulgaris |
| | | Dandelion | Taraxacum officinale |
| | 409 | Marshmallow | Althaea officinalis |
| | | Gotu kola | Centella asiatica |
| | | Stinging nettles | Urtica dioica |
| **Pittaja** | 205 | Gokshura | Tribulus terrestris |
| | 402 | Coriander | Coriandrum sativum |
| | | Cumin | Cumimum cyminum |
| | | Fennel | Foeniculum vulgare |
| | 405 | Burdock | Arctium lappa |
| | | Yellow dock | Rumex crispus |
| | | Milk Thistle | Silybum marianum |
| | 407 | Turmeric | Curcuma longa |
| | | Barberry | Berberis vulgaris |
| | | Dandelion | Taraxacum officinale |
| | 409 | Marshmallow | Althaea officinalis |
| | | Gotu kola | Centella asiatica |
| | | Stinging nettles | Urtica dioica |
| **Kaphaja** | 205 | Gokshura | Tribulus terrestris |
| | 403 | Ginger | Zingiber officinale |
| | | Cumin | Cumimum cyminum |
| | | Fenugreek | Trigonella foenum-graecum |
| | 406 | Myrrh | Commiphora myrrha |
| | | Elecampane | Inula helenium |
| | | Yellow dock | Rumex crispus |
| | 407 | Turmeric | Curcuma longa |
| | | Barberry | Berberis vulgaris |
| | | Dandelion | Taraxacum officinale |
| | 409 | Marshmallow | Althaea officinalis |
| | | Gotu kola | Centella asiatica |
| | | Stinging nettles | Urtica dioica |

| Dosha | Low Dose | High Dose |
|-------|----------|-----------|
| Vata | 1 of each X2 per day before meals | 2 of each X2 per day before meals |
| Pitta | 1 of each X2 per day with meals | 2 of each X2 per day with meals |
| Kapha | 2 of each X2 per day after meals | 3 of each X2 per day after meals |

## Description:
See the description under Prostate disorders.

Use the Vataja herbs if Vata is predominant in the Vikriti (imbalance) with a Vata Vikriti diet / lifestyle.

Use the Pittaja herbs if Pitta is predominant in the Vikriti (imbalance) with a Pitta Vikriti diet / lifestyle.

Use the Kaphaja herbs if Kapha is predominant in the Vikriti (imbalance) with a Kapha Vikriti diet / lifestyle.

# Inflammation (skin)

| Dosha | Code | Common Name | Latin Name |
|---|---|---|---|
| **Vataja** | 401 | Cumin | Cumimum cyminum |
| | | Fennel | Foeniculum vulgare |
| | | Cardamom | Elettaria cardamomum |
| | 405 | Burdock | Arctium lappa |
| | | Yellow dock | Rumex crispus |
| | | Milk Thistle | Silybum marianum |
| | 407 | Turmeric | Curcuma longa |
| | | Barberry | Berberis vulgaris |
| | | Dandelion | Taraxacum officinale |
| | 409 | Marshmallow | Althaea officinalis |
| | | Gotu kola | Centella asiatica |
| | | Stinging nettles | Urtica dioica |
| **Pittaja** | 402 | Coriander | Coriandrum sativum |
| | | Cumin | Cumimum cyminum |
| | | Fennel | Foeniculum vulgare |
| | 405 | Burdock | Arctium lappa |
| | | Yellow dock | Rumex crispus |
| | | Milk Thistle | Silybum marianum |
| | 407 | Turmeric | Curcuma longa |
| | | Barberry | Berberis vulgaris |
| | | Dandelion | Taraxacum officinale |
| | 409 | Marshmallow | Althaea officinalis |
| | | Gotu kola | Centella asiatica |
| | | Stinging nettles | Urtica dioica |
| **Kaphaja** | 403 | Ginger | Zingiber officinale |
| | | Cumin | Cumimum cyminum |
| | | Fenugreek | Trigonella foenum-graecum |
| | 405 | Burdock | Arctium lappa |
| | | Yellow dock | Rumex crispus |
| | | Milk Thistle | Silybum marianum |
| | 407 | Turmeric | Curcuma longa |
| | | Barberry | Berberis vulgaris |
| | | Dandelion | Taraxacum officinale |
| | 409 | Marshmallow | Althaea officinalis |
| | | Gotu kola | Centella asiatica |
| | | Stinging nettles | Urtica dioica |

| Dosha | Low Dose | High Dose |
|-------|----------|-----------|
| Vata | 1 of each X2 per day before meals | 2 of each X2 per day before meals |
| Pitta | 1 of each X2 per day with meals | 2 of each X2 per day with meals |
| Kapha | 2 of each X2 per day after meals | 3 of each X2 per day after meals |

## Description:

These herbal blends can be used when Pitta invades Rasa Dhatu and causes the typical symptomology of Pitta; inflammation, burning, heat, redness, etc., on the skin. These are specific blends to use according to this Pitta Roga condition. There is a slight effect on reducing Ama. If there is a high level of Ama showing up in diagnosis it is better to use the 'Ama' blends to lower Ama and stop the cause of Ama formation. This is usually better to do before the treatment of inflammation in the skin. Duration of use should be limited to three weeks for Vata Prakriti; eight weeks for Pitta Prakriti; and four weeks for Kapha Prakriti.

Any Dosha can cause this pathology by increasing Pitta Dosha. As the main goal of these blends is to control Pitta lifestyle and diet should be used to reduce the causal Dosha. Diet alone is very important in the treatment of this disorder. A vegan diet would be the best if possible for the patient. Diet should follow Pitta Vikriti (no sour, acid, fermented, etc., foods) for the patient during the duration of the treatment, and then diet should go back to the Prakriti of the patient after the disorder is controlled.

Use the Vataja herbs if Vata is predominant in the Vikriti (imbalance) with a Vata Vikriti diet / lifestyle.

Use the Pittaja herbs if Pitta is predominant in the Vikriti (imbalance) with a Pitta Vikriti diet / lifestyle.

Use the Kaphaja herbs if Kapha is predominant in the Vikriti (imbalance) with a Kapha Vikriti diet / lifestyle.

## Inflammation (urinary system)

| Dosha | Code | Common Name | Latin Name |
|---|---|---|---|
| **Vataja** | 205 | Gokshura | Tribulus terrestris |
| | 402 | Coriander | Coriandrum sativum |
| | | Cumin | Cumimum cyminum |
| | | Fennel | Foeniculum vulgare |
| | 405 | Burdock | Arctium lappa |
| | | Yellow dock | Rumex crispus |
| | | Milk Thistle | Silybum marianum |
| | 409 | Marshmallow | Althaea officinalis |
| | | Gotu kola | Centella asiatica |
| | | Stinging nettles | Urtica dioica |
| **Pittaja** | 205 | Gokshura | Tribulus terrestris |
| | 402 | Coriander | Coriandrum sativum |
| | | Cumin | Cumimum cyminum |
| | | Fennel | Foeniculum vulgare |
| | 405 | Burdock | Arctium lappa |
| | | Yellow dock | Rumex crispus |
| | | Milk Thistle | Silybum marianum |
| | 409 | Marshmallow | Althaea officinalis |
| | | Gotu kola | Centella asiatica |
| | | Stinging nettles | Urtica dioica |
| **Kaphaja** | 205 | Gokshura | Tribulus terrestris |
| | 209 | Punarnava | Boerhaavia diffusa |
| | 402 | Coriander | Coriandrum sativum |
| | | Cumin | Cumimum cyminum |
| | | Fennel | Foeniculum vulgare |
| | 405 | Burdock | Arctium lappa |
| | | Yellow dock | Rumex crispus |
| | | Milk Thistle | Silybum marianum |

| Dosha | Low Dose | High Dose |
|---|---|---|
| **Vata** | 1 of each X2 per day before meals | 2 of each X2 per day before meals |
| **Pitta** | 1 of each X2 per day with meals | 2 of each X2 per day with meals |
| **Kapha** | 2 of each X2 per day after meals | 3 of each X2 per day after meals |

## Description:

These herbal blends can be used as an anti-inflammatory for the whole urinary system including urethra, bladder and kidneys (Mutravaha Srota). Very often inflammation is caused from an imbalance in the colon or an excessive amount of Ama in the colon.

Either one will create a bacterial imbalance in the flora that will affect the bladder by proximity. Other causes are poor hygiene, excessive sex, not drinking enough liquids or drinking too much alcohol. For women, vaginal flora should also be monitored. This is a classic Pitta Roga problem that often plagues Pitta Prakriti people.

Functionally any Dosha can cause this problem as the Dosha disrupts the function of Agni and then Ama is created. The main cause of urinary tract inflammation is Ama according to Ayurveda. Structurally the whole urinary system is under the control of Kapha Dosha. Thus, we often see Kapha implicated in the disorders of this system.

Use the Vataja herbs if Vata is predominant in the Vikriti (imbalance) with a Vata Vikriti diet / lifestyle.

Use the Pittaja herbs if Pitta is predominant in the Vikriti (imbalance) with a Pitta Vikriti diet / lifestyle.

Use the Kaphaja herbs if Kapha is predominant in the Vikriti (imbalance) with a Kapha Vikriti diet / lifestyle.

## Insomnia

| Dosha | Code | Common Name | Latin Name |
|-------|------|-------------|------------|
| Vataja | 210 | Shankhpushpi | Convolvulus pluricaulis |
| | 401 | Cumin | Cumimum cyminum |
| | | Fennel | Foeniculum vulgare |
| | | Cardamom | Elettaria cardamomum |
| | 410 | Passion flower | Passiflora incarnata |
| | | Skullcap | Scutellaria lateriflora |
| | | Gotu kola | Centella asiatica |
| Pittaja | 210 | Shankhpushpi | Convolvulus pluricaulis |
| | 402 | Coriander | Coriandrum sativum |
| | | Cumin | Cumimum cyminum |
| | | Fennel | Foeniculum vulgare |
| | 410 | Passion flower | Passiflora incarnata |
| | | Skullcap | Scutellaria lateriflora |
| | | Gotu kola | Centella asiatica |
| Kaphaja | 210 | Shankhpushpi | Convolvulus pluricaulis |
| | 403 | Ginger | Zingiber officinale |
| | | Cumin | Cumimum cyminum |
| | | Fenugreek | Trigonella foenum-graecum |
| | 410 | Passion flower | Passiflora incarnata |
| | | Skullcap | Scutellaria lateriflora |
| | | Gotu kola | Centella asiatica |

| Dosha | Low Dose | High Dose |
|-------|----------|-----------|
| Vata | 1 of each X2 per day before meals | 2 of each X2 per day before meals |
| Pitta | 1 of each X2 per day with meals | 2 of each X2 per day with meals |
| Kapha | 2 of each X2 per day after meals | 3 of each X2 per day after meals |

## Description:

Insomnia is a symptom of a sleeping disorder characterized by persistent difficulty falling asleep or staying awake despite the opportunity to sleep. Insomnia is a symptom, not a stand-alone diagnosis or a disease. By definition, insomnia is 'difficulty initiating or maintaining sleep or both' and it may be due to inadequate quality or quantity of sleep. It is typically followed by functional impairment while awake. Insomniacs have been known to complain about being unable to close their eyes or 'rest their mind' for more than a few minutes at a time. Both organic and non-organic insomnia constitute a sleep disorder. An estimated 50 to 70 million Americans suffer from insomnia on a regular basis each year. Insomnia occurs 1.4 times more commonly in women than in men.

These herbal blends can be used for all forms of insomnia and work to control the movement of Vata Dosha in Majjavaha Srota. This disorder can be classified as Vata Roga by function as Vata is using Majjavaha Srota. As Kapha Dosha controls the structure it is common to find some form of Kapha disorder in insomnia; usually an insufficient amount. It typically takes 10 to 14 days for these blends to reach their full effect. The herbs are Sattvic to balance the psychological functioning of the mind and are safe to take for long periods of time up to twelve months.

Lifestyle changes need to be made in order for the herbal blends to work. Daily Abhyanga is considered a good support to this treatment; use Vata reducing oils in this case to help develop the correct movement of Vata. Ayurvedic therapies such as Nadishodhana Pranayama, mantra, yoga asana, mild exercise and relaxation are indicated. Diet should follow the Prakriti of the patient.

Use the Vataja herbs if Vata is predominant in the Prakriti with a Vata Prakriti diet / lifestyle.

Use the Pittaja herbs if Pitta is predominant in the Prakriti with a Pitta Prakriti diet / lifestyle.

Use the Kaphaja herbs if Kapha is predominant in the Prakriti with a Kapha Prakriti diet / lifestyle.

## Irregular menstruation

| Dosha | Code | Common Name | Latin Name |
|---|---|---|---|
| Vataja | 211 | Shatavari | Asparagus racemosus |
| | 403 | Ginger | Zingiber officinale |
| | | Cumin | Cumimum cyminum |
| | | Fenugreek | Trigonella foenum-graecum |
| | 404 | Angelica | Angelica archangelica |
| | | Wild yam | Dioscorea villosa |
| | | Valerian | Valeriana officinalis |
| | 408 | Vitex | Vitex agnus-castus |
| | | Black cohosh | Cimicifuga racemosa |
| | | Cramp bark | Viburnum opulus |
| Pittaja | 211 | Shatavari | Asparagus racemosus |
| | 402 | Coriander | Coriandrum sativum |
| | | Cumin | Cumimum cyminum |
| | | Fennel | Foeniculum vulgare |
| | 405 | Burdock | Arctium lappa |
| | | Yellow dock | Rumex crispus |
| | | Milk Thistle | Silybum marianum |
| | 408 | Vitex | Vitex agnus-castus |
| | | Black cohosh | Cimicifuga racemosa |
| | | Cramp bark | Viburnum opulus |
| Kaphaja | 211 | Shatavari | Asparagus racemosus |
| | 403 | Ginger | Zingiber officinale |
| | | Cumin | Cumimum cyminum |
| | | Fenugreek | Trigonella foenum-graecum |
| | 404 | Angelica | Angelica archangelica |
| | | Wild yam | Dioscorea villosa |
| | | Valerian | Valeriana officinalis |
| | 408 | Vitex | Vitex agnus-castus |
| | | Black cohosh | Cimicifuga racemosa |
| | | Cramp bark | Viburnum opulus |

| Dosha | Low Dose | High Dose |
|---|---|---|
| Vata | 1 of each X2 per day before meals | 2 of each X2 per day before meals |
| Pitta | 1 of each X2 per day with meals | 2 of each X2 per day with meals |
| Kapha | 2 of each X2 per day after meals | 3 of each X2 per day after meals |

## Description:

Irregular menstruation symptoms are Vata Roga as Apana Vayu controls the release of menstruation and Prana Vayu controls endocrine function generally. As menstruation fluid is an Upadhatu of Rasa Dhatu and Kapha, and the uterus / vagina are under the control of Pitta and Rakta Dhatu, any Dosha can cause menstruation irregularities functionally.

Remember the following points about menstruation (Artava):

- Kapha controls the fluid through Rasa Dhatu (Upadhatu)
- Kapha controls the growth hormones through Shukra Dhatu
- Pitta controls the uterus and gives color to the fluid through Rakta Dhatu
- Pitta controls hormone levels in the blood through liver function & Rakta Dhatu
- Vata controls all cycles in time & endocrine function through Prana Vayu
- Vata controls the release of menstrual fluid through Apana Vayu
- Vata controls non-growth hormones in general through different polarities of Prana / Apana, Samana / Vyana and Udana / Apana
- Vata controls both Kapha and Pitta

All three Doshas need to be evaluated. A history should be written down to assess the root cause and which Dosha was disturbed first. What, where, how long, when in the cycle and the resulting feeling or symptom that comes with disruption should be noted down. It is important to write this down chronologically and get clear on the overall situation of the cycle as it will help to establish a therapeutic goal and treatment approach. Remember, even a slight discomfort or mood swing is indicative of Dosha imbalance in Ayurveda and should be remedied as soon as possible, especially for young women.

Use the Vataja herbs if Vata is predominant in the Vikriti (imbalance) with a Vata Vikriti diet / lifestyle.

Use the Pittaja herbs if Pitta is predominant in the Vikriti (imbalance) with a Pitta Vikriti diet / lifestyle.

Use the Kaphaja herbs if Kapha is predominant in the Vikriti (imbalance) with a Kapha Vikriti diet / lifestyle.

# Irritable bowel syndrome (IBS)

| Dosha | Code | Common Name | Latin Name |
|---|---|---|---|
| Vataja | 401 | Cumin | Cumimum cyminum |
| | | Fennel | Foeniculum vulgare |
| | | Cardamom | Elettaria cardamomum |
| | 404 | Angelica | Angelica archangelica |
| | | Wild yam | Dioscorea villosa |
| | | Valerian | Valeriana officinalis |
| | 407 | Turmeric | Curcuma longa |
| | | Barberry | Berberis vulgaris |
| | | Dandelion | Taraxacum officinale |
| | 409 | Marshmallow | Althaea officinalis |
| | | Gotu kola | Centella asiatica |
| | | Stinging nettles | Urtica dioica |
| Pittaja | 402 | Coriander | Coriandrum sativum |
| | | Cumin | Cumimum cyminum |
| | | Fennel | Foeniculum vulgare |
| | 404 | Angelica | Angelica archangelica |
| | | Wild yam | Dioscorea villosa |
| | | Valerian | Valeriana officinalis |
| | 407 | Turmeric | Curcuma longa |
| | | Barberry | Berberis vulgaris |
| | | Dandelion | Taraxacum officinale |
| | 409 | Marshmallow | Althaea officinalis |
| | | Gotu kola | Centella asiatica |
| | | Stinging nettles | Urtica dioica |
| Kaphaja | 403 | Ginger | Zingiber officinale |
| | | Cumin | Cumimum cyminum |
| | | Fenugreek | Trigonella foenum-graecum |
| | 404 | Angelica | Angelica archangelica |
| | | Wild yam | Dioscorea villosa |
| | | Valerian | Valeriana officinalis |
| | 407 | Turmeric | Curcuma longa |
| | | Barberry | Berberis vulgaris |
| | | Dandelion | Taraxacum officinale |

| Dosha | Low Dose | High Dose |
|---|---|---|
| Vata | 1 of each X2 per day before meals | 2 of each X2 per day before meals |
| Pitta | 1 of each X2 per day with meals | 2 of each X2 per day with meals |
| Kapha | 2 of each X2 per day after meals | 3 of each X2 per day after meals |

## Description:

These herbal blends can be used to remove Ama from the gastrointestinal tract. It is anti-inflammatory and will heal any wounds to the mucus membrane. According to Ayurveda IBS (Irritable Bowel Syndrome) diverticulitis, colitis and other painful digestive problems that are due to lesions or infections to the mucus membranes in the digestive system are caused by Ama. These blends remove Ama, reduce infection, stop pain and inflammation. It is advised to use These blends for at least three months for the best effect. Normally it takes six to twelve months to cure a chronic problem. These blends will give the patient fairly fast relief – in about five to seven days they should experience a reduction in symptoms in most cases.

The diet should be changed to an anti-Ama diet appropriate for the Prakriti of the person. If possible coffee, carbonated drinks, alcohol, sugar and red meat should be removed from the diet. A vegetarian diet would be best.

Use the Vataja herbs if Vata is predominant in the Vikriti (imbalance) with a Vata Prakriti diet / lifestyle.

Use the Pittaja herbs if Pitta is predominant in the Vikriti (imbalance) with a Pitta Prakriti diet / lifestyle.

Use the Kaphaja herbs if Kapha is predominant in the Vikriti (imbalance) with a Kapha Prakriti diet / lifestyle.

## Kidney disorders

| Dosha | Code | Common Name | Latin Name |
|---|---|---|---|
| Vataja | 205 | Gokshura | Tribulus terrestris |
| | 401 | Cumin | Cumimum cyminum |
| | | Fennel | Foeniculum vulgare |
| | | Cardamom | Elettaria cardamomum |
| | 407 | Turmeric | Curcuma longa |
| | | Barberry | Berberis vulgaris |
| | | Dandelion | Taraxacum officinale |
| | 409 | Marshmallow | Althaea officinalis |
| | | Gotu kola | Centella asiatica |
| | | Stinging nettles | Urtica dioica |
| Pittaja | 205 | Gokshura | Tribulus terrestris |
| | 208 | Manjishta | Rubia cordifolia |
| | 402 | Coriander | Coriandrum sativum |
| | | Cumin | Cumimum cyminum |
| | | Fennel | Foeniculum vulgare |
| | 407 | Turmeric | Curcuma longa |
| | | Barberry | Berberis vulgaris |
| | | Dandelion | Taraxacum officinale |
| | 409 | Marshmallow | Althaea officinalis |
| | | Gotu kola | Centella asiatica |
| | | Stinging nettles | Urtica dioica |
| Kaphaja | 205 | Gokshura | Tribulus terrestris |
| | 208 | Manjishta | Rubia cordifolia |
| | 403 | Ginger | Zingiber officinale |
| | | Cumin | Cumimum cyminum |
| | | Fenugreek | Trigonella foenum-graecum |
| | 407 | Turmeric | Curcuma longa |
| | | Barberry | Berberis vulgaris |
| | | Dandelion | Taraxacum officinale |
| | 409 | Marshmallow | Althaea officinalis |
| | | Gotu kola | Centella asiatica |
| | | Stinging nettles | Urtica dioica |

| Dosha | Low Dose | High Dose |
|---|---|---|
| Vata | 1 of each X2 per day before meals | 2 of each X2 per day before meals |
| Pitta | 1 of each X2 per day with meals | 2 of each X2 per day with meals |
| Kapha | 2 of each X2 per day after meals | 3 of each X2 per day after meals |

## Description:

Diseases of the kidney are diverse, but individuals with kidney diseases often display similar clinical symptoms. Common symptoms involving the kidneys include the nephritic and nephrotic syndromes, renal cysts, acute kidney injury, chronic kidney disease, urinary tract infection, nephrolithiasis, and urinary tract obstruction. Although they are not normally harmful, kidney stones can be painful. The kidneys participate in homeostasis regulating acid-base balance (pH), electrolyte concentrations, extracellular fluid volume, and blood pressure. The kidneys accomplish these homeostatic functions both independently and in conjunction with other organs and glands, particularly those of the endocrine system.

These herbal blends can be used to strengthen the kidneys, bladder, urethra and adrenal glands. The kidneys support the adrenal glands according to Ayurveda. Therefore, these blends are also important to use for patients who have taken cortisone medications or birth control pills for long periods of time (more than two years – after six years more than 60% of patients will show adrenal insufficiency).

As secondary Vata organ by function the kidneys often 'dry out' due to high Vata conditions (Vata Vriddhi). As Kapha organs by structure the kidneys get congested and weakened from overwork or strain on Meda Dhatu. Overweight conditions put heavy strain on the kidneys as do high stress lifestyles; equally the excessive use of chemical medications damage the kidneys and adrenal glands.

These blends will also tend to dissolve kidney stones. They can be used for long periods of time up to twelve months. If there are no clear pathology or symptomology for the patient, then use the herbal blends according to Vikriti. Change the consumption of liquids – avoid acidic or carbonated drinks, fermented liquids, coffee, tea, etc. Diet should follow the Vikriti of the patient.

Use the Vataja herbs if Vata is predominant in the Vikriti (imbalance) with a Vata Vikriti diet / lifestyle.

Use the Pittaja herbs if Pitta is predominant in the Vikriti (imbalance) with a Pitta Vikriti diet / lifestyle.

Use the Kaphaja herbs if Kapha is predominant in the Vikriti (imbalance) with a Kapha Vikriti diet / lifestyle.

# Kidney stones

| Dosha | Code | Common Name | Latin Name |
|---|---|---|---|
| **Vataja** | 205 | Gokshura | Tribulus terrestris |
| | 401 | Cumin | Cumimum cyminum |
| | | Fennel | Foeniculum vulgare |
| | | Cardamom | Elettaria cardamomum |
| | 407 | Turmeric | Curcuma longa |
| | | Barberry | Berberis vulgaris |
| | | Dandelion | Taraxacum officinale |
| | 409 | Marshmallow | Althaea officinalis |
| | | Gotu kola | Centella asiatica |
| | | Stinging nettles | Urtica dioica |
| **Pittaja** | 205 | Gokshura | Tribulus terrestris |
| | 208 | Manjishta | Rubia cordifolia |
| | 402 | Coriander | Coriandrum sativum |
| | | Cumin | Cumimum cyminum |
| | | Fennel | Foeniculum vulgare |
| | 407 | Turmeric | Curcuma longa |
| | | Barberry | Berberis vulgaris |
| | | Dandelion | Taraxacum officinale |
| | 409 | Marshmallow | Althaea officinalis |
| | | Gotu kola | Centella asiatica |
| | | Stinging nettles | Urtica dioica |
| **Kaphaja** | 205 | Gokshura | Tribulus terrestris |
| | 208 | Manjishta | Rubia cordifolia |
| | 403 | Ginger | Zingiber officinale |
| | | Cumin | Cumimum cyminum |
| | | Fenugreek | Trigonella foenum-graecum |
| | 407 | Turmeric | Curcuma longa |
| | | Barberry | Berberis vulgaris |
| | | Dandelion | Taraxacum officinale |
| | 409 | Marshmallow | Althaea officinalis |
| | | Gotu kola | Centella asiatica |
| | | Stinging nettles | Urtica dioica |

| Dosha | Low Dose | High Dose |
|---|---|---|
| **Vata** | 1 of each X2 per day before meals | 2 of each X2 per day before meals |
| **Pitta** | 1 of each X2 per day with meals | 2 of each X2 per day with meals |
| **Kapha** | 2 of each X2 per day after meals | 3 of each X2 per day after meals |

**Description:**
See the description under Kidney disorders. Follow the diet and lifestyle according to Vikriti.

Use the Vataja herbs if Vata is predominant in the Vikriti (imbalance) with a Vata Vikriti diet / lifestyle.

Use the Pittaja herbs if Pitta is predominant in the Vikriti (imbalance) with a Pitta Vikriti diet / lifestyle.

Use the Kaphaja herbs if Kapha is predominant in the Vikriti (imbalance) with a Kapha Vikriti diet / lifestyle.

## Lactation (lack of)

| Dosha | Code | Common Name | Latin Name |
|---|---|---|---|
| Vataja | 211<br>401 | Shatavari<br>Cumin<br>Fennel<br>Cardamom | Asparagus racemosus<br>Cumimum cyminum<br>Foeniculum vulgare<br>Elettaria cardamomum |
| Pittaja | 211<br>402 | Shatavari<br>Coriander<br>Cumin<br>Fennel | Asparagus racemosus<br>Coriandrum sativum<br>Cumimum cyminum<br>Foeniculum vulgare |
| Kaphaja | 211<br>401 | Shatavari<br>Cumin<br>Fennel<br>Cardamom | Asparagus racemosus<br>Cumimum cyminum<br>Foeniculum vulgare<br>Elettaria cardamomum |

| Dosha | Low Dose | High Dose |
|---|---|---|
| Vata | 1 of each X2 per day before meals | 2 of each X2 per day before meals |
| Pitta | 1 of each X2 per day with meals | 2 of each X2 per day with meals |
| Kapha | 2 of each X2 per day after meals | 3 of each X2 per day after meals |

## Description:

This is a symptomatic herbal blend that has a galactagogue action as per Prakriti type. Care should be given to assess the state of Rasa Dhatu and Kapha Dosha. If needed *Vitex agnus-castus* can be used as a Mother Tincture at a dose of 30 drops X3 per day in addition to these herbal blends.

Use the Vataja herbs if Vata is predominant in the Prakriti with a Vata Prakriti diet / lifestyle.

Use the Pittaja herbs if Pitta is predominant in the Prakriti with a Pitta Prakriti diet / lifestyle.

Use the Kaphaja herbs if Kapha is predominant in the Prakriti with a Kapha Prakriti diet / lifestyle.

## Leucorrhea

| Dosha | Code | Common Name | Latin Name |
|---|---|---|---|
| **Vataja** | 212 | Pau d'arco | Tabebuia impetiginosa |
| | 401 | Cumin | Cumimum cyminum |
| | | Fennel | Foeniculum vulgare |
| | | Cardamom | Elettaria cardamomum |
| | 404 | Angelica | Angelica archangelica |
| | | Wild yam | Dioscorea villosa |
| | | Valerian | Valeriana officinalis |
| | 407 | Turmeric | Curcuma longa |
| | | Barberry | Berberis vulgaris |
| | | Dandelion | Taraxacum officinale |
| | 408 | Vitex | Vitex agnus-castus |
| | | Black cohosh | Cimicifuga racemosa |
| | | Cramp bark | Viburnum opulus |
| **Pittaja** | 212 | Pau d'arco | Tabebuia impetiginosa |
| | 402 | Coriander | Coriandrum sativum |
| | | Cumin | Cumimum cyminum |
| | | Fennel | Foeniculum vulgare |
| | 405 | Burdock | Arctium lappa |
| | | Yellow dock | Rumex crispus |
| | | Milk Thistle | Silybum marianum |
| | 407 | Turmeric | Curcuma longa |
| | | Barberry | Berberis vulgaris |
| | | Dandelion | Taraxacum officinale |
| | 408 | Vitex | Vitex agnus-castus |
| | | Black cohosh | Cimicifuga racemosa |
| | | Cramp bark | Viburnum opulus |
| **Kaphaja** | 212 | Pau d'arco | Tabebuia impetiginosa |
| | 403 | Ginger | Zingiber officinale |
| | | Cumin | Cumimum cyminum |
| | | Fenugreek | Trigonella foenum-graecum |
| | 406 | Myrrh | Commiphora myrrha |
| | | Elecampane | Inula helenium |
| | | Yellow dock | Rumex crispus |
| | 407 | Turmeric | Curcuma longa |
| | | Barberry | Berberis vulgaris |
| | | Dandelion | Taraxacum officinale |
| | 408 | Vitex | Vitex agnus-castus |
| | | Black cohosh | Cimicifuga racemosa |
| | | Cramp bark | Viburnum opulus |

| Dosha | Low Dose | High Dose |
|-------|----------|-----------|
| Vata | 1 of each X2 per day before meals | 2 of each X2 per day before meals |
| Pitta | 1 of each X2 per day with meals | 2 of each X2 per day with meals |
| Kapha | 2 of each X2 per day after meals | 3 of each X2 per day after meals |

## Description:

These herbal blends can be used for all types of leucorrhea. This is basically Kapha Roga that can be caused by Vata, Pitta or Kapha. Verify that there is not a chronic digestive problem. An imbalance in the colon will provoke leucorrhea; in other words, this is usually an Ama condition in the colon that causes an increase in bacteria, vaginal or intestinal. If this is the case begin with herbal blends under 'Ama' to lower the Ama in the digestive system before beginning with this formula. Excessive sexual intercourse, or poor hygiene can also be a factor if there is no Ama present. These herbal blends can be used for a period of one to three months.

The diet should be changed to an anti-Ama diet appropriate for the Prakriti of the person. Coffee, carbonated drinks, alcohol and sugar should be removed from the diet as well as red meat. A vegan diet would be the best if possible. Lifestyle and diet should follow the Vikriti of the patient after the Anti-Ama diet has been completed.

Use the Vataja herbs if Vata is predominant in the Vikriti (imbalance) with a Vata Vikriti diet / lifestyle.

Use the Pittaja herbs if Pitta is predominant in the Vikriti (imbalance) with a Pitta Vikriti diet / lifestyle.

Use the Kaphaja herbs if Kapha is predominant in the Vikriti (imbalance) with a Kapha Vikriti diet / lifestyle.

## Liver disorders (cirrhosis, necrosis, hepatitis AB)

| Dosha | Code | Common Name | Latin Name |
|---|---|---|---|
| **Vataja** | 206 | Guduchi | Tinospora cordifolia |
| | 207 | Haritaki | Terminalia chebula |
| | 401 | Cumin | Cumimum cyminum |
| | | Fennel | Foeniculum vulgare |
| | | Cardamom | Elettaria cardamomum |
| | 407 | Turmeric | Curcuma longa |
| | | Barberry | Berberis vulgaris |
| | | Dandelion | Taraxacum officinale |
| **Pittaja** | 206 | Guduchi | Tinospora cordifolia |
| | 207 | Haritaki | Terminalia chebula |
| | 402 | Coriander | Coriandrum sativum |
| | | Cumin | Cumimum cyminum |
| | | Fennel | Foeniculum vulgare |
| | 405 | Burdock | Arctium lappa |
| | | Yellow dock | Rumex crispus |
| | | Milk Thistle | Silybum marianum |
| | 407 | Turmeric | Curcuma longa |
| | | Barberry | Berberis vulgaris |
| | | Dandelion | Taraxacum officinale |
| **Kaphaja** | 206 | Guduchi | Tinospora cordifolia |
| | 207 | Haritaki | Terminalia chebula |
| | 403 | Ginger | Zingiber officinale |
| | | Cumin | Cumimum cyminum |
| | | Fenugreek | Trigonella foenum-graecum |
| | 405 | Burdock | Arctium lappa |
| | | Yellow dock | Rumex crispus |
| | | Milk Thistle | Silybum marianum |
| | 407 | Turmeric | Curcuma longa |
| | | Barberry | Berberis vulgaris |
| | | Dandelion | Taraxacum officinale |

| Dosha | Low Dose | High Dose |
|---|---|---|
| **Vata** | 1 of each X2 per day before meals | 2 of each X2 per day before meals |
| **Pitta** | 1 of each X2 per day with meals | 2 of each X2 per day with meals |
| **Kapha** | 2 of each X2 per day after meals | 3 of each X2 per day after meals |

## Description:

These herbal blends can be used for all forms of liver disorders (cirrhosis, necrosis, hepatitis, etc.). These blends will work on both

Sama and Nirama conditions, e.g., with or without Ama. This is a Pitta Roga condition and the blends works primarily on Rakta Dhatu. These blends act as tonic to the liver and at the same time remove Ama and/or the pathogen, such as the hepatitis virus. These blends are both reducing and tonic to the Pitta areas and tissues of the body. Vata Prakriti people need to limit the use of these blends to a two-month period that can be repeated in cycles of two-months herbs /one-month no herbs /two-months herbs /one-month no herbs for a period of up to twelve months. There is no restriction for Pitta or Kapha Prakriti types on the duration of using these herbal blends. A typical treatment should last six months or longer to cure the problem. For chronic conditions expect a year of treatment.

If there is no clear pathology or symptomology for the patient, then use these blends according to Vikriti. An anti-Pitta diet is important to follow for all types modified as per Prakriti. Sugar, oils and alcohol should be removed from the diet. A vegetarian or vegan diet is best when treating the liver.

Use the Vataja herbs if Vata is predominant in the Vikriti (imbalance) with a Pitta Prakriti diet / lifestyle.

Use the Pittaja herbs if Pitta is predominant in the Vikriti (imbalance) with a Pitta Vikriti diet / lifestyle.

Use the Kaphaja herbs if Kapha is predominant in the Vikriti (imbalance) with a Pitta Prakriti diet / lifestyle.

## Low appetite

| Dosha | Code | Common Name | Latin Name |
|---|---|---|---|
| Vataja | 401 | Cumin | Cumimum cyminum |
| | | Fennel | Foeniculum vulgare |
| | | Cardamom | Elettaria cardamomum |
| | 404 | Angelica | Angelica archangelica |
| | | Wild yam | Dioscorea villosa |
| | | Valerian | Valeriana officinalis |
| Pittaja | 402 | Coriander | Coriandrum sativum |
| | | Cumin | Cumimum cyminum |
| | | Fennel | Foeniculum vulgare |
| | 405 | Burdock | Arctium lappa |
| | | Yellow dock | Rumex crispus |
| | | Milk Thistle | Silybum marianum |
| Kaphaja | 403 | Ginger | Zingiber officinale |
| | | Cumin | Cumimum cyminum |
| | | Fenugreek | Trigonella foenum-graecum |
| | 406 | Myrrh | Commiphora myrrha |
| | | Elecampane | Inula helenium |
| | | Yellow dock | Rumex crispus |

| Dosha | Low Dose | High Dose |
|---|---|---|
| Vata | 1 of each X2 per day before meals | 2 of each X2 per day before meals |
| Pitta | 1 of each X2 per day with meals | 2 of each X2 per day with meals |
| Kapha | 2 of each X2 per day after meals | 3 of each X2 per day after meals |

## Description:

Low appetite is called Munda Agni in Ayurveda. It is a Kapha Roga and can be caused by any Dosha. Treatment should follow the Vikriti of the patient.

Use the Vataja herbs if Vata is predominant in the Vikriti (imbalance) with a Vata Vikriti diet / lifestyle.

Use the Pittaja herbs if Pitta is predominant in the Vikriti (imbalance) with a Pitta Vikriti diet / lifestyle.

Use the Kaphaja herbs if Kapha is predominant in the Vikriti (imbalance) with a Kapha Vikriti diet / lifestyle.

## Low immunity

| Dosha | Code | Common Name | Latin Name |
|---|---|---|---|
| Vataja | 203 | Ashwagandha | Withania somnifera |
| | 206 | Guduchi | Tinospora cordifolia |
| | 211 | Shatavari | Asparagus racemosus |
| | 301 | Amalaki | Emblica officinalis |
| | | Bibhitaki | Terminalia belerica |
| | | Haritaki | Terminalia chebula |
| Pittaja | 201 | Amalaki | Emblica officinalis |
| | 206 | Guduchi | Tinospora cordifolia |
| | 211 | Shatavari | Asparagus racemosus |
| | 301 | Amalaki | Emblica officinalis |
| | | Bibhitaki | Terminalia belerica |
| | | Haritaki | Terminalia chebula |
| Kaphaja | 203 | Ashwagandha | Withania somnifera |
| | 206 | Guduchi | Tinospora cordifolia |
| | 209 | Punarnava | Boerhaavia diffusa |
| | 301 | Amalaki | Emblica officinalis |
| | | Bibhitaki | Terminalia belerica |
| | | Haritaki | Terminalia chebula |

| Dosha | Low Dose | High Dose |
|---|---|---|
| Vata | 1 of each X2 per day before meals | 2 of each X2 per day before meals |
| Pitta | 1 of each X2 per day with meals | 2 of each X2 per day with meals |
| Kapha | 2 of each X2 per day after meals | 3 of each X2 per day after meals |

## Description:

Immunity is the result of Dosha equilibrium. When the Dosha are functioning correctly there is correct Dhatu formation, good Bala (vitality) and stamina. Agni is stable and no toxins or Ama is formed. The final result of a balanced Dosha function is called Ojas. Low immunity is the opposite of the above description and is complicated. Immune function includes many different Dhatus, Srotas and Agni, it is much more than just low Ojas. If Ojas is low it is due to a number of existing problems that have not been diagnosed and corrected.

The first thing to do as a practitioner is to correct the function of Agni and remove Ama; Agni is first line of defense for the immune system. Next the herbal blends that are given here can be used with a Vikriti diet and lifestyle for the patient.

Use the Vataja herbs if Vata is predominant in the Vikriti (imbalance) with a Vata Vikriti diet / lifestyle.

Use the Pittaja herbs if Pitta is predominant in the Vikriti (imbalance) with a Pitta Vikriti diet / lifestyle.

Use the Kaphaja herbs if Kapha is predominant in the Vikriti (imbalance) with a Kapha Vikriti diet / lifestyle.

## Low Ojas

| Dosha | Code | Common Name | Latin Name |
|---|---|---|---|
| **Vataja** | 203 | Ashwagandha | Withania somnifera |
| | 206 | Guduchi | Tinospora cordifolia |
| | 211 | Shatavari | Asparagus racemosus |
| | 301 | Amalaki | Emblica officinalis |
| | | Bibhitaki | Terminalia belerica |
| | | Haritaki | Terminalia chebula |
| **Pittaja** | 201 | Amalaki | Emblica officinalis |
| | 206 | Guduchi | Tinospora cordifolia |
| | 211 | Shatavari | Asparagus racemosus |
| | 301 | Amalaki | Emblica officinalis |
| | | Bibhitaki | Terminalia belerica |
| | | Haritaki | Terminalia chebula |
| **Kaphaja** | 203 | Ashwagandha | Withania somnifera |
| | 206 | Guduchi | Tinospora cordifolia |
| | 209 | Punarnava | Boerhaavia diffusa |
| | 301 | Amalaki | Emblica officinalis |
| | | Bibhitaki | Terminalia belerica |
| | | Haritaki | Terminalia chebula |

| Dosha | Low Dose | High Dose |
|---|---|---|
| **Vata** | 1 of each X2 per day before meals | 2 of each X2 per day before meals |
| **Pitta** | 1 of each X2 per day with meals | 2 of each X2 per day with meals |
| **Kapha** | 2 of each X2 per day after meals | 3 of each X2 per day after meals |

### Description:
See the description under 'Low immunity'.

Use the Vataja herbs if Vata is predominant in the Vikriti (imbalance) with a Vata Vikriti diet / lifestyle.

Use the Pittaja herbs if Pitta is predominant in the Vikriti (imbalance) with a Pitta Vikriti diet / lifestyle.

Use the Kaphaja herbs if Kapha is predominant in the Vikriti (imbalance) with a Kapha Vikriti diet / lifestyle.

## Lumbago

| Dosha | Code | Common Name | Latin Name |
|---|---|---|---|
| **Vataja** | 401 | Cumin | Cumimum cyminum |
| | | Fennel | Foeniculum vulgare |
| | | Cardamom | Elettaria cardamomum |
| | 406 | Myrrh | Commiphora myrrha |
| | | Elecampane | Inula helenium |
| | | Yellow dock | Rumex crispus |
| | 410 | Passion flower | Passiflora incarnata |
| | | Skullcap | Scutellaria lateriflora |
| | | Gotu kola | Centella asiatica |
| **Pittaja** | 402 | Coriander | Coriandrum sativum |
| | | Cumin | Cumimum cyminum |
| | | Fennel | Foeniculum vulgare |
| | 406 | Myrrh | Commiphora myrrha |
| | | Elecampane | Inula helenium |
| | | Yellow dock | Rumex crispus |
| | 410 | Passion flower | Passiflora incarnata |
| | | Skullcap | Scutellaria lateriflora |
| | | Gotu kola | Centella asiatica |
| **Kaphaja** | 403 | Ginger | Zingiber officinale |
| | | Cumin | Cumimum cyminum |
| | | Fenugreek | Trigonella foenum-graecum |
| | 406 | Myrrh | Commiphora myrrha |
| | | Elecampane | Inula helenium |
| | | Yellow dock | Rumex crispus |
| | 410 | Passion flower | Passiflora incarnata |
| | | Skullcap | Scutellaria lateriflora |
| | | Gotu kola | Centella asiatica |

| Dosha | Low Dose | High Dose |
|---|---|---|
| **Vata** | 1 of each X2 per day before meals | 2 of each X2 per day before meals |
| **Pitta** | 1 of each X2 per day with meals | 2 of each X2 per day with meals |
| **Kapha** | 2 of each X2 per day after meals | 3 of each X2 per day after meals |

## Description:

This is a symptomatic blend of herbs to strengthen Asthi Dhatu and reduce nerve pain from congested Vata (Vyana Vayu). The cause of the problem should be diagnosed and corrected if possible. External treatments with oil and heat should be used (Snehana and Svedhana) as per Prakriti, but diet and lifestyle should follow Vikriti. This is a

Vata Roga disorder as Vata Dosha controls Asthi Dhatu. Functionally pain is also a Vataja problem.

Use the Vataja herbs if Vata is predominant in the Vikriti (imbalance) with a Vata Vikriti diet / lifestyle.

Use the Pittaja herbs if Pitta is predominant in the Vikriti (imbalance) with a Pitta Vikriti diet / lifestyle.

Use the Kaphaja herbs if Kapha is predominant in the Vikriti (imbalance) with a Kapha Vikriti diet / lifestyle.

## Lung congestion

| Dosha | Code | Common Name | Latin Name |
|---|---|---|---|
| Vataja | 403 | Ginger | Zingiber officinale |
| | | Cumin | Cumimum cyminum |
| | | Fenugreek | Trigonella foenum-graecum |
| | 406 | Myrrh | Commiphora myrrha |
| | | Elecampane | Inula helenium |
| | | Yellow dock | Rumex crispus |
| Pittaja | 402 | Coriander | Coriandrum sativum |
| | | Cumin | Cumimum cyminum |
| | | Fennel | Foeniculum vulgare |
| | 406 | Myrrh | Commiphora myrrha |
| | | Elecampane | Inula helenium |
| | | Yellow dock | Rumex crispus |
| Kaphaja | 403 | Ginger | Zingiber officinale |
| | | Cumin | Cumimum cyminum |
| | | Fenugreek | Trigonella foenum-graecum |
| | 406 | Myrrh | Commiphora myrrha |
| | | Elecampane | Inula helenium |
| | | Yellow dock | Rumex crispus |

| Dosha | Low Dose | High Dose |
|---|---|---|
| Vata | 1 of each X2 per day before meals | 2 of each X2 per day before meals |
| Pitta | 1 of each X2 per day with meals | 2 of each X2 per day with meals |
| Kapha | 2 of each X2 per day after meals | 3 of each X2 per day after meals |

### Description:

Lung congestion is a Kapha Roga problem located in a Kapha Dhatu, e.g., Rasa Dhatu. Functionally Vata can cause this through dryness, etc., and Pitta through heat / inflammation. Hence, any Dosha can cause this problem functionally. These herbal blends work symptomatically to remove the excess Kapha Dosha. Diet and lifestyle should be used to stop the causal Dosha from increasing.

Use the Vataja herbs if Vata is predominant in the Vikriti (imbalance) with a Vata Vikriti diet / lifestyle.

Use the Pittaja herbs if Pitta is predominant in the Vikriti (imbalance) with a Pitta Vikriti diet / lifestyle.

Use the Kaphaja herbs if Kapha is predominant in the Vikriti (imbalance) with a Kapha Vikriti diet / lifestyle.

## Lung disorders

| Dosha | Code | Common Name | Latin Name |
|---|---|---|---|
| Vataja | 211 | Shatavari | Asparagus racemosus |
| | 403 | Ginger | Zingiber officinale |
| | | Cumin | Cumimum cyminum |
| | | Fenugreek | Trigonella foenum-graecum |
| | 406 | Myrrh | Commiphora myrrha |
| | | Elecampane | Inula helenium |
| | | Yellow dock | Rumex crispus |
| Pittaja | 211 | Shatavari | Asparagus racemosus |
| | 402 | Coriander | Coriandrum sativum |
| | | Cumin | Cumimum cyminum |
| | | Fennel | Foeniculum vulgare |
| | 406 | Myrrh | Commiphora myrrha |
| | | Elecampane | Inula helenium |
| | | Yellow dock | Rumex crispus |
| Kaphaja | 211 | Shatavari | Asparagus racemosus |
| | 403 | Ginger | Zingiber officinale |
| | | Cumin | Cumimum cyminum |
| | | Fenugreek | Trigonella foenum-graecum |
| | 406 | Myrrh | Commiphora myrrha |
| | | Elecampane | Inula helenium |
| | | Yellow dock | Rumex crispus |

| Dosha | Low Dose | High Dose |
|---|---|---|
| Vata | 1 of each X2 per day before meals | 2 of each X2 per day before meals |
| Pitta | 1 of each X2 per day with meals | 2 of each X2 per day with meals |
| Kapha | 2 of each X2 per day after meals | 3 of each X2 per day after meals |

## Description:

These herbal blends can be used to rejuvenate the lungs when they have been weakened from disease, pollution, smoking or medication. The blends are a general tonic to strengthen and rejuvenate the lungs from any physical problem and support Rasa Dhatu. Lung problems are Kapha Roga issues as Kapha controls Rasa Dhatu. If there is a psychosomatic aspect to the lung condition add the blend 410 to the above recommendations. These herbal blends should be used for at least three months and are safe to use for long periods of time up to one year. Use this formula according to Vikriti.

Use the Vataja herbs if Vata is predominant in the Vikriti (imbalance) with a Vata Vikriti diet / lifestyle.

Use the Pittaja herbs if Pitta is predominant in the Vikriti (imbalance) with a Pitta Vikriti diet / lifestyle.

Use the Kaphaja herbs if Kapha is predominant in the Vikriti (imbalance) with a Kapha Vikriti diet / lifestyle.

# Lupus

| Dosha | Code | Common Name | Latin Name |
|---|---|---|---|
| Vataja | 207 | Haritaki | Terminalia chebula |
| | 208 | Manjishta | Rubia cordifolia |
| | 212 | Pau d'arco | Tabebuia impetiginosa |
| | 401 | Cumin | Cumimum cyminum |
| | | Fennel | Foeniculum vulgare |
| | | Cardamom | Elettaria cardamomum |
| Pittaja | 207 | Haritaki | Terminalia chebula |
| | 208 | Manjishta | Rubia cordifolia |
| | 212 | Pau d'arco | Tabebuia impetiginosa |
| | 402 | Coriander | Coriandrum sativum |
| | | Cumin | Cumimum cyminum |
| | | Fennel | Foeniculum vulgare |
| Kaphaja | 207 | Haritaki | Terminalia chebula |
| | 208 | Manjishta | Rubia cordifolia |
| | 212 | Pau d'arco | Tabebuia impetiginosa |
| | 403 | Ginger | Zingiber officinale |
| | | Cumin | Cumimum cyminum |
| | | Fenugreek | Trigonella foenum-graecum |

| Dosha | Low Dose | High Dose |
|---|---|---|
| Vata | 1 of each X2 per day before meals | 2 of each X2 per day before meals |
| Pitta | 1 of each X2 per day with meals | 2 of each X2 per day with meals |
| Kapha | 2 of each X2 per day after meals | 3 of each X2 per day after meals |

## Description:

Lupus is a chronic inflammatory disease that occurs when the body's immune system attacks its own tissues and organs (autoimmune disorder). Inflammation caused by lupus can affect many different body systems — including the joints, skin, kidneys, blood cells, brain, heart and lungs. Lupus can be difficult to diagnose because its signs and symptoms often mimic those of other ailments. The cause for lupus is unknown and it is considered to be incurable.

Nine of every ten occurrences of lupus are in females, researchers have looked at the relationship between estrogen and lupus. Many women have more lupus symptoms before menstrual periods and/or during pregnancy when estrogen production is high.

Ayurveda views autoimmune disorders as a breakdown of normal homeostasis which is controlled by the three Doshas. All factors that disrupt the normal Dosha function can be causal factors. Modern medicine generally agrees that environment, chemicals (medical or industrial), genetics, hormones and stress are factors, though how these factors trigger lupus is not known. In Ayurveda, all of these factors disrupt normal Dosha function, Agni and thus result in Ama formation. Therefore, treatment protocol consists of balancing Dosha, Agni and removing Ama. Additionally, if symptoms are worse before menstruation then herbal support to balance the cycle is indicated. This can be done by adding product number 408 to the above blends.

Due to the inflammatory nature of lupus it is classified as Pitta Roga in Ayurveda. Functionally any Dosha can cause this disorder. In my clinical practice, I have had excellent results in controlling and removing most symptoms associated with lupus. This is done by using a lifestyle and diet as per Vikriti and supporting this with the above herbal blends. Avoiding possible trigger factors is important during the first year of treatment.

For more information on lupus see: http://www.lupus.org

Use the Vataja herbs if Vata is predominant in the Vikriti (imbalance) with a Vata Vikriti diet / lifestyle.
Use the Pittaja herbs if Pitta is predominant in the Vikriti (imbalance) with a Pitta Vikriti diet / lifestyle.
Use the Kaphaja herbs if Kapha is predominant in the Vikriti (imbalance) with a Kapha Vikriti diet / lifestyle.

For more information on autoimmune disorders refer to: *Ayurvedic Medicine for Westerners, Application of Ayurvedic Treatments Throughout Life* (Volume 5), chapter 16

## Lymphatic congestion

| Dosha | Code | Common Name | Latin Name |
|---|---|---|---|
| **Vataja** | 401 | Cumin | Cumimum cyminum |
| | | Fennel | Foeniculum vulgare |
| | | Cardamom | Elettaria cardamomum |
| | 405 | Burdock | Arctium lappa |
| | | Yellow dock | Rumex crispus |
| | | Milk Thistle | Silybum marianum |
| | 407 | Turmeric | Curcuma longa |
| | | Barberry | Berberis vulgaris |
| | | Dandelion | Taraxacum officinale |
| **Pittaja** | 402 | Coriander | Coriandrum sativum |
| | | Cumin | Cumimum cyminum |
| | | Fennel | Foeniculum vulgare |
| | 405 | Burdock | Arctium lappa |
| | | Yellow dock | Rumex crispus |
| | | Milk Thistle | Silybum marianum |
| | 407 | Turmeric | Curcuma longa |
| | | Barberry | Berberis vulgaris |
| | | Dandelion | Taraxacum officinale |
| **Kaphaja** | 403 | Ginger | Zingiber officinale |
| | | Cumin | Cumimum cyminum |
| | | Fenugreek | Trigonella foenum-graecum |
| | 405 | Burdock | Arctium lappa |
| | | Yellow dock | Rumex crispus |
| | | Milk Thistle | Silybum marianum |
| | 407 | Turmeric | Curcuma longa |
| | | Barberry | Berberis vulgaris |
| | | Dandelion | Taraxacum officinale |

| Dosha | Low Dose | High Dose |
|---|---|---|
| **Vata** | 1 of each X2 per day before meals | 2 of each X2 per day before meals |
| **Pitta** | 1 of each X2 per day with meals | 2 of each X2 per day with meals |
| **Kapha** | 2 of each X2 per day after meals | 3 of each X2 per day after meals |

## Description:

Lymphatic congestion is Kapha Roga both functionally and by structure (Rasa Dhatu). Any Dosha can cause Kapha to increase in the lymphatic system and care should be taken to understand the cause of this problem. These herbal blends are basically symptomatic to clear and remove congestion in Rasa Dhatu.

Use the Vataja herbs if Vata is predominant in the Vikriti (imbalance) with a Vata Vikriti diet / lifestyle.

Use the Pittaja herbs if Pitta is predominant in the Vikriti (imbalance) with a Pitta Vikriti diet / lifestyle.

Use the Kaphaja herbs if Kapha is predominant in the Vikriti (imbalance) with a Kapha Vikriti diet / lifestyle.

## Malabsorption syndrome

| Dosha | Code | Common Name | Latin Name |
|---|---|---|---|
| Vataja | 202 | Arjuna | Terminalia arjuna |
| | 207 | Haritaki | Terminalia chebula |
| | 301 | Amalaki | Emblica officinalis |
| | | Bibhitaki | Terminalia belerica |
| | | Haritaki | Terminalia chebula |
| Pittaja | 202 | Arjuna | Terminalia arjuna |
| | 301 | Amalaki | Emblica officinalis |
| | | Bibhitaki | Terminalia belerica |
| | | Haritaki | Terminalia chebula |
| Kaphaja | 202 | Arjuna | Terminalia arjuna |
| | 207 | Haritaki | Terminalia chebula |
| | 301 | Amalaki | Emblica officinalis |
| | | Bibhitaki | Terminalia belerica |
| | | Haritaki | Terminalia chebula |

| Dosha | Low Dose | High Dose |
|---|---|---|
| Vata | 1 of each X2 per day before meals | 2 of each X2 per day before meals |
| Pitta | 1 of each X2 per day with meals | 2 of each X2 per day with meals |
| Kapha | 2 of each X2 per day after meals | 3 of each X2 per day after meals |

## Description:

Malabsorption syndrome refers to a number of disorders in which the intestines are not able to adequately absorb certain nutrients into the bloodstream. Malabsorption can impede the absorption of macronutrients (proteins, carbohydrates, and fats), micronutrients (vitamins and minerals), or both. The main symptom is chronic fatigue that persists in spite of dietary and lifestyle changes.

Ayurveda considered this to be a disorder of Agni and is often associated with Ama. Any Dosha can cause this syndrome. Treatment, diet and lifestyle should follow Vikriti.

Use the Vataja herbs if Vata is predominant in the Vikriti (imbalance) with a Vata Vikriti diet / lifestyle.

Use the Pittaja herbs if Pitta is predominant in the Vikriti (imbalance) with a Pitta Vikriti diet / lifestyle.

Use the Kaphaja herbs if Kapha is predominant in the Vikriti (imbalance) with a Kapha Vikriti diet / lifestyle.

## Memory loss

| Dosha | Code | Common Name | Latin Name |
|---|---|---|---|
| Vataja | 204 | Bramhi | Bacopa monnieri |
| Pittaja | 204 | Bramhi | Bacopa monnieri |
| Kaphaja | 204 | Bramhi | Bacopa monnieri |

| Dosha | Low Dose | High Dose |
|---|---|---|
| Vata | 1 of each X2 per day before meals | 2 of each X2 per day before meals |
| Pitta | 1 of each X2 per day with meals | 2 of each X2 per day with meals |
| Kapha | 2 of each X2 per day after meals | 3 of each X2 per day after meals |

### Description:

Memory loss can be due to a number of reasons in Ayurveda. The most notable cause, after old age, is a malfunction of Vata Dosha in the mind. Prana Vayu is responsible for mental functions and any long-term disruption of Vata will eventually create problems with this sub-Dosha. This treatment is a classic remedy to increase Sattva and stability in the mind and is considered to be balanced for all Doshas. Nadishodhana pranayama is an important therapy to use with normal anti-stress lifestyle as per Prakriti.

Use the Vataja herbs if Vata is predominant in the Prakriti with a Vata Prakriti diet / lifestyle.

Use the Pittaja herbs if Pitta is predominant in the Prakriti with a Pitta Prakriti diet / lifestyle.

Use the Kaphaja herbs if Kapha is predominant in the Prakriti with a Kapha Prakriti diet / lifestyle.

## Menopause

| Dosha | Code | Common Name | Latin Name |
|---|---|---|---|
| Vataja | 211 | Shatavari | Asparagus racemosus |
| | 401 | Cumin | Cumimum cyminum |
| | | Fennel | Foeniculum vulgare |
| | | Cardamom | Elettaria cardamomum |
| | 404 | Angelica | Angelica archangelica |
| | | Wild yam | Dioscorea villosa |
| | | Valerian | Valeriana officinalis |
| | 408 | Vitex | Vitex agnus-castus |
| | | Black cohosh | Cimicifuga racemosa |
| | | Cramp bark | Viburnum opulus |
| Pittaja | 208 | Manjishta | Rubia cordifolia |
| | 211 | Shatavari | Asparagus racemosus |
| | 402 | Coriander | Coriandrum sativum |
| | | Cumin | Cumimum cyminum |
| | | Fennel | Foeniculum vulgare |
| | 408 | Vitex | Vitex agnus-castus |
| | | Black cohosh | Cimicifuga racemosa |
| | | Cramp bark | Viburnum opulus |
| Kaphaja | 211 | Shatavari | Asparagus racemosus |
| | 403 | Ginger | Zingiber officinale |
| | | Cumin | Cumimum cyminum |
| | | Fenugreek | Trigonella foenum-graecum |
| | 404 | Angelica | Angelica archangelica |
| | | Wild yam | Dioscorea villosa |
| | | Valerian | Valeriana officinalis |
| | 408 | Vitex | Vitex agnus-castus |
| | | Black cohosh | Cimicifuga racemosa |
| | | Cramp bark | Viburnum opulus |

| Dosha | Low Dose | High Dose |
|---|---|---|
| Vata | 1 of each X2 per day before meals | 2 of each X2 per day before meals |
| Pitta | 1 of each X2 per day with meals | 2 of each X2 per day with meals |
| Kapha | 2 of each X2 per day after meals | 3 of each X2 per day after meals |

## Description:

In Ayurveda, any signs of perimenopause or menopause relate directly to an increase of Vata Dosha. Thus, the first step in treatment is to balance Vata, then Agni and remove any Ama that may be present. The next step would be analyzing the state of Shukra

Dhatu. If there are obvious signs of high Vata or low Kapha in Shukra then it should be nourished and strengthened with Rasayana medications. The most basic way to do this is through diet and exercise. Of course, all the other six Dhatus must be nourished before the food essence reaches the seventh level of Shukra Dhatu, so one must start with the basic essential therapy; diet. Once the diet is stable herbs can be taken to strengthen Shukra directly.

The main approach in Ayurveda is one of tonics and strengthening the body; supporting the body or Brimhana therapies. Not of disease treatment – as menopause is not an illness – it is a form of Vata Vriddhi which explains why some women do not have any symptoms. Be very clear, just by balancing Vata most or all of menopausal symptoms can disappear.

These herbal blends can be used for all symptoms of perimenopause or menopause. The herbs work to support the endocrine system and balance the functions of both Vata and Pitta that are responsible for the majority of symptoms. These blends can be used safely for up to five years according to Vikriti. A diet that removes all stimulants (coffee, alcohol, etc.) is recommended. Many women note that by stopping coffee, wine or other stimulants the symptoms reduce or disappear; this is because these substances increase and aggravate Vata Dosha.

The physical things that can be done are to exercise regularly, eat a natural diet, and begin to rejuvenate the body with herbs. Many symptoms like hot flashes will disappear from diet alone. The combination of a natural diet low in protein and regular exercise can be as effective as HRT. Lifestyle and diet should follow the Prakriti of the patient.

Use the Vataja herbs if Vata is predominant in the Prakriti with a Vata Prakriti diet / lifestyle.

Use the Pittaja herbs if Pitta is predominant in the Prakriti with a Pitta Prakriti diet / lifestyle.

Use the Kaphaja herbs if Kapha is predominant in the Prakriti with a Kapha Prakriti diet / lifestyle.

## Menorrhagia (excessive)

| Dosha | Code | Common Name | Latin Name |
|---|---|---|---|
| Vataja | 202 | Arjuna | Terminalia arjuna |
| | 401 | Cumin | Cumimum cyminum |
| | | Fennel | Foeniculum vulgare |
| | | Cardamom | Elettaria cardamomum |
| | 407 | Turmeric | Curcuma longa |
| | | Barberry | Berberis vulgaris |
| | | Dandelion | Taraxacum officinale |
| Pittaja | 202 | Arjuna | Terminalia arjuna |
| | 402 | Coriander | Coriandrum sativum |
| | | Cumin | Cumimum cyminum |
| | | Fennel | Foeniculum vulgare |
| | 407 | Turmeric | Curcuma longa |
| | | Barberry | Berberis vulgaris |
| | | Dandelion | Taraxacum officinale |
| Kaphaja | 202 | Arjuna | Terminalia arjuna |
| | 403 | Ginger | Zingiber officinale |
| | | Cumin | Cumimum cyminum |
| | | Fenugreek | Trigonella foenum-graecum |
| | 407 | Turmeric | Curcuma longa |
| | | Barberry | Berberis vulgaris |
| | | Dandelion | Taraxacum officinale |

| Dosha | Low Dose | High Dose |
|---|---|---|
| Vata | 1 of each X2 per day before meals | 2 of each X2 per day before meals |
| Pitta | 1 of each X2 per day with meals | 2 of each X2 per day with meals |
| Kapha | 2 of each X2 per day after meals | 3 of each X2 per day after meals |

## Description:

There are a number of reasons why menorrhagia occurs. Sometimes this can indicate more severe problems. Care should be used in treating menorrhagia and the root cause should be identified. Menorrhagia can be from hormonal imbalances or as a part of perimenopause. It is primarily a Pitta Roga problem as it involves the uterus, blood circulation and menstrual flow. Abortions, miscarriages, endometriosis, and IUD's can all be potential causes to menorrhagia.

Lifestyle and diet should follow a Pitta Vikriti program for everyone and the herbal blends should be taken according to Vikriti. Any Dosha can cause this disorder and disrupt the function of Pitta.

Use the Vataja herbs if Vata is predominant in the Vikriti (imbalance) with a Pitta Vikriti diet / lifestyle.

Use the Pittaja herbs if Pitta is predominant in the Vikriti (imbalance) with a Pitta Vikriti diet / lifestyle.

Use the Kaphaja herbs if Kapha is predominant in the Vikriti (imbalance) with a Pitta Vikriti diet / lifestyle.

## Menstrual cramps

| Dosha | Code | Common Name | Latin Name |
|---|---|---|---|
| Vataja | 211 | Shatavari | Asparagus racemosus |
| | 401 | Cumin | Cumimum cyminum |
| | | Fennel | Foeniculum vulgare |
| | | Cardamom | Elettaria cardamomum |
| | 404 | Angelica | Angelica archangelica |
| | | Wild yam | Dioscorea villosa |
| | | Valerian | Valeriana officinalis |
| | 408 | Vitex | Vitex agnus-castus |
| | | Black cohosh | Cimicifuga racemosa |
| | | Cramp bark | Viburnum opulus |
| Pittaja | 208 | Manjishta | Rubia cordifolia |
| | 211 | Shatavari | Asparagus racemosus |
| | 402 | Coriander | Coriandrum sativum |
| | | Cumin | Cumimum cyminum |
| | | Fennel | Foeniculum vulgare |
| | 408 | Vitex | Vitex agnus-castus |
| | | Black cohosh | Cimicifuga racemosa |
| | | Cramp bark | Viburnum opulus |
| Kaphaja | 211 | Shatavari | Asparagus racemosus |
| | 403 | Ginger | Zingiber officinale |
| | | Cumin | Cumimum cyminum |
| | | Fenugreek | Trigonella foenum-graecum |
| | 404 | Angelica | Angelica archangelica |
| | | Wild yam | Dioscorea villosa |
| | | Valerian | Valeriana officinalis |
| | 408 | Vitex | Vitex agnus-castus |
| | | Black cohosh | Cimicifuga racemosa |
| | | Cramp bark | Viburnum opulus |

| Dosha | Low Dose | High Dose |
|---|---|---|
| Vata | 1 of each X2 per day before meals | 2 of each X2 per day before meals |
| Pitta | 1 of each X2 per day with meals | 2 of each X2 per day with meals |
| Kapha | 2 of each X2 per day after meals | 3 of each X2 per day after meals |

## Description:

Cramps and pain before or during menstruation are an imbalance of Vata Dosha and relate directly to Apana Vayu. Pain is a result of Vata constriction in the Srotamsi and is more prone to happen in Vata Prakriti or Vata dual type constitutions, but can manifest in any constitution. Treatment is generally long-term and the herbal blends work to balance Vata and improve circulation of Apana Vayu with heating, analgesic herbs. This disorder involves both the Apana and Vyana Vayus in the Srotamsi. The menstruation channel (Artavavaha Srota) will be disturbed by this and can affect Pitta. Excess Kapha can constrict Vata as well by moving from Rasa Dhatu into Artavavaha Srota, creating pressure, reducing flow or blockage, all of which will manifest as cramps or pain. Treatments should follow Vikriti for the patient.

Use the Vataja herbs if Vata is predominant in the Vikriti (imbalance) with a Vata Vikriti diet / lifestyle.

Use the Pittaja herbs if Pitta is predominant in the Vikriti (imbalance) with a Pitta Vikriti diet / lifestyle.

Use the Kaphaja herbs if Kapha is predominant in the Vikriti (imbalance) with a Kapha Vikriti diet / lifestyle.

## Menstrual disorders

| Dosha | Code | Common Name | Latin Name |
|---|---|---|---|
| Vataja | 208 | Manjishta | Rubia cordifolia |
| | 211 | Shatavari | Asparagus racemosus |
| | 401 | Cumin | Cumimum cyminum |
| | | Fennel | Foeniculum vulgare |
| | | Cardamom | Elettaria cardamomum |
| | 404 | Angelica | Angelica archangelica |
| | | Wild yam | Dioscorea villosa |
| | | Valerian | Valeriana officinalis |
| | 408 | Vitex | Vitex agnus-castus |
| | | Black cohosh | Cimicifuga racemosa |
| | | Cramp bark | Viburnum opulus |
| Pittaja | 208 | Manjishta | Rubia cordifolia |
| | 211 | Shatavari | Asparagus racemosus |
| | 402 | Coriander | Coriandrum sativum |
| | | Cumin | Cumimum cyminum |
| | | Fennel | Foeniculum vulgare |
| | 408 | Vitex | Vitex agnus-castus |
| | | Black cohosh | Cimicifuga racemosa |
| | | Cramp bark | Viburnum opulus |
| Kaphaja | 202 | Arjuna | Terminalia arjuna |
| | 208 | Manjishta | Rubia cordifolia |
| | 403 | Ginger | Zingiber officinale |
| | | Cumin | Cumimum cyminum |
| | | Fenugreek | Trigonella foenum-graecum |
| | 404 | Angelica | Angelica archangelica |
| | | Wild yam | Dioscorea villosa |
| | | Valerian | Valeriana officinalis |
| | 408 | Vitex | Vitex agnus-castus |
| | | Black cohosh | Cimicifuga racemosa |
| | | Cramp bark | Viburnum opulus |

| Dosha | Low Dose | High Dose |
|---|---|---|
| Vata | 1 of each X2 per day before meals | 2 of each X2 per day before meals |
| Pitta | 1 of each X2 per day with meals | 2 of each X2 per day with meals |
| Kapha | 2 of each X2 per day after meals | 3 of each X2 per day after meals |

## Description:

Ayurveda views menstruation problems as a combination of several factors. First, by importance is Vata and then Pitta and Kapha

Doshas. it must be stressed that good health is the basis of a trouble-free cycle and bad health is going to affect the menstruation cycle. In this context, regular physical exercise and good food play an important role. It is naive to believe that taking herbs and not exercising or eating well will bring your patient health. An overall lifestyle should be adapted in conjunction with these herbal blends. Hence, these herbs are to help balance the overall health and the Doshas that are behind the symptoms and may not reduce an acute symptom immediately. These blends should be taken as per Vikriti for at least three months and not more than one year.

Use the Vataja herbs if Vata is predominant in the Vikriti (imbalance) with a Vata Vikriti diet / lifestyle.

Use the Pittaja herbs if Pitta is predominating in the Vikriti (imbalance)   with a Pitta Vikriti diet / lifestyle.

Use the Kaphaja herbs if Kapha is predominant in the Vikriti (imbalance) with a Kapha Vikriti diet / lifestyle.

## Mental debility

| Dosha | Code | Common Name | Latin Name |
|-------|------|-------------|------------|
| Vataja | 204 | Bramhi | Bacopa monnieri |
| | 210 | Shankhpushpi | Convolvulus pluricaulis |
| | 401 | Cumin | Cumimum cyminum |
| | | Fennel | Foeniculum vulgare |
| | | Cardamom | Elettaria cardamomum |
| | 410 | Passion flower | Passiflora incarnata |
| | | Skullcap | Scutellaria lateriflora |
| | | Gotu kola | Centella asiatica |
| Pittaja | 204 | Bramhi | Bacopa monnieri |
| | 210 | Shankhpushpi | Convolvulus pluricaulis |
| | 402 | Coriander | Coriandrum sativum |
| | | Cumin | Cumimum cyminum |
| | | Fennel | Foeniculum vulgare |
| | 410 | Passion flower | Passiflora incarnata |
| | | Skullcap | Scutellaria lateriflora |
| | | Gotu kola | Centella asiatica |
| Kaphaja | 204 | Bramhi | Bacopa monnieri |
| | 210 | Shankhpushpi | Convolvulus pluricaulis |
| | 403 | Ginger | Zingiber officinale |
| | | Cumin | Cumimum cyminum |
| | | Fenugreek | Trigonella foenum-graecum |
| | 410 | Passion flower | Passiflora incarnata |
| | | Skullcap | Scutellaria lateriflora |
| | | Gotu kola | Centella asiatica |

| Dosha | Low Dose | High Dose |
|-------|----------|-----------|
| Vata | 1 of each X2 per day before meals | 2 of each X2 per day before meals |
| Pitta | 1 of each X2 per day with meals | 2 of each X2 per day with meals |
| Kapha | 2 of each X2 per day after meals | 3 of each X2 per day after meals |

## Description:
Like memory loss mental debility is a disorder of Prana Vayu and Vata Dosha in general. Mental debility is more serious and so additional herbs have been added to control the movement of Vata. Lifestyle and diet need to be modified in order for this disorder to be cured. Nadishodhana pranayama is a basic part of the treatment.

Use the Vataja herbs if Vata is predominant in the Vikriti (imbalance) with a Vata Vikriti diet / lifestyle.

Use the Pittaja herbs if Pitta is predominant in the Vikriti (imbalance) with a Pitta Vikriti diet / lifestyle.

Use the Kaphaja herbs if Kapha is predominant in the Vikriti (imbalance) with a Kapha Vikriti diet / lifestyle.

## Migraines

| Dosha | Code | Common Name | Latin Name |
|---|---|---|---|
| Vataja | 401 | Cumin | Cumimum cyminum |
| | | Fennel | Foeniculum vulgare |
| | | Cardamom | Elettaria cardamomum |
| | 404 | Angelica | Angelica archangelica |
| | | Wild yam | Dioscorea villosa |
| | | Valerian | Valeriana officinalis |
| | 407 | Turmeric | Curcuma longa |
| | | Barberry | Berberis vulgaris |
| | | Dandelion | Taraxacum officinale |
| Pittaja | 402 | Coriander | Coriandrum sativum |
| | | Cumin | Cumimum cyminum |
| | | Fennel | Foeniculum vulgare |
| | 405 | Burdock | Arctium lappa |
| | | Yellow dock | Rumex crispus |
| | | Milk Thistle | Silybum marianum |
| | 407 | Turmeric | Curcuma longa |
| | | Barberry | Berberis vulgaris |
| | | Dandelion | Taraxacum officinale |
| Kaphaja | 403 | Ginger | Zingiber officinale |
| | | Cumin | Cumimum cyminum |
| | | Fenugreek | Trigonella foenum-graecum |
| | 406 | Myrrh | Commiphora myrrha |
| | | Elecampane | Inula helenium |
| | | Yellow dock | Rumex crispus |
| | 407 | Turmeric | Curcuma longa |
| | | Barberry | Berberis vulgaris |
| | | Dandelion | Taraxacum officinale |

| Dosha | Low Dose | High Dose |
|---|---|---|
| Vata | 1 of each X2 per day before meals | 2 of each X2 per day before meals |
| Pitta | 1 of each X2 per day with meals | 2 of each X2 per day with meals |
| Kapha | 2 of each X2 per day after meals | 3 of each X2 per day after meals |

## Description:

Migraines and headaches can be from three distinct sources, functional, digestive or hormonal. Functional can include nerve compression due to accidents or tissue degeneration. This treatment is specific for digestive or metabolic migraines that are due to Dosha malfunction. Once Doshas are disrupted then Agni gets affected and

Ama is formed. Any of the three Doshas can cause this problem when mixed with Ama. As the problem is located in Rakta Dhatu and Raktavahasrota it can be classified as Pitta Roga by structure or location. This treatment should follow Vikriti and will need at least one month of treatment to give full results. See the indications below for headaches due to Dosha Vriddhi:

- Vataja – quick onset, sharp, throbbing pain, on the side of the head, pain can move around, intensity can be variable, irregular symptoms
- Pittaja – onset in one or more hours, light sensitive, increasing with day light – decreasing at night, pain behind the eyes and forehead area, regular symptoms
- Kaphaja – slow onset, up to one day before, dull, deep pain in the back of the head, or inside the head, regular symptoms

Use the Vataja herbs if Vata is predominant in the Vikriti (imbalance) with a Vata Vikriti diet / lifestyle.

Use the Pittaja herbs if Pitta is predominant in the Vikriti (imbalance) with a Pitta Vikriti diet / lifestyle.

Use the Kaphaja herbs if Kapha is predominant in the Vikriti (imbalance) with a Kapha Vikriti diet / lifestyle.

# Migrating joint pain

| Dosha | Code | Common Name | Latin Name |
|---|---|---|---|
| Vataja | 401 | Cumin | Cumimum cyminum |
| | | Fennel | Foeniculum vulgare |
| | | Cardamom | Elettaria cardamomum |
| | 404 | Angelica | Angelica archangelica |
| | | Wild yam | Dioscorea villosa |
| | | Valerian | Valeriana officinalis |
| | 408 | Vitex | Vitex agnus-castus |
| | | Black cohosh | Cimicifuga racemosa |
| | | Cramp bark | Viburnum opulus |
| Pittaja | 402 | Coriander | Coriandrum sativum |
| | | Cumin | Cumimum cyminum |
| | | Fennel | Foeniculum vulgare |
| | 404 | Angelica | Angelica archangelica |
| | | Wild yam | Dioscorea villosa |
| | | Valerian | Valeriana officinalis |
| | 408 | Vitex | Vitex agnus-castus |
| | | Black cohosh | Cimicifuga racemosa |
| | | Cramp bark | Viburnum opulus |
| Kaphaja | 403 | Ginger | Zingiber officinale |
| | | Cumin | Cumimum cyminum |
| | | Fenugreek | Trigonella foenum-graecum |
| | 404 | Angelica | Angelica archangelica |
| | | Wild yam | Dioscorea villosa |
| | | Valerian | Valeriana officinalis |
| | 408 | Vitex | Vitex agnus-castus |
| | | Black cohosh | Cimicifuga racemosa |
| | | Cramp bark | Viburnum opulus |

| Dosha | Low Dose | High Dose |
|---|---|---|
| Vata | 1 of each X2 per day before meals | 2 of each X2 per day before meals |
| Pitta | 1 of each X2 per day with meals | 2 of each X2 per day with meals |
| Kapha | 2 of each X2 per day after meals | 3 of each X2 per day after meals |

## Description:

Migrating joint pain is a Vata Roga problem both by function and location in structure. These herbal blends treat Vata Dosha and can be used for any kind of variable or migrating pain that manifests in Mamsa Dhatu or Asthi Dhatu. These kinds of variable pain generally show some kind of developing pathology, or symptoms of an existing pathology. Before giving these blends make sure that you are not ignoring some other problem. Use these blends when there is no obvious other kind of problem that could be causing the pain. The herbs have a mild tonic effect on the tissues, but have a stronger tonic effect on Vata through pain control by the use of analgesic herbs. It does remove Ama to some extent from the Srotas that nourish these Dhatus. This formula should be used for at least two months to realize its full effects. It is safe to use for periods up to one year

Use the Vataja herbs if Vata is predominant in the Vikriti (imbalance) with a Vata Vikriti diet / lifestyle.

Use the Pittaja herbs if Pitta is predominant in the Vikriti (imbalance) with a Pitta Vikriti diet / lifestyle.

Use the Kaphaja herbs if Kapha is predominant in the Vikriti (imbalance) with a Kapha Vikriti diet / lifestyle.

## Multiple scleroses

| Dosha | Code | Common Name | Latin Name |
|---|---|---|---|
| Vataja | 203 | Ashwagandha | Withania somnifera |
| | 205 | Gokshura | Tribulus terrestris |
| | 401 | Cumin | Cumimum cyminum |
| | | Fennel | Foeniculum vulgare |
| | | Cardamom | Elettaria cardamomum |
| | 404 | Angelica | Angelica archangelica |
| | | Wild yam | Dioscorea villosa |
| | | Valerian | Valeriana officinalis |
| Pittaja | 203 | Ashwagandha | Withania somnifera |
| | 205 | Gokshura | Tribulus terrestris |
| | 402 | Coriander | Coriandrum sativum |
| | | Cumin | Cumimum cyminum |
| | | Fennel | Foeniculum vulgare |
| | 405 | Burdock | Arctium lappa |
| | | Yellow dock | Rumex crispus |
| | | Milk Thistle | Silybum marianum |
| Kaphaja | 203 | Ashwagandha | Withania somnifera |
| | 205 | Gokshura | Tribulus terrestris |
| | 403 | Ginger | Zingiber officinale |
| | | Cumin | Cumimum cyminum |
| | | Fenugreek | Trigonella foenum-graecum |
| | 405 | Burdock | Arctium lappa |
| | | Yellow dock | Rumex crispus |
| | | Milk Thistle | Silybum marianum |

| Dosha | Low Dose | High Dose |
|---|---|---|
| Vata | 1 of each X2 per day before meals | 2 of each X2 per day before meals |
| Pitta | 1 of each X2 per day with meals | 2 of each X2 per day with meals |
| Kapha | 2 of each X2 per day after meals | 3 of each X2 per day after meals |

## Description:

Multiple sclerosis (MS) is an inflammatory disease in which the fatty myelin sheaths around the axons of the brain and spinal cord are damaged, leading to demyelination and scarring as well as a broad spectrum of signs and symptoms. Disease onset usually occurs in young adults, and it is more common in females. MS affects the ability of nerve cells in the brain and spinal cord to communicate with each other.

There is no known cure for MS. Treatments attempt to return function after an attack, prevent new attacks, and prevent disability. MS medications can have adverse effects or be poorly tolerated, and many patients pursue alternative treatments.

Ayurveda views this pathology as one that involves two Doshas; Pitta and Kapha. Pitta as the manager of heat in the body attacks the nerve sheaths (Majja Dhatu) that are controlled by Kapha. This disease is usually classified as Kapha Roga because Majja Dhatu is under the control of Kapha and is being damaged; functionally it is Pittaja. Causes of this pathology are considered to be due to an excess of Dosha accumulation mixed with Ama or non-digested food. Different mixes of Dosha and Ama cause different manifestations of this disease. Any Dosha can cause this pathology by increasing or aggravating Pitta and forcing Pitta into Majja Dhatu.

The Ayurvedic point of view that Ama is the main causal factor behind autoimmune disorders cannot be forgotten or ignored. MS is classified as an autoimmune disease because the body's immune system attacks and damages the myelin. This occurs because Ama is attached to the nerve tissue and the immune response tries to remove it. This results in the immunity attacking the nerve tissue which has difficulty to separate from the Ama that has attached to the myelin sheath.

Multiple Sclerosis is classified as a difficult disease to cure, but curable in early stages. MS becomes incurable after the nerve myelin is lost or damaged beyond the body's ability to repair it. Then it moves into the third category of impossible to cure, but possible to manage. MS is best treated in the first two years as it is still possible to reverse the pathology. Depending on the person it can still be curable up to ten years. In most cases, it becomes impossible to cure after ten years, but it is possible to manage the disorder.

The primary form of therapy is lifestyle and diet. Herbs can help as a support to remove Ama and balance Dosha. Remove all drugs, stimulants, coffee, cigarettes and alcohol from the diet. A Vegan diet for the first year of treatment is best, or a vegetarian diet if vegan is not possible. A Vata reducing lifestyle is best to control MS, otherwise follow the Vikriti of the patient. Regularity in the lifestyle and a reduction of stress factors is very, very important.

The main treatment for MS in India is Panchakarma. If time and money allow this treatment option then it should be considered after diet and lifestyle changes have been implemented.

Use the Vataja herbs if Vata is predominant in the Vikriti (imbalance) with a Vata Vikriti diet / lifestyle.

Use the Pittaja herbs if Pitta is predominant in the Vikriti (imbalance) with a Pitta Vikriti diet and Vata Vikriti lifestyle.

Use the Kaphaja herbs if Kapha is predominant in the Vikriti (imbalance) with a Kapha Vikriti diet and Vata Vikriti lifestyle.

For more information on Multiple Sclerosis refer to: *Ayurvedic Medicine for Westerners, Application of Ayurvedic Treatments Throughout Life* (Volume 5), chapter 16

## Muscle cramps

| Dosha | Code | Common Name | Latin Name |
|-------|------|-------------|------------|
| **Vataja** | 401 | Cumin | Cumimum cyminum |
| | | Fennel | Foeniculum vulgare |
| | | Cardamom | Elettaria cardamomum |
| | 408 | Vitex | Vitex agnus-castus |
| | | Black cohosh | Cimicifuga racemosa |
| | | Cramp bark | Viburnum opulus |
| | 410 | Passion flower | Passiflora incarnata |
| | | Skullcap | Scutellaria lateriflora |
| | | Gotu kola | Centella asiatica |
| **Pittaja** | 402 | Coriander | Coriandrum sativum |
| | | Cumin | Cumimum cyminum |
| | | Fennel | Foeniculum vulgare |
| | 408 | Vitex | Vitex agnus-castus |
| | | Black cohosh | Cimicifuga racemosa |
| | | Cramp bark | Viburnum opulus |
| | 410 | Passion flower | Passiflora incarnata |
| | | Skullcap | Scutellaria lateriflora |
| | | Gotu kola | Centella asiatica |
| **Kaphaja** | 403 | Ginger | Zingiber officinale |
| | | Cumin | Cumimum cyminum |
| | | Fenugreek | Trigonella foenum-graecum |
| | 408 | Vitex | Vitex agnus-castus |
| | | Black cohosh | Cimicifuga racemosa |
| | | Cramp bark | Viburnum opulus |
| | 410 | Passion flower | Passiflora incarnata |
| | | Skullcap | Scutellaria lateriflora |
| | | Gotu kola | Centella asiatica |

| Dosha | Low Dose | High Dose |
|-------|----------|-----------|
| **Vata** | 1 of each X2 per day before meals | 2 of each X2 per day before meals |
| **Pitta** | 1 of each X2 per day with meals | 2 of each X2 per day with meals |
| **Kapha** | 2 of each X2 per day after meals | 3 of each X2 per day after meals |

## Description:

Muscle cramps and pain are due to Vata not moving freely in the Srotamsi. These kinds of disorders are classified as Vata Roga by function and Kapha Roga by location as Kapha controls Mamsa Dhatu. The herbal blends support a correct function of Vata in Mamsa Dhatu and are therefore somewhat symptomatic. Care should be given in diagnosis to evaluate the cause of the cramping and Vata Vriddhi that provokes the pain. External treatments with oil and heat are highly recommended (Snehana and Svedhana). These can be done locally with oil and hot water bottle, or generally with Abhyanga and a hot shower or hot bath to help the oil be absorbed. Usually a Vata pacifying oil is used such as Vatashamaka, Balashwagandha, Bala, or Dashamula is used. If none of these are available use organic sesame oil.

Use the Vataja herbs if Vata is predominant in the Vikriti (imbalance) with a Vata Vikriti diet / lifestyle.

Use the Pittaja herbs if Pitta is predominant in the Vikriti (imbalance) with a Pitta Vikriti diet / lifestyle.

Use the Kaphaja herbs if Kapha is predominant in the Vikriti (imbalance) with a Kapha Vikriti diet / lifestyle.

## Nausea

| Dosha | Code | Common Name | Latin Name |
|-------|------|-------------|------------|
| **Vataja** | 207 | Haritaki | Terminalia chebula |
| | 401 | Cumin | Cumimum cyminum |
| | | Fennel | Foeniculum vulgare |
| | | Cardamom | Elettaria cardamomum |
| | 404 | Angelica | Angelica archangelica |
| | | Wild yam | Dioscorea villosa |
| | | Valerian | Valeriana officinalis |
| **Pittaja** | 201 | Amalaki | Emblica officinalis |
| | 402 | Coriander | Coriandrum sativum |
| | | Cumin | Cumimum cyminum |
| | | Fennel | Foeniculum vulgare |
| | 407 | Turmeric | Curcuma longa |
| | | Barberry | Berberis vulgaris |
| | | Dandelion | Taraxacum officinale |
| **Kaphaja** | 207 | Haritaki | Terminalia chebula |
| | 403 | Ginger | Zingiber officinale |
| | | Cumin | Cumimum cyminum |
| | | Fenugreek | Trigonella foenum-graecum |
| | 407 | Turmeric | Curcuma longa |
| | | Barberry | Berberis vulgaris |
| | | Dandelion | Taraxacum officinale |

| Dosha | Low Dose | High Dose |
|-------|----------|-----------|
| **Vata** | 1 of each X2 per day before meals | 2 of each X2 per day before meals |
| **Pitta** | 1 of each X2 per day with meals | 2 of each X2 per day with meals |
| **Kapha** | 2 of each X2 per day after meals | 3 of each X2 per day after meals |

## Description:

Nausea is notable stomach discomfort, heaviness and the sensation of wanting to vomit. In Ayurveda, this is a Kapha Roga problem that can be caused by any Dosha functionally. It is considered to be a problem of Munda Agni, or low Agni function typical of Kapha Vriddhi. Viral or bacterial infections can also cause a feeling of nausea, so it is important to find the cause. If no cause is apparent use these herbal blends to correct Dosha and Agni functions as per Vikriti.

Use the Vataja herbs if Vata is predominant in the Vikriti (imbalance) with a Vata Vikriti diet / lifestyle.

Use the Pittaja herbs if Pitta is predominant in the Vikriti (imbalance) with a Pitta Vikriti diet / lifestyle.

Use the Kaphaja herbs if Kapha is predominant in the Vikriti (imbalance) with a Kapha Vikriti diet / lifestyle.

## Nephritis

| Dosha | Code | Common Name | Latin Name |
|---|---|---|---|
| **Vataja** | 209 | Punarnava | Boerhaavia diffusa |
| | 401 | Cumin | Cumimum cyminum |
| | | Fennel | Foeniculum vulgare |
| | | Cardamom | Elettaria cardamomum |
| | 407 | Turmeric | Curcuma longa |
| | | Barberry | Berberis vulgaris |
| | | Dandelion | Taraxacum officinale |
| | 409 | Marshmallow | Althaea officinalis |
| | | Gotu kola | Centella asiatica |
| | | Stinging nettles | Urtica dioica |
| **Pittaja** | 205 | Gokshura | Tribulus terrestris |
| | 402 | Coriander | Coriandrum sativum |
| | | Cumin | Cumimum cyminum |
| | | Fennel | Foeniculum vulgare |
| | 407 | Turmeric | Curcuma longa |
| | | Barberry | Berberis vulgaris |
| | | Dandelion | Taraxacum officinale |
| | 409 | Marshmallow | Althaea officinalis |
| | | Gotu kola | Centella asiatica |
| | | Stinging nettles | Urtica dioica |
| **Kaphaja** | 209 | Punarnava | Boerhaavia diffusa |
| | 403 | Ginger | Zingiber officinale |
| | | Cumin | Cumimum cyminum |
| | | Fenugreek | Trigonella foenum-graecum |
| | 407 | Turmeric | Curcuma longa |
| | | Barberry | Berberis vulgaris |
| | | Dandelion | Taraxacum officinale |
| | 409 | Marshmallow | Althaea officinalis |
| | | Gotu kola | Centella asiatica |
| | | Stinging nettles | Urtica dioica |

| Dosha | Low Dose | High Dose |
|---|---|---|
| **Vata** | 1 of each X2 per day before meals | 2 of each X2 per day before meals |
| **Pitta** | 1 of each X2 per day with meals | 2 of each X2 per day with meals |
| **Kapha** | 2 of each X2 per day after meals | 3 of each X2 per day after meals |

## Description:

Nephritis is an inflammation of the kidney, which causes impaired kidney function. Nephritis can be due to a variety of causes, including kidney disease, autoimmune disease and infection. It is a serious condition and should be diagnosed by professionals to ascertain the cause. These herbal blends are symptomatic in approach to reduce inflammation in Mutravaha Srota. These herbs will help to rejuvenate the kidneys when in early states of pathology.

As the kidneys are part of Meda Dhatu and Kapha controls Meda most kidney disorders are classified as Kapha Roga. Functionally, Vata is using the kidneys and urinary system so many kidney disorders are functionally Vataja. Because nephritis is an inflammation of the kidneys Pitta is involved, perhaps it is even the cause of the pathology. Hence, from a functional point of view, this problem is usually a mix of both Vataja and Pittaja – determining which of the two is the cause will allow for a faster recovery time and a more efficient treatment through diet and lifestyle.

Use the Vataja herbs if Vata is predominant in the Vikriti (imbalance) with a Vata Vikriti diet / lifestyle.

Use the Pittaja herbs if Pitta is predominant in the Vikriti (imbalance) with a Pitta Vikriti diet / lifestyle.

Use the Kaphaja herbs if Kapha is predominant in the Vikriti (imbalance) with a Kapha Vikriti diet / lifestyle.

## Nerve pain

| Dosha | Code | Common Name | Latin Name |
|---|---|---|---|
| **Vataja** | 203 | Ashwagandha | Withania somnifera |
| | 204 | Bramhi | Bacopa monnieri |
| | 401 | Cumin | Cumimum cyminum |
| | | Fennel | Foeniculum vulgare |
| | | Cardamom | Elettaria cardamomum |
| | 404 | Angelica | Angelica archangelica |
| | | Wild yam | Dioscorea villosa |
| | | Valerian | Valeriana officinalis |
| **Pittaja** | 203 | Ashwagandha | Withania somnifera |
| | 204 | Bramhi | Bacopa monnieri |
| | 402 | Coriander | Coriandrum sativum |
| | | Cumin | Cumimum cyminum |
| | | Fennel | Foeniculum vulgare |
| | 410 | Passion flower | Passiflora incarnata |
| | | Skullcap | Scutellaria lateriflora |
| | | Gotu kola | Centella asiatica |
| **Kaphaja** | 203 | Ashwagandha | Withania somnifera |
| | 204 | Bramhi | Bacopa monnieri |
| | 403 | Ginger | Zingiber officinale |
| | | Cumin | Cumimum cyminum |
| | | Fenugreek | Trigonella foenum-graecum |
| | 410 | Passion flower | Passiflora incarnata |
| | | Skullcap | Scutellaria lateriflora |
| | | Gotu kola | Centella asiatica |

| Dosha | Low Dose | High Dose |
|---|---|---|
| **Vata** | 1 of each X2 per day before meals | 2 of each X2 per day before meals |
| **Pitta** | 1 of each X2 per day with meals | 2 of each X2 per day with meals |
| **Kapha** | 2 of each X2 per day after meals | 3 of each X2 per day after meals |

## Description:
See the description under Neuralgia.

Use the Vataja herbs if Vata is predominant in the Vikriti (imbalance) with a Vata Vikriti diet / lifestyle.

Use the Pittaja herbs if Pitta is predominant in the Vikriti (imbalance) with a Pitta Vikriti diet / lifestyle.

Use the Kaphaja herbs if Kapha is predominant in the Vikriti (imbalance) with a Kapha Vikriti diet / lifestyle.

## Nervous disorders

| Dosha | Code | Common Name | Latin Name |
|-------|------|-------------|------------|
| Vataja | 204 | Bramhi | Bacopa monnieri |
| | 207 | Haritaki | Terminalia chebula |
| | 210 | Shankhpushpi | Convolvulus pluricaulis |
| | 301 | Amalaki | Emblica officinalis |
| | | Bibhitaki | Terminalia belerica |
| | | Haritaki | Terminalia chebula |
| | 410 | Passion flower | Passiflora incarnata |
| | | Skullcap | Scutellaria lateriflora |
| | | Gotu kola | Centella asiatica |
| Pittaja | 201 | Amalaki | Emblica officinalis |
| | 204 | Bramhi | Bacopa monnieri |
| | 210 | Shankhpushpi | Convolvulus pluricaulis |
| | 301 | Amalaki | Emblica officinalis |
| | | Bibhitaki | Terminalia belerica |
| | | Haritaki | Terminalia chebula |
| | 410 | Passion flower | Passiflora incarnata |
| | | Skullcap | Scutellaria lateriflora |
| | | Gotu kola | Centella asiatica |
| Kaphaja | 204 | Bramhi | Bacopa monnieri |
| | 209 | Punarnava | Boerhaavia diffusa |
| | 210 | Shankhpushpi | Convolvulus pluricaulis |
| | 301 | Amalaki | Emblica officinalis |
| | | Bibhitaki | Terminalia belerica |
| | | Haritaki | Terminalia chebula |
| | 410 | Passion flower | Passiflora incarnata |
| | | Skullcap | Scutellaria lateriflora |
| | | Gotu kola | Centella asiatica |

| Dosha | Low Dose | High Dose |
|-------|----------|-----------|
| Vata | 1 of each X2 per day before meals | 2 of each X2 per day before meals |
| Pitta | 1 of each X2 per day with meals | 2 of each X2 per day with meals |
| Kapha | 2 of each X2 per day after meals | 3 of each X2 per day after meals |

## Description:

Nervous disorders are Vataja by function and Kapha Roga conditions by structure (Majja Dhatu). In general, it is important to treat both Vata functionally and Majja Dhatu (Kapha) or the structure. Lifestyle therapies to control Vata are very important, most critical is the practice of Nadishodhana pranayama daily. These herbal blends control the movement of Vata and help maintain the structure. Treatment should follow Vikriti of the patient. Nervous disorders are due to Dosha Vriddhi and external stress factors. Effort should be made to reduce stress factors both physically and emotionally.

Nervous disorders should not be confused with neurological disorders that are diseases of the central and peripheral nervous system. In other words, the brain, spinal cord, cranial nerves, peripheral nerves, nerve roots, autonomic nervous system, neuromuscular junction, and muscles. These disorders include Epilepsy, Alzheimer disease (dementias), cerebrovascular diseases including stroke, migraine and other headache disorders, Multiple Sclerosis, Parkinson's disease, neuro-infections, brain tumors, traumatic disorders of the nervous system such as brain trauma, and neurological disorders as a result of malnutrition. Examples of symptoms include paralysis, muscle weakness, poor coordination, loss of sensation, seizures, confusion, pain and altered levels of consciousness. There are more than 600 neurologic diseases.

Use the Vataja herbs if Vata is predominant in the Vikriti (imbalance) with a Vata Vikriti diet / lifestyle.

Use the Pittaja herbs if Pitta is predominant in the Vikriti (imbalance) with a Pitta Vikriti diet and Vata lifestyle.

Use the Kaphaja herbs if Kapha is predominant in the Vikriti (imbalance) with a Kapha Vikriti diet and Vata lifestyle.

## Neuralgia

| Dosha | Code | Common Name | Latin Name |
|---|---|---|---|
| Vataja | 203 | Ashwagandha | Withania somnifera |
| | 204 | Bramhi | Bacopa monnieri |
| | 401 | Cumin | Cumimum cyminum |
| | | Fennel | Foeniculum vulgare |
| | | Cardamom | Elettaria cardamomum |
| | 404 | Angelica | Angelica archangelica |
| | | Wild yam | Dioscorea villosa |
| | | Valerian | Valeriana officinalis |
| Pittaja | 203 | Ashwagandha | Withania somnifera |
| | 204 | Bramhi | Bacopa monnieri |
| | 402 | Coriander | Coriandrum sativum |
| | | Cumin | Cumimum cyminum |
| | | Fennel | Foeniculum vulgare |
| | 410 | Passion flower | Passiflora incarnata |
| | | Skullcap | Scutellaria lateriflora |
| | | Gotu kola | Centella asiatica |
| Kaphaja | 203 | Ashwagandha | Withania somnifera |
| | 204 | Bramhi | Bacopa monnieri |
| | 403 | Ginger | Zingiber officinale |
| | | Cumin | Cumimum cyminum |
| | | Fenugreek | Trigonella foenum-graecum |
| | 410 | Passion flower | Passiflora incarnata |
| | | Skullcap | Scutellaria lateriflora |
| | | Gotu kola | Centella asiatica |

| Dosha | Low Dose | High Dose |
|---|---|---|
| Vata | 1 of each X2 per day before meals | 2 of each X2 per day before meals |
| Pitta | 1 of each X2 per day with meals | 2 of each X2 per day with meals |
| Kapha | 2 of each X2 per day after meals | 3 of each X2 per day after meals |

## Description:

There are a variety of different forms of Neuralgia depending on the cause. Generally, the term is used to indicate varying degrees of nerve pain. It can either be part of another pathology or an independent disorder. The nerve tissue is under the control of Kapha Dosha in Majja Dhatu. Vata uses these tissues to carry out its function of communication and movement. When Vata is obstructed in some way the body feels this as pain. When Pitta is implicated then the nerve tissue becomes inflamed and the pathology becomes more complicated.

Ayurveda tries to understand the cause of neuralgia according to Dosha. Usually the Vikriti will indicate the causal Dosha, but not always. Lifestyle and diet are very important for these herbal treatments to work effectively. Nadishodhana pranayama is an important part of the treatment as is daily Abhyanga treatments followed by hot shower or bath (Snehana / Svedhana).

Use the Vataja herbs if Vata is predominant in the Vikriti (imbalance) with a Vata Vikriti diet / lifestyle.

Use the Pittaja herbs if Pitta is predominant in the Vikriti (imbalance) with a Pitta Vikriti diet / lifestyle.

Use the Kaphaja herbs if Kapha is predominant in the Vikriti (imbalance) with a Kapha Vikriti diet / lifestyle.

## Obesity (dietary)

| Dosha | Code | Common Name | Latin Name |
|---|---|---|---|
| Vataja | 209 | Punarnava | Boerhaavia diffusa |
| | 401 | Cumin | Cumimum cyminum |
| | | Fennel | Foeniculum vulgare |
| | | Cardamom | Elettaria cardamomum |
| | 406 | Myrrh | Commiphora myrrha |
| | | Elecampane | Inula helenium |
| | | Yellow dock | Rumex crispus |
| | 407 | Turmeric | Curcuma longa |
| | | Barberry | Berberis vulgaris |
| | | Dandelion | Taraxacum officinale |
| Pittaja | 209 | Punarnava | Boerhaavia diffusa |
| | 402 | Coriander | Coriandrum sativum |
| | | Cumin | Cumimum cyminum |
| | | Fennel | Foeniculum vulgare |
| | 405 | Burdock | Arctium lappa |
| | | Yellow dock | Rumex crispus |
| | | Milk Thistle | Silybum marianum |
| | 406 | Myrrh | Commiphora myrrha |
| | | Elecampane | Inula helenium |
| | | Yellow dock | Rumex crispus |
| Kaphaja | 209 | Punarnava | Boerhaavia diffusa |
| | 403 | Ginger | Zingiber officinale |
| | | Cumin | Cumimum cyminum |
| | | Fenugreek | Trigonella foenum-graecum |
| | 406 | Myrrh | Commiphora myrrha |
| | | Elecampane | Inula helenium |
| | | Yellow dock | Rumex crispus |
| | 407 | Turmeric | Curcuma longa |
| | | Barberry | Berberis vulgaris |
| | | Dandelion | Taraxacum officinale |

| Dosha | Low Dose | High Dose |
|---|---|---|
| Vata | 1 of each X2 per day before meals | 2 of each X2 per day before meals |
| Pitta | 1 of each X2 per day with meals | 2 of each X2 per day with meals |
| Kapha | 2 of each X2 per day after meals | 3 of each X2 per day after meals |

## Description:

These herbal blends can be used to help patients who are trying to lose weight due to dietary causes. For obesity that is due to endocrine imbalance add the blend number 408 to the above herbs. These blends will remove Ama from the Srotamsi and increase Dhatu Agni. They work directly on Meda Dhatu and help to restore normal metabolism in the first four Dhatus. These blends should be used for a minimum of three months and are safe for long term use of up to twelve months.

Use these herbal blends according to Vikriti. Diet is extremely important in the treatment of this disorder. A vegetarian diet would be good, a Vegan diet would be the best if possible for the patient. Diet should follow the Prakriti of the patient, but they should use the strict Vikriti diet as per their constitution. This means if you are Pitta Prakriti use the Pitta Vikriti diet; if you are Kapha Prakriti use the Kapha Vikriti diet, etc. The herbal blends should be given according to Vikriti as already noted above. Removal of red meat, sugar and refined oils are important for these blends to work correctly. Exercise for a minimum of thirty minutes per day is absolutely necessary, longer periods are better to reduce weight, but should not exceed one hour per day. Working with a professional trainer is a good idea when trying to increase the duration of exercise.

If there are psychological issues around food it is advised to recommend the patient to see a psychologist specializing in food or dietary disorders. This is a special field of study and difficult. Professional help may be necessary to cure the patient of poor eating habits.

Use the Vataja herbs if Vata is predominant in the Vikriti (imbalance) with a Vata Vikriti diet / lifestyle.

Use the Pittaja herbs if Pitta is predominant in the Vikriti (imbalance) with a Pitta Vikriti diet / lifestyle.

Use the Kaphaja herbs if Kapha is predominant in the Vikriti (imbalance) with a Kapha Vikriti diet / lifestyle.

## Oedema (Edema)

| Dosha | Code | Common Name | Latin Name |
|---|---|---|---|
| Vataja | 209 | Punarnava | Boerhaavia diffusa |
| | 403 | Ginger | Zingiber officinale |
| | | Cumin | Cumimum cyminum |
| | | Fenugreek | Trigonella foenum-graecum |
| | 409 | Marshmallow | Althaea officinalis |
| | | Gotu kola | Centella asiatica |
| | | Stinging nettles | Urtica dioica |
| Pittaja | 209 | Punarnava | Boerhaavia diffusa |
| | 402 | Coriander | Coriandrum sativum |
| | | Cumin | Cumimum cyminum |
| | | Fennel | Foeniculum vulgare |
| | 409 | Marshmallow | Althaea officinalis |
| | | Gotu kola | Centella asiatica |
| | | Stinging nettles | Urtica dioica |
| Kaphaja | 209 | Punarnava | Boerhaavia diffusa |
| | 403 | Ginger | Zingiber officinale |
| | | Cumin | Cumimum cyminum |
| | | Fenugreek | Trigonella foenum-graecum |
| | 409 | Marshmallow | Althaea officinalis |
| | | Gotu kola | Centella asiatica |
| | | Stinging nettles | Urtica dioica |

| Dosha | Low Dose | High Dose |
|---|---|---|
| Vata | 1 of each X2 per day before meals | 2 of each X2 per day before meals |
| Pitta | 1 of each X2 per day with meals | 2 of each X2 per day with meals |
| Kapha | 2 of each X2 per day after meals | 3 of each X2 per day after meals |

## Description:

See the description under Edema.

Use the Vataja herbs if Vata is predominant in the Vikriti (imbalance) with a Vata Vikriti diet / lifestyle.

Use the Pittaja herbs if Pitta is predominant in the Vikriti (imbalance) with a Pitta Vikriti diet / lifestyle.

Use the Kaphaja herbs if Kapha is predominant in the Vikriti (imbalance) with a Kapha Vikriti diet / lifestyle.

## Old age

| Dosha | Code | Common Name | Latin Name |
|---|---|---|---|
| **Vataja** | 203 | Ashwagandha | Withania somnifera |
| | 204 | Bramhi | Bacopa monnieri |
| | 211 | Shatavari | Asparagus racemosus |
| | 301 | Amalaki | Emblica officinalis |
| | | Bibhitaki | Terminalia belerica |
| | | Haritaki | Terminalia chebula |
| **Pittaja** | 203 | Ashwagandha | Withania somnifera |
| | 204 | Bramhi | Bacopa monnieri |
| | 211 | Shatavari | Asparagus racemosus |
| | 301 | Amalaki | Emblica officinalis |
| | | Bibhitaki | Terminalia belerica |
| | | Haritaki | Terminalia chebula |
| **Kaphaja** | 203 | Ashwagandha | Withania somnifera |
| | 204 | Bramhi | Bacopa monnieri |
| | 211 | Shatavari | Asparagus racemosus |
| | 301 | Amalaki | Emblica officinalis |
| | | Bibhitaki | Terminalia belerica |
| | | Haritaki | Terminalia chebula |

| Dosha | Low Dose | High Dose |
|---|---|---|
| **Vata** | 1 of each X2 per day before meals | 2 of each X2 per day before meals |
| **Pitta** | 1 of each X2 per day with meals | 2 of each X2 per day with meals |
| **Kapha** | 2 of each X2 per day after meals | 3 of each X2 per day after meals |

## Description:

These herbal blends are classic Rasayana remedies to delay aging. According to the Caraka Samhita everybody should start taking Rasayana herbs from the age of forty to delay the aging process. Hence, it is better to start taking Rasayana herbs before really needing them in order to build up the Bala and Ojas. It is fine to use these blends if there is a small amount of Ama. However, if there appears to be a lot of Ama, fatigue, headaches, or other signs of Ama the patient should first use the 'Ama' formula in this book with a reducing anti-Ama diet. As old age is not a pathology the therapies for diet and lifestyle (as well as herbal) should follow Prakriti.

Rasayana treatments for the elderly (from sixty-five years old) follow the same logic as Rasayanas in general. The primary point with the elderly is to go slowly and to support Agni and the digestive system more than would be necessary with an adult between the ages of sixteen and sixty-five. Keep in mind that the whole metabolism slows down and elderly people get tired quicker and have less stamina than younger people. Therefore, the treatments and doses should account for these changes.

Use the Vataja herbs if Vata is predominant in the Prakriti with a Vata Prakriti diet / lifestyle.

Use the Pittaja herbs if Pitta is predominant in the Prakriti with a Pitta Prakriti diet / lifestyle.

Use the Kaphaja herbs if Kapha is predominant in the Prakriti with a Kapha Prakriti diet / lifestyle.

## Osteoarthritis

| Dosha | Code | Common Name | Latin Name |
|---|---|---|---|
| **Vataja** | 401 | Cumin | Cumimum cyminum |
| | | Fennel | Foeniculum vulgare |
| | | Cardamom | Elettaria cardamomum |
| | 404 | Angelica | Angelica archangelica |
| | | Wild yam | Dioscorea villosa |
| | | Valerian | Valeriana officinalis |
| | 407 | Turmeric | Curcuma longa |
| | | Barberry | Berberis vulgaris |
| | | Dandelion | Taraxacum officinale |
| **Pittaja** | 402 | Coriander | Coriandrum sativum |
| | | Cumin | Cumimum cyminum |
| | | Fennel | Foeniculum vulgare |
| | 405 | Burdock | Arctium lappa |
| | | Yellow dock | Rumex crispus |
| | | Milk Thistle | Silybum marianum |
| | 407 | Turmeric | Curcuma longa |
| | | Barberry | Berberis vulgaris |
| | | Dandelion | Taraxacum officinale |
| **Kaphaja** | 403 | Ginger | Zingiber officinale |
| | | Cumin | Cumimum cyminum |
| | | Fenugreek | Trigonella foenum-graecum |
| | 406 | Myrrh | Commiphora myrrha |
| | | Elecampane | Inula helenium |
| | | Yellow dock | Rumex crispus |
| | 407 | Turmeric | Curcuma longa |
| | | Barberry | Berberis vulgaris |
| | | Dandelion | Taraxacum officinale |

| Dosha | Low Dose | High Dose |
|---|---|---|
| **Vata** | 1 of each X2 per day before meals | 2 of each X2 per day before meals |
| **Pitta** | 1 of each X2 per day with meals | 2 of each X2 per day with meals |
| **Kapha** | 2 of each X2 per day after meals | 3 of each X2 per day after meals |

## Description:

Osteoarthritis (OA) is sometimes called degenerative joint disease, or degenerative arthritis, is the most common chronic degenerative condition of the joints. It occurs when the protective cartilage on the ends of the bones wears down over time. Although osteoarthritis can damage any joint in the body, the disorder most commonly affects joints in the hands, knees, hips, neck and spine.

In Ayurveda, this is a Vata Roga pathology caused by Ama. Its name in Sanskrit is *Amavata*. As there are many different types of these joint disorders many of the treatments are the same. Ayurveda also recognizes a disease caused by the vitiation of Vata and Rakta (Pitta) called *Vatarakta*; it includes burning painful joints and gout. Ama disorders need to be treated with Shodhana therapies in order to remove the cause. If the disease is treated before the Dhatu is damaged there can be full recovery. If the pathology is treated after the Dhatu is damaged it is only possible to stop the pathology from further development. Note that once the structure, or Dhatu, is damaged it is not possible to repair. Early treatment is imperative to avoid structural damage to the body. If possible Panchakarma is the best treatment option.

Lifestyle and diet should follow Vikriti, a vegetarian diet is best for this condition. If there is strong pain or inflammation, then the Mother Tincture of *Harpagophytum procumbens* (Devil's claw) can be taken with these herbal blends. Dose is 30 drops X3 per day before meals for three to four weeks.

Use the Vataja herbs if Vata is predominant in the Vikriti (imbalance) with a Vata Vikriti diet / lifestyle.

Use the Pittaja herbs if Pitta is predominant in the Vikriti (imbalance) with a Pitta Vikriti diet / lifestyle.

Use the Kaphaja herbs if Kapha is predominant in the Vikriti (imbalance) with a Kapha Vikriti diet / lifestyle.

## Osteoporosis

| Dosha | Code | Common Name | Latin Name |
|---|---|---|---|
| **Vataja** | 203 | Ashwagandha | Withania somnifera |
| | 207 | Haritaki | Terminalia chebula |
| | 401 | Cumin | Cumimum cyminum |
| | | Fennel | Foeniculum vulgare |
| | | Cardamom | Elettaria cardamomum |
| | 404 | Angelica | Angelica archangelica |
| | | Wild yam | Dioscorea villosa |
| | | Valerian | Valeriana officinalis |
| **Pittaja** | 203 | Ashwagandha | Withania somnifera |
| | 207 | Haritaki | Terminalia chebula |
| | 402 | Coriander | Coriandrum sativum |
| | | Cumin | Cumimum cyminum |
| | | Fennel | Foeniculum vulgare |
| | 405 | Burdock | Arctium lappa |
| | | Yellow dock | Rumex crispus |
| | | Milk Thistle | Silybum marianum |
| **Kaphaja** | 203 | Ashwagandha | Withania somnifera |
| | 207 | Haritaki | Terminalia chebula |
| | 403 | Ginger | Zingiber officinale |
| | | Cumin | Cumimum cyminum |
| | | Fenugreek | Trigonella foenum-graecum |
| | 404 | Angelica | Angelica archangelica |
| | | Wild yam | Dioscorea villosa |
| | | Valerian | Valeriana officinalis |

| Dosha | Low Dose | High Dose |
|---|---|---|
| **Vata** | 1 of each X2 per day before meals | 2 of each X2 per day before meals |
| **Pitta** | 1 of each X2 per day with meals | 2 of each X2 per day with meals |
| **Kapha** | 2 of each X2 per day after meals | 3 of each X2 per day after meals |

## Description:

Osteoporosis is a progressive bone disease that is characterized by a decrease in bone mass and density which can lead to an increased risk of fracture. In osteoporosis, the bone mineral density is reduced. It is a Vata Roga condition by both function and structure (Asthi Dhatu). In Ayurveda, the main treatment is diet and lifestyle. A number of studies (e.g., Riggs, 1986) have shown that a low protein diet increases bone density, thus a vegan diet, high in whole grains is generally the best therapeutic choice to increase bone density. Dairy products do have calcium, but this mineral is used in the digestion of animal proteins, resulting in a neutral level of body calcium (neither gain nor loss).

Ayurveda traditionally classifies osteoporosis as low Majja Pāka – reduced Majja Dhatu (bone marrow). As Majja hydrates and maintains Asthi Dhatu this is logical. Therefore, Rasayana herbs can be used to build up Majja Dhatu. This does not mean that we cannot use herbs and diet to add minerals to the bones, but it adds an important aspect of hydrating the bones through bone marrow. Essentially, Ayurveda views this disorder as a 'drying out' of the bones, meaning the loss of minerals is due to dehydration of the bones as Vata increases with age or due to lifestyle.

Use the Vataja herbs if Vata is predominant in the Vikriti (imbalance) with a Vata Vikriti diet / lifestyle.

Use the Pittaja herbs if Pitta is predominant in the Vikriti (imbalance) with a Pitta Vikriti diet / lifestyle.

Use the Kaphaja herbs if Kapha is predominant in the Vikriti (imbalance) with a Kapha Vikriti diet / lifestyle.

## Overwork

| Dosha | Code | Common Name | Latin Name |
|---|---|---|---|
| Vataja | 203 | Ashwagandha | Withania somnifera |
| | 204 | Bramhi | Bacopa monnieri |
| | 211 | Shatavari | Asparagus racemosus |
| | 401 | Cumin | Cumimum cyminum |
| | | Fennel | Foeniculum vulgare |
| | | Cardamom | Elettaria cardamomum |
| Pittaja | 203 | Ashwagandha | Withania somnifera |
| | 204 | Bramhi | Bacopa monnieri |
| | 211 | Shatavari | Asparagus racemosus |
| | 402 | Coriander | Coriandrum sativum |
| | | Cumin | Cumimum cyminum |
| | | Fennel | Foeniculum vulgare |
| Kaphaja | 203 | Ashwagandha | Withania somnifera |
| | 204 | Bramhi | Bacopa monnieri |
| | 211 | Shatavari | Asparagus racemosus |
| | 403 | Ginger | Zingiber officinale |
| | | Cumin | Cumimum cyminum |
| | | Fenugreek | Trigonella foenum-graecum |

| Dosha | Low Dose | High Dose |
|---|---|---|
| Vata | 1 of each X2 per day before meals | 2 of each X2 per day before meals |
| Pitta | 1 of each X2 per day with meals | 2 of each X2 per day with meals |
| Kapha | 2 of each X2 per day after meals | 3 of each X2 per day after meals |

## Description:

Overwork reduces Bala and Ojas. These herbal blends are classic Rasayana remedies to build up Ojas.

Use the Vataja herbs if Vata is predominant in the Vikriti (imbalance) with a Vata Vikriti diet / lifestyle.

Use the Pittaja herbs if Pitta is predominant in the Vikriti (imbalance) with a Pitta Vikriti diet / lifestyle.

Use the Kaphaja herbs if Kapha is predominant in the Vikriti (imbalance) with a Kapha Vikriti diet / lifestyle.

## Palpitations

| Dosha | Code | Common Name | Latin Name |
|-------|------|-------------|------------|
| Vataja | 202 | Arjuna | Terminalia arjuna |
| | 203 | Ashwagandha | Withania somnifera |
| | 210 | Shankhpushpi | Convolvulus pluricaulis |
| | 301 | Amalaki | Emblica officinalis |
| | | Bibhitaki | Terminalia belerica |
| | | Haritaki | Terminalia chebula |
| Pittaja | 201 | Amalaki | Emblica officinalis |
| | 202 | Arjuna | Terminalia arjuna |
| | 210 | Shankhpushpi | Convolvulus pluricaulis |
| | 301 | Amalaki | Emblica officinalis |
| | | Bibhitaki | Terminalia belerica |
| | | Haritaki | Terminalia chebula |
| Kaphaja | 202 | Arjuna | Terminalia arjuna |
| | 209 | Punarnava | Boerhaavia diffusa |
| | 210 | Shankhpushpi | Convolvulus pluricaulis |
| | 301 | Amalaki | Emblica officinalis |
| | | Bibhitaki | Terminalia belerica |
| | | Haritaki | Terminalia chebula |

| Dosha | Low Dose | High Dose |
|-------|----------|-----------|
| Vata | 1 of each X2 per day before meals | 2 of each X2 per day before meals |
| Pitta | 1 of each X2 per day with meals | 2 of each X2 per day with meals |
| Kapha | 2 of each X2 per day after meals | 3 of each X2 per day after meals |

## Description:

Heart palpitations are a Vata Roga condition and functionally are Vataja. Pitta Dosha controls the heart (Rakta Dhatu) and Kapha controls the heart muscle (Mamsa Dhatu). All three Doshas are implicated in heart function so any of them can cause heart disorders. These herbal blends work to control Vyana Vayu, the form of Vata that controls the heart beat and circulation. Lifestyle should follow Vata Vikriti including daily use of Nadishodhana pranayama. Diet can follow Vikriti or Prakriti depending on the overall health of the patient. Heart palpitations are often the result of overwork or prolonged periods of stress, both of which create chronic Vata Vriddhi conditions. Treatment needs to look at the whole lifestyle and try to remove major stress factors, irregular habits and strive to sleep and eat at regular times in the day and night.

Use the Vataja herbs if Vata is predominant in the Vikriti (imbalance) with a Vata Vikriti diet / lifestyle.

Use the Pittaja herbs if Pitta is predominant in the Vikriti (imbalance) with a Pitta Vikriti diet and a Vata Vikriti lifestyle.

Use the Kaphaja herbs if Kapha is predominant in the Vikriti (imbalance) with a Kapha Vikriti diet and a Vata Vikriti lifestyle.

## Paralysis

| Dosha | Code | Common Name | Latin Name |
|---|---|---|---|
| Vataja | 204 | Bramhi | Bacopa monnieri |
| | 210 | Shankhpushpi | Convolvulus pluricaulis |
| | 401 | Cumin | Cumimum cyminum |
| | | Fennel | Foeniculum vulgare |
| | | Cardamom | Elettaria cardamomum |
| Pittaja | 204 | Bramhi | Bacopa monnieri |
| | 210 | Shankhpushpi | Convolvulus pluricaulis |
| | 402 | Coriander | Coriandrum sativum |
| | | Cumin | Cumimum cyminum |
| | | Fennel | Foeniculum vulgare |
| Kaphaja | 204 | Bramhi | Bacopa monnieri |
| | 210 | Shankhpushpi | Convolvulus pluricaulis |
| | 403 | Ginger | Zingiber officinale |
| | | Cumin | Cumimum cyminum |
| | | Fenugreek | Trigonella foenum-graecum |

| Dosha | Low Dose | High Dose |
|---|---|---|
| Vata | 1 of each X2 per day before meals | 2 of each X2 per day before meals |
| Pitta | 1 of each X2 per day with meals | 2 of each X2 per day with meals |
| Kapha | 2 of each X2 per day after meals | 3 of each X2 per day after meals |

**Description:**
Paralysis is the loss of the ability to move (and sometimes to feel) in a part of, or all of the body, typically as a result of illness, poison, or injury. There are more than 600 neurologic diseases. The WHO estimated in 2006 that neurological disorders and their direct consequences affect as many as one billion people worldwide. Paralysis is often a symptom of a complex neurologic pathology, although it can be an individual disorder by itself, or due to injury. Correct diagnosis is important to understand the casual factors.

This is a Vata Roga condition and these herbal blends are working symptomatically on restoring the correct movement to Vata Dosha. It is very important that the patient is diagnosed and treated by health care professionals, and if possible that the cause of the disorder is determined. The treatment of choice in Ayurveda for paralysis is Panchakarma. Lifestyle and diet play an important part in treatment. Daily oil and heat (Snehana and Svedhana) therapies should be given to the patient to control Vata.

Use the Vataja herbs if Vata is predominant in the Vikriti (imbalance) with a Vata Vikriti diet / lifestyle.

Use the Pittaja herbs if Pitta is predominant in the Vikriti (imbalance) with a Pitta Vikriti diet / lifestyle.

Use the Kaphaja herbs if Kapha is predominant in the Vikriti (imbalance) with a Kapha Vikriti diet / lifestyle.

## Parkinson's disease

| Dosha | Code | Common Name | Latin Name |
|---|---|---|---|
| Vataja | 203 | Ashwagandha | Withania somnifera |
| | 204 | Bramhi | Bacopa monnieri |
| | 211 | Shatavari | Asparagus racemosus |
| | 301 | Amalaki | Emblica officinalis |
| | | Bibhitaki | Terminalia belerica |
| | | Haritaki | Terminalia chebula |
| Pittaja | 203 | Ashwagandha | Withania somnifera |
| | 204 | Bramhi | Bacopa monnieri |
| | 211 | Shatavari | Asparagus racemosus |
| | 301 | Amalaki | Emblica officinalis |
| | | Bibhitaki | Terminalia belerica |
| | | Haritaki | Terminalia chebula |
| Kaphaja | 203 | Ashwagandha | Withania somnifera |
| | 204 | Bramhi | Bacopa monnieri |
| | 211 | Shatavari | Asparagus racemosus |
| | 301 | Amalaki | Emblica officinalis |
| | | Bibhitaki | Terminalia belerica |
| | | Haritaki | Terminalia chebula |

| Dosha | Low Dose | High Dose |
|---|---|---|
| Vata | 1 of each X2 per day before meals | 2 of each X2 per day before meals |
| Pitta | 1 of each X2 per day with meals | 2 of each X2 per day with meals |
| Kapha | 2 of each X2 per day after meals | 3 of each X2 per day after meals |

## Description:

Parkinson's disease (PD) is a degenerative disorder of the central nervous system. A number of environmental factors have been associated with an increased risk of Parkinson's including: pesticide exposure, head injuries, and living in the country or farming. Rural environments and the drinking of well-water may be risks as they are indirect measures of exposure to pesticides. Implicated chemicals include insecticides, primarily chlorpyrifos and organochlorines and pesticides, such as rotenone or paraquat, and some herbicides may also be implicated. Heavy metals exposure is a possible risk factor by accumulating in the midbrain tissue.

In Ayurveda Parkinson's disease is classified as a Vata Roga condition. It is a Vata Vriddhi disorder that views Vata increasing in Majja Dhatu and Majjavaha Srota. This is a Vata Roga disorder by function as Vata dries out the structure of Majja. It is also important to reduce Ama from the Srotamsi and stabilize the digestive system. As modern medicine has noted a number of environment agrochemicals that cause Parkinson's disease it is important to use Langhana therapies with, or prior to, using Rasayana therapies. The removal of Ama and chemical toxins is perhaps the best prevention of this disorder; use the 'Ama' blends if in doubt before using these herbal blends. Panchakarma would be advised for those patients at risk. Treatment is basically Rasayana for all types of patients; follow the Vikriti indications for diet, lifestyle and herbs.

Use the Vataja herbs if Vata is predominant in the Vikriti (imbalance) with a Vata Vikriti diet / lifestyle.

Use the Pittaja herbs if Pitta is predominant in the Vikriti (imbalance) with a Pitta Vikriti diet / lifestyle.

Use the Kaphaja herbs if Kapha is predominant in the Vikriti (imbalance) with a Kapha Vikriti diet / lifestyle.

## Peptic ulcers

| Dosha | Code | Common Name | Latin Name |
|---|---|---|---|
| Vataja | 201 | Amalaki | Emblica officinalis |
| | 211 | Shatavari | Asparagus racemosus |
| | 401 | Cumin | Cumimum cyminum |
| | | Fennel | Foeniculum vulgare |
| | | Cardamom | Elettaria cardamomum |
| | 404 | Angelica | Angelica archangelica |
| | | Wild yam | Dioscorea villosa |
| | | Valerian | Valeriana officinalis |
| Pittaja | 201 | Amalaki | Emblica officinalis |
| | 211 | Shatavari | Asparagus racemosus |
| | 402 | Coriander | Coriandrum sativum |
| | | Cumin | Cumimum cyminum |
| | | Fennel | Foeniculum vulgare |
| | 405 | Burdock | Arctium lappa |
| | | Yellow dock | Rumex crispus |
| | | Milk Thistle | Silybum marianum |
| Kaphaja | 201 | Amalaki | Emblica officinalis |
| | 211 | Shatavari | Asparagus racemosus |
| | 402 | Coriander | Coriandrum sativum |
| | | Cumin | Cumimum cyminum |
| | | Fennel | Foeniculum vulgare |
| | 404 | Angelica | Angelica archangelica |
| | | Wild yam | Dioscorea villosa |
| | | Valerian | Valeriana officinalis |

| Dosha | Low Dose | High Dose |
|---|---|---|
| Vata | 1 of each X2 per day before meals | 2 of each X2 per day before meals |
| Pitta | 1 of each X2 per day with meals | 2 of each X2 per day with meals |
| Kapha | 2 of each X2 per day after meals | 3 of each X2 per day after meals |

## Description:

Peptic ulcer disease (PUD), also known as a stomach ulcer, is a break in the lining of the stomach, first part of the small intestine, or occasionally the lower esophagus. An ulcer in the stomach is known as a gastric ulcer while that in the first part of the intestines is known as a duodenal ulcer. The most common symptoms are waking at night with upper abdominal pain or upper abdominal pain that improves with eating. The pain is often described as a burning or dull ache. Other symptoms include belching, vomiting, weight loss, or poor appetite.

This is a Pitta Roga disorder and can be caused by either Vata or Pitta; this pathology is rarely caused by Kapha as it is a Tikshna Agni disorder. It is Vataja when there are psychosomatic links (e.g., stress, etc.) that trigger the crisis. It is a Pittaja problem when there are signs of Tikshna Agni due to diet or emotions like frustration.

Diet should follow a Pitta Vikriti for all types with a lifestyle that controls Vata. Nadishodhana pranayama is very useful as well.

Use the Vataja herbs if Vata is predominant in the Vikriti (imbalance) with a Pitta Vikriti diet and a Vata Vikriti lifestyle.

Use the Pittaja herbs if Pitta is predominant in the Vikriti (imbalance) with a Pitta Vikriti diet and a Vata Vikriti lifestyle.

Use the Kaphaja herbs if Kapha is predominant in the Vikriti (imbalance) with a Pitta Vikriti diet and a Vata Vikriti lifestyle.

## Pleurisy

| Dosha | Code | Common Name | Latin Name |
|---|---|---|---|
| Vataja | 211 | Shatavari | Asparagus racemosus |
| | 403 | Ginger | Zingiber officinale |
| | | Cumin | Cumimum cyminum |
| | | Fenugreek | Trigonella foenum-graecum |
| | 406 | Myrrh | Commiphora myrrha |
| | | Elecampane | Inula helenium |
| | | Yellow dock | Rumex crispus |
| Pittaja | 211 | Shatavari | Asparagus racemosus |
| | 402 | Coriander | Coriandrum sativum |
| | | Cumin | Cumimum cyminum |
| | | Fennel | Foeniculum vulgare |
| | 406 | Myrrh | Commiphora myrrha |
| | | Elecampane | Inula helenium |
| | | Yellow dock | Rumex crispus |
| Kaphaja | 211 | Shatavari | Asparagus racemosus |
| | 403 | Ginger | Zingiber officinale |
| | | Cumin | Cumimum cyminum |
| | | Fenugreek | Trigonella foenum-graecum |
| | 406 | Myrrh | Commiphora myrrha |
| | | Elecampane | Inula helenium |
| | | Yellow dock | Rumex crispus |

| Dosha | Low Dose | High Dose |
|---|---|---|
| Vata | 1 of each X2 per day before meals | 2 of each X2 per day before meals |
| Pitta | 1 of each X2 per day with meals | 2 of each X2 per day with meals |
| Kapha | 2 of each X2 per day after meals | 3 of each X2 per day after meals |

## Description:

Pleurisy is a condition involving inflammation of the tissue layers (pleura) lining the lungs and inner chest wall. Pleurisy is often associated with the accumulation of fluid between the two layers of pleura, known as pleural effusion. Pleurisy is caused by a variety of conditions such as virus infection, bacterial infections, pulmonary embolism, sickle cell anemia, chemotherapy, radiotherapy, HIV, AIDS and autoimmune disorders to name a few.

Pleurisy is a serious condition and is classified as Kapha Roga in Ayurveda because Kapha controls the lungs (Rasa Dhatu). Functionally it is Pittaja due to the inflammation of the pleura. But can be caused by any of the Doshas which increase Pitta, either mixed with Ama or not (Sama / Nirama). Pleurisy is dangerous and should be treated by a primary care practitioner before using these herbal blends. In some cases hospitalization may be necessary. These herbal blends are mainly designed to help the lungs to regenerate after an allopathic treatment, even though they will reduce mild inflammatory conditions. These blends can be used at any time after Pleurisy to strengthen the lungs and to avoid a relapse. I do not recommend mixing these herbs with an allopathic treatment. Diet and lifestyle should support the herbal treatment as per Vikriti.

Use the Vataja herbs if Vata is predominant in the Vikriti (imbalance) with a Vata Vikriti diet / lifestyle.

Use the Pittaja herbs if Pitta is predominant in the Vikriti (imbalance) with a Pitta Vikriti diet / lifestyle.

Use the Kaphaja herbs if Kapha is predominant in the Vikriti (imbalance) with a Kapha Vikriti diet / lifestyle.

## PMS (Premenstrual syndrome)

| Dosha | Code | Common Name | Latin Name |
|---|---|---|---|
| Vataja | 211 | Shatavari | Asparagus racemosus |
| | 403 | Ginger | Zingiber officinale |
| | | Cumin | Cumimum cyminum |
| | | Fenugreek | Trigonella foenum-graecum |
| | 404 | Angelica | Angelica archangelica |
| | | Wild yam | Dioscorea villosa |
| | | Valerian | Valeriana officinalis |
| | 408 | Vitex | Vitex agnus-castus |
| | | Black cohosh | Cimicifuga racemosa |
| | | Cramp bark | Viburnum opulus |
| Pittaja | 211 | Shatavari | Asparagus racemosus |
| | 402 | Coriander | Coriandrum sativum |
| | | Cumin | Cumimum cyminum |
| | | Fennel | Foeniculum vulgare |
| | 404 | Angelica | Angelica archangelica |
| | | Wild yam | Dioscorea villosa |
| | | Valerian | Valeriana officinalis |
| | 408 | Vitex | Vitex agnus-castus |
| | | Black cohosh | Cimicifuga racemosa |
| | | Cramp bark | Viburnum opulus |
| Kaphaja | 211 | Shatavari | Asparagus racemosus |
| | 403 | Ginger | Zingiber officinale |
| | | Cumin | Cumimum cyminum |
| | | Fenugreek | Trigonella foenum-graecum |
| | 404 | Angelica | Angelica archangelica |
| | | Wild yam | Dioscorea villosa |
| | | Valerian | Valeriana officinalis |
| | 408 | Vitex | Vitex agnus-castus |
| | | Black cohosh | Cimicifuga racemosa |
| | | Cramp bark | Viburnum opulus |

| Dosha | Low Dose | High Dose |
|---|---|---|
| Vata | 1 of each X2 per day before meals | 2 of each X2 per day before meals |
| Pitta | 1 of each X2 per day with meals | 2 of each X2 per day with meals |
| Kapha | 2 of each X2 per day after meals | 3 of each X2 per day after meals |

## Description:

Premenstrual syndrome is Vata Roga by function. These herbal blends can be used for all forms of premenstrual problems. They work to control Apana Vayu and also support Shukra Dhatu through phytosteroids action. Cramps, depression and other typical symptoms are addressed through the reduction of the function of Vata Dosha in various Srotamsi. The endocrine system will receive a broad range of support from these blends allowing the body to choose the phytosteroids it needs to produce any hormones that may be deficient. These blends are balanced and can be used for six to twelve months without problem. For longer periods of use the patient needs to be assessed monthly or bi-monthly. Many women suffer from abdominal bloating and breast tenderness before their menstruation. It is important to reduce salt, and to reduce all foods containing salt. It would speed up the therapeutic response if cheese, red meat, dairy products, alcohol and coffee were reduced or stopped during the beginning of the treatment.

Use the Vataja herbs if Vata is predominant in the Vikriti (imbalance) with a Vata Vikriti diet / lifestyle.

Use the Pittaja herbs if Pitta is predominant in the Vikriti (imbalance) with a Pitta Vikriti diet / lifestyle.

Use the Kaphaja herbs if Kapha is predominant in the Vikriti (imbalance) with a Kapha Vikriti diet / lifestyle.

For more information on Ayurvedic Gynecology refer to: *Ayurvedic Medicine for Westerners, Application of Ayurvedic Treatments Throughout Life* (Volume 5), chapter 8

## Pneumonia

| Dosha | Code | Common Name | Latin Name |
|-------|------|-------------|------------|
| Vataja | 211 | Shatavari | Asparagus racemosus |
| | 403 | Ginger | Zingiber officinale |
| | | Cumin | Cumimum cyminum |
| | | Fenugreek | Trigonella foenum-graecum |
| | 406 | Myrrh | Commiphora myrrha |
| | | Elecampane | Inula helenium |
| | | Yellow dock | Rumex crispus |
| Pittaja | 211 | Shatavari | Asparagus racemosus |
| | 402 | Coriander | Coriandrum sativum |
| | | Cumin | Cumimum cyminum |
| | | Fennel | Foeniculum vulgare |
| | 406 | Myrrh | Commiphora myrrha |
| | | Elecampane | Inula helenium |
| | | Yellow dock | Rumex crispus |
| Kaphaja | 211 | Shatavari | Asparagus racemosus |
| | 403 | Ginger | Zingiber officinale |
| | | Cumin | Cumimum cyminum |
| | | Fenugreek | Trigonella foenum-graecum |
| | 406 | Myrrh | Commiphora myrrha |
| | | Elecampane | Inula helenium |
| | | Yellow dock | Rumex crispus |

| Dosha | Low Dose | High Dose |
|-------|----------|-----------|
| Vata | 1 of each X2 per day before meals | 2 of each X2 per day before meals |
| Pitta | 1 of each X2 per day with meals | 2 of each X2 per day with meals |
| Kapha | 2 of each X2 per day after meals | 3 of each X2 per day after meals |

## Description:

Pneumonia is an inflammatory condition of the lung and is a Pitta Roga problem by function and located in a Kapha Dhatu, e.g., Rasa Dhatu. Hence, it can be classified as Kapha Roga by location or structure. Functionally Vata can aggravate Pitta through dryness, and Kapha through congestion. Hence, any Dosha can cause pneumonia. These herbal blends work symptomatically to remove the excess Pitta Dosha from the lungs and to strengthen the lung tissue, helping them to recover from illness. Diet and lifestyle should be used to stop the causal Dosha from increasing, or Vikriti.

Use the Vataja herbs if Vata is predominant in the Vikriti (imbalance) with a Vata Vikriti diet / lifestyle.

Use the Pittaja herbs if Pitta is predominant in the Vikriti (imbalance) with a Pitta Vikriti diet / lifestyle.

Use the Kaphaja herbs if Kapha is predominant in the Vikriti (imbalance) with a Kapha Vikriti diet / lifestyle.

## Poisoning

| Dosha | Code | Common Name | Latin Name |
|-------|------|-------------|------------|
| Vataja | 204 | Bramhi | Bacopa monnieri |
| | 206 | Guduchi | Tinospora cordifolia |
| | 212 | Pau d'arco | Tabebuia impetiginosa |
| | 301 | Amalaki | Emblica officinalis |
| | | Bibhitaki | Terminalia belerica |
| | | Haritaki | Terminalia chebula |
| Pittaja | 204 | Bramhi | Bacopa monnieri |
| | 206 | Guduchi | Tinospora cordifolia |
| | 212 | Pau d'arco | Tabebuia impetiginosa |
| | 301 | Amalaki | Emblica officinalis |
| | | Bibhitaki | Terminalia belerica |
| | | Haritaki | Terminalia chebula |
| Kaphaja | 204 | Bramhi | Bacopa monnieri |
| | 206 | Guduchi | Tinospora cordifolia |
| | 212 | Pau d'arco | Tabebuia impetiginosa |
| | 301 | Amalaki | Emblica officinalis |
| | | Bibhitaki | Terminalia belerica |
| | | Haritaki | Terminalia chebula |

| Dosha | Low Dose | High Dose |
|-------|----------|-----------|
| Vata | 1 of each X2 per day before meals | 2 of each X2 per day before meals |
| Pitta | 1 of each X2 per day with meals | 2 of each X2 per day with meals |
| Kapha | 2 of each X2 per day after meals | 3 of each X2 per day after meals |

## Description:
In today's world poisoning, can mean any toxic substance that damages or poisons the body. This could mean a scorpion bite or herbicide chemicals. In essence, any substance that is damaging the body can be termed as a kind of 'poison'. These herbal blends are known in Ayurveda to remove poisons from the tissues and help restore normal functions to the digestion. These herbal blends work best when accompanied by a Detoxifying Diet or Anti-Ama Diet. Eating light, easy to digest food helps the body to remove toxins. Obviously, these herbs are not a substitution for emergency care if the poisoning is acute, in the USA use the internet to find the emergency number near you at this address: http://www.poison.org/

Use the Vataja herbs if Vata is predominant in the Vikriti (imbalance) with a Vata Vikriti diet / lifestyle.

Use the Pittaja herbs if Pitta is predominant in the Vikriti (imbalance) with a Pitta Vikriti diet / lifestyle.

Use the Kaphaja herbs if Kapha is predominant in the Vikriti (imbalance) with a Kapha Vikriti diet / lifestyle.

## Post-natal care

| Dosha | Code | Common Name | Latin Name |
|-------|------|-------------|------------|
| **Vataja** | 211 | Shatavari | Asparagus racemosus |
| | 301 | Amalaki | Emblica officinalis |
| | | Bibhitaki | Terminalia belerica |
| | | Haritaki | Terminalia chebula |
| **Pittaja** | 211 | Shatavari | Asparagus racemosus |
| | 301 | Amalaki | Emblica officinalis |
| | | Bibhitaki | Terminalia belerica |
| | | Haritaki | Terminalia chebula |
| **Kaphaja** | 211 | Shatavari | Asparagus racemosus |
| | 301 | Amalaki | Emblica officinalis |
| | | Bibhitaki | Terminalia belerica |
| | | Haritaki | Terminalia chebula |

| Dosha | Low Dose | High Dose |
|-------|----------|-----------|
| **Vata** | 1 of each X2 per day before meals | 2 of each X2 per day before meals |
| **Pitta** | 1 of each X2 per day with meals | 2 of each X2 per day with meals |
| **Kapha** | 2 of each X2 per day after meals | 3 of each X2 per day after meals |

## Description:

Foremost in postpartum therapies is oil massage on the whole body, focusing on the abdomen and trunk area – this can be self-massage. Another woman (family, friend, or therapist if no other option is there) should massage the new mother's whole body especially the back, thighs, legs and abdomen several times a week for two or three weeks if possible. This is ideal and helps the mother recover much quicker from birthing.

The mother should be given Vata reducing herbs (see above) and a nourishing diet (Vata Prakriti diet) that is sweet in taste and promote body weight and milk production. The *Dashamula* formula is useful for this period of time, especially in a massage oil or as a Basti (enema) preparation. The herb of choice for most women due to its beneficial all around supportive action is Shatavari (*Asparagus racemosus*). It literally does everything that a new mother needs as it supports both her and her baby. In these herbal blends Shatavari is mixed with Triphala to help digestion and assimilation of nutrients. Lifestyle should also follow Vata Prakriti.

Use the Vataja herbs if Vata is predominant in the Vikriti (imbalance) with a Vata Prakriti diet / lifestyle.

Use the Pittaja herbs if Pitta is predominant in the Vikriti (imbalance) with a Vata Prakriti diet / lifestyle.

Use the Kaphaja herbs if Kapha is predominant in the Vikriti (imbalance) with a Vata Prakriti diet / lifestyle.

## Premature ejaculation

| Dosha | Code | Common Name | Latin Name |
|---|---|---|---|
| **Vataja** | 203 | Ashwagandha | Withania somnifera |
| | 211 | Shatavari | Asparagus racemosus |
| | 301 | Amalaki | Emblica officinalis |
| | | Bibhitaki | Terminalia belerica |
| | | Haritaki | Terminalia chebula |
| | 401 | Cumin | Cumimum cyminum |
| | | Fennel | Foeniculum vulgare |
| | | Cardamom | Elettaria cardamomum |
| **Pittaja** | 203 | Ashwagandha | Withania somnifera |
| | 211 | Shatavari | Asparagus racemosus |
| | 301 | Amalaki | Emblica officinalis |
| | | Bibhitaki | Terminalia belerica |
| | | Haritaki | Terminalia chebula |
| | 402 | Coriander | Coriandrum sativum |
| | | Cumin | Cumimum cyminum |
| | | Fennel | Foeniculum vulgare |
| **Kaphaja** | 203 | Ashwagandha | Withania somnifera |
| | 211 | Shatavari | Asparagus racemosus |
| | 301 | Amalaki | Emblica officinalis |
| | | Bibhitaki | Terminalia belerica |
| | | Haritaki | Terminalia chebula |
| | 403 | Ginger | Zingiber officinale |
| | | Cumin | Cumimum cyminum |
| | | Fenugreek | Trigonella foenum-graecum |

| Dosha | Low Dose | High Dose |
|---|---|---|
| **Vata** | 1 of each X2 per day before meals | 2 of each X2 per day before meals |
| **Pitta** | 1 of each X2 per day with meals | 2 of each X2 per day with meals |
| **Kapha** | 2 of each X2 per day after meals | 3 of each X2 per day after meals |

## Description:

Premature ejaculation (PE) occurs when a man experiences orgasm and expels semen soon after sexual contact and with minimal penile stimulation. It has also been called early ejaculation. Definitions include: 'ejaculation which always or nearly always occurs prior to or within about one minute.' Men's typical ejaculatory latency is approximately 4–8 minutes. It can include ejaculation without contact or physical stimulation.

This is a Vata Roga problem linked to the polarity of Prana / Apana Vayu. Vata controls ejaculation (Apana) and is linked to the mind (Prana). An overstimulation of the mind (Prana) causes an overstimulation of the penis (Apana) and often causes PE. There are many variations of this function, the other Doshas have minor roles. Treatment focus is on Vata first and then Kapha and Shukra Dhatu second. Treatment should follow Vikriti with daily Nadishodhana pranayama as part of lifestyle. Removal of drugs and stimulants like coffee and alcohol accelerate therapeutic results.

Use the Vataja herbs if Vata is predominant in the Vikriti (imbalance) with a Vata Vikriti diet / lifestyle.

Use the Pittaja herbs if Pitta is predominant in the Vikriti (imbalance) with a Pitta Vikriti diet / lifestyle.

Use the Kaphaja herbs if Kapha is predominant in the Vikriti (imbalance) with a Kapha Vikriti diet / lifestyle.

For more information on Men's Health in Ayurveda refer to: *Ayurvedic Medicine for Westerners, Application of Ayurvedic Treatments Throughout Life* (Volume 5), chapter 12

## Premenstrual disorders (PMS)

| Dosha | Code | Common Name | Latin Name |
|---|---|---|---|
| Vataja | 211 | Shatavari | Asparagus racemosus |
| | 403 | Ginger | Zingiber officinale |
| | | Cumin | Cumimum cyminum |
| | | Fenugreek | Trigonella foenum-graecum |
| | 404 | Angelica | Angelica archangelica |
| | | Wild yam | Dioscorea villosa |
| | | Valerian | Valeriana officinalis |
| | 408 | Vitex | Vitex agnus-castus |
| | | Black cohosh | Cimicifuga racemosa |
| | | Cramp bark | Viburnum opulus |
| Pittaja | 211 | Shatavari | Asparagus racemosus |
| | 402 | Coriander | Coriandrum sativum |
| | | Cumin | Cumimum cyminum |
| | | Fennel | Foeniculum vulgare |
| | 404 | Angelica | Angelica archangelica |
| | | Wild yam | Dioscorea villosa |
| | | Valerian | Valeriana officinalis |
| | 408 | Vitex | Vitex agnus-castus |
| | | Black cohosh | Cimicifuga racemosa |
| | | Cramp bark | Viburnum opulus |
| Kaphaja | 211 | Shatavari | Asparagus racemosus |
| | 403 | Ginger | Zingiber officinale |
| | | Cumin | Cumimum cyminum |
| | | Fenugreek | Trigonella foenum-graecum |
| | 404 | Angelica | Angelica archangelica |
| | | Wild yam | Dioscorea villosa |
| | | Valerian | Valeriana officinalis |
| | 408 | Vitex | Vitex agnus-castus |
| | | Black cohosh | Cimicifuga racemosa |
| | | Cramp bark | Viburnum opulus |

| Dosha | Low Dose | High Dose |
|---|---|---|
| Vata | 1 of each X2 per day before meals | 2 of each X2 per day before meals |
| Pitta | 1 of each X2 per day with meals | 2 of each X2 per day with meals |
| Kapha | 2 of each X2 per day after meals | 3 of each X2 per day after meals |

## Description:
See the description under PMS.

Use the Vataja herbs if Vata is predominant in the Vikriti (imbalance) with a Vata Vikriti diet / lifestyle.

Use the Pittaja herbs if Pitta is predominant in the Vikriti (imbalance) with a Pitta Vikriti diet / lifestyle.

Use the Kaphaja herbs if Kapha is predominant in the Vikriti (imbalance) with a Kapha Vikriti diet / lifestyle.

## Prostate disorders

| Dosha | Code | Common Name | Latin Name |
|-------|------|-------------|------------|
| **Vataja** | 205 | Gokshura | Tribulus terrestris |
| | 401 | Cumin | Cumimum cyminum |
| | | Fennel | Foeniculum vulgare |
| | | Cardamom | Elettaria cardamomum |
| | 407 | Turmeric | Curcuma longa |
| | | Barberry | Berberis vulgaris |
| | | Dandelion | Taraxacum officinale |
| | 409 | Marshmallow | Althaea officinalis |
| | | Gotu kola | Centella asiatica |
| | | Stinging nettles | Urtica dioica |
| **Pittaja** | 205 | Gokshura | Tribulus terrestris |
| | 402 | Coriander | Coriandrum sativum |
| | | Cumin | Cumimum cyminum |
| | | Fennel | Foeniculum vulgare |
| | 405 | Burdock | Arctium lappa |
| | | Yellow dock | Rumex crispus |
| | | Milk Thistle | Silybum marianum |
| | 407 | Turmeric | Curcuma longa |
| | | Barberry | Berberis vulgaris |
| | | Dandelion | Taraxacum officinale |
| | 409 | Marshmallow | Althaea officinalis |
| | | Gotu kola | Centella asiatica |
| | | Stinging nettles | Urtica dioica |
| **Kaphaja** | 205 | Gokshura | Tribulus terrestris |
| | 403 | Ginger | Zingiber officinale |
| | | Cumin | Cumimum cyminum |
| | | Fenugreek | Trigonella foenum-graecum |
| | 406 | Myrrh | Commiphora myrrha |
| | | Elecampane | Inula helenium |
| | | Yellow dock | Rumex crispus |
| | 407 | Turmeric | Curcuma longa |
| | | Barberry | Berberis vulgaris |
| | | Dandelion | Taraxacum officinale |
| | 409 | Marshmallow | Althaea officinalis |
| | | Gotu kola | Centella asiatica |
| | | Stinging nettles | Urtica dioica |

| Dosha | Low Dose | High Dose |
|-------|----------|-----------|
| Vata | 1 of each X2 per day before meals | 2 of each X2 per day before meals |
| Pitta | 1 of each X2 per day with meals | 2 of each X2 per day with meals |
| Kapha | 2 of each X2 per day after meals | 3 of each X2 per day after meals |

## Description:

The prostate is a compound tubuloalveolar exocrine gland of the male reproductive system that is sponge like in structure. Structurally it is under the control of Kapha and Shukra Dhatu. Functionally it is controlled by Vata Dosha and is part of two Srotamsi; Mutravaha Srota and Shukravaha Srota. Apana Vayu is the main form of Vata to function in the prostate. There are two common disorders of the prostate:

- Prostatitis is inflammation of the prostate gland. There are different forms of prostatitis, each with different causes and outcomes. Acute prostatitis and chronic bacterial prostatitis are treated with antibiotics; chronic non-bacterial prostatitis or male chronic pelvic pain syndrome, which comprises about 95% of prostatitis diagnoses. In chronic cases, it can also cause pain after ejaculation.

- Benign prostatic hyperplasia (BPH) occurs in older men; the prostate often enlarges to the point where urination becomes difficult. Symptoms include needing to go to the toilet often (frequency) or taking a while to get started (hesitancy). If the prostate grows too large it may constrict the urethra and impede the flow of urine, making urination difficult and painful and in extreme cases completely impossible. It can also cause pain after ejaculation.

Causes of prostate disorders are lifestyle habits such as smoking, poor dietary intake, sedentary habits, the use of illegal drugs and steroid medications. Stress and overwork can also be a factor in some patients. In Ayurveda, the main cause of disorders in the prostate is due to Ama accumulation and a lack of exercise. The prostate is a spongy gland located below the bladder. Hence, it has a tendency to accumulate Ama from the urinary system as well as the rectum. Typically, prostate disorders start after fifty years of age and become epidemic after fifty-five years of age in men.

The reason why this is happening on such a large scale is due to lifestyle and dietary habits. When men sit for long periods of time the Ama accumulated in the body will 'settle' in the lowest point; when sitting, this is the prostate gland. So, our modern, sedentary lifestyle is a main cause of prostate issues. Of course, if the diet is good (means digestible) then there is no Ama building up the systems of evacuation like the bladder and colon. Each Dosha can cause pathology in the prostate. Here are the main indications:

- Vataja – stress, anxiety, variable symptoms, variable flow of urine, pain after ejaculation
- Pittaja – stress, burning, regular symptoms, low flow of urine, dripping, pain after ejaculation
- Kaphaja – depression, dull aching, regular symptoms, low flow of urine, dripping

In Ayurveda, the main treatment is to change lifestyle habits to increase exercise and reduce stress. Next is to change the diet from heavy animal based foods to favor a plant based diet. Obviously, the liquids intake should be modified to remove coffee, tea, all forms of alcohol, carbonated drinks and chemical drinks (sodas). When this is done then results are rapid. With these blends the patient can optionally add the tincture of *Serenoa serrulata* (Saw palmetto) at 20 drops X 3 per day throughout the treatment.

Prevention is the best medicine. If the advice here is followed then most prostate disorders can be avoided, including cancer. Cancer cells love inflamed tissues and having an environment that is in a constant low-grade inflammatory response is a perfect environment for cancer cells to explode.

Use the Vataja herbs if Vata is predominant in the Vikriti (imbalance) with a Vata Vikriti diet / lifestyle.
Use the Pittaja herbs if Pitta is predominant in the Vikriti (imbalance) with a Pitta Vikriti diet / lifestyle.
Use the Kaphaja herbs if Kapha is predominant in the Vikriti (imbalance) with a Kapha Vikriti diet / lifestyle.

For more information on Men's Health in Ayurveda refer to: *Ayurvedic Medicine for Westerners, Application of Ayurvedic Treatments Throughout Life* (Volume 5), chapter 12

## Prostatitis

| Dosha | Code | Common Name | Latin Name |
|---|---|---|---|
| **Vataja** | 205 | Gokshura | Tribulus terrestris |
| | 401 | Cumin | Cumimum cyminum |
| | | Fennel | Foeniculum vulgare |
| | | Cardamom | Elettaria cardamomum |
| | 407 | Turmeric | Curcuma longa |
| | | Barberry | Berberis vulgaris |
| | | Dandelion | Taraxacum officinale |
| | 409 | Marshmallow | Althaea officinalis |
| | | Gotu kola | Centella asiatica |
| | | Stinging nettles | Urtica dioica |
| **Pittaja** | 205 | Gokshura | Tribulus terrestris |
| | 402 | Coriander | Coriandrum sativum |
| | | Cumin | Cumimum cyminum |
| | | Fennel | Foeniculum vulgare |
| | 405 | Burdock | Arctium lappa |
| | | Yellow dock | Rumex crispus |
| | | Milk Thistle | Silybum marianum |
| | 407 | Turmeric | Curcuma longa |
| | | Barberry | Berberis vulgaris |
| | | Dandelion | Taraxacum officinale |
| | 409 | Marshmallow | Althaea officinalis |
| | | Gotu kola | Centella asiatica |
| | | Stinging nettles | Urtica dioica |
| **Kaphaja** | 205 | Gokshura | Tribulus terrestris |
| | 403 | Ginger | Zingiber officinale |
| | | Cumin | Cumimum cyminum |
| | | Fenugreek | Trigonella foenum-graecum |
| | 406 | Myrrh | Commiphora myrrha |
| | | Elecampane | Inula helenium |
| | | Yellow dock | Rumex crispus |
| | 407 | Turmeric | Curcuma longa |
| | | Barberry | Berberis vulgaris |
| | | Dandelion | Taraxacum officinale |
| | 409 | Marshmallow | Althaea officinalis |
| | | Gotu kola | Centella asiatica |
| | | Stinging nettles | Urtica dioica |

| Dosha | Low Dose | High Dose |
|-------|----------|-----------|
| Vata | 1 of each X2 per day before meals | 2 of each X2 per day before meals |
| Pitta | 1 of each X2 per day with meals | 2 of each X2 per day with meals |
| Kapha | 2 of each X2 per day after meals | 3 of each X2 per day after meals |

## Description:
See the description under Prostate disorders.

Use the Vataja herbs if Vata is predominant in the Vikriti (imbalance) with a Vata Vikriti diet / lifestyle.

Use the Pittaja herbs if Pitta is predominant in the Vikriti (imbalance) with a Pitta Vikriti diet / lifestyle.

Use the Kaphaja herbs if Kapha is predominant in the Vikriti (imbalance) with a Kapha Vikriti diet / lifestyle.

## Psoriasis

| Dosha | Code | Common Name | Latin Name |
|-------|------|-------------|------------|
| **Vataja** | 212 | Pau d'arco | Tabebuia impetiginosa |
| | 401 | Cumin | Cumimum cyminum |
| | | Fennel | Foeniculum vulgare |
| | | Cardamom | Elettaria cardamomum |
| | 404 | Angelica | Angelica archangelica |
| | | Wild yam | Dioscorea villosa |
| | | Valerian | Valeriana officinalis |
| | 407 | Turmeric | Curcuma longa |
| | | Barberry | Berberis vulgaris |
| | | Dandelion | Taraxacum officinale |
| | 409 | Marshmallow | Althaea officinalis |
| | | Gotu kola | Centella asiatica |
| | | Stinging nettles | Urtica dioica |
| **Pittaja** | 212 | Pau d'arco | Tabebuia impetiginosa |
| | 402 | Coriander | Coriandrum sativum |
| | | Cumin | Cumimum cyminum |
| | | Fennel | Foeniculum vulgare |
| | 405 | Burdock | Arctium lappa |
| | | Yellow dock | Rumex crispus |
| | | Milk Thistle | Silybum marianum |
| | 407 | Turmeric | Curcuma longa |
| | | Barberry | Berberis vulgaris |
| | | Dandelion | Taraxacum officinale |
| | 409 | Marshmallow | Althaea officinalis |
| | | Gotu kola | Centella asiatica |
| | | Stinging nettles | Urtica dioica |
| **Kaphaja** | 212 | Pau d'arco | Tabebuia impetiginosa |
| | 403 | Ginger | Zingiber officinale |
| | | Cumin | Cumimum cyminum |
| | | Fenugreek | Trigonella foenum-graecum |
| | 405 | Burdock | Arctium lappa |
| | | Yellow dock | Rumex crispus |
| | | Milk Thistle | Silybum marianum |
| | 407 | Turmeric | Curcuma longa |
| | | Barberry | Berberis vulgaris |
| | | Dandelion | Taraxacum officinale |
| | 409 | Marshmallow | Althaea officinalis |
| | | Gotu kola | Centella asiatica |
| | | Stinging nettles | Urtica dioica |

| Dosha | Low Dose | High Dose |
|-------|----------|-----------|
| Vata | 1 of each X2 per day before meals | 2 of each X2 per day before meals |
| Pitta | 1 of each X2 per day with meals | 2 of each X2 per day with meals |
| Kapha | 2 of each X2 per day after meals | 3 of each X2 per day after meals |

## Description:

Psoriasis is a chronic, non-contagious autoimmune disease which affects the skin and joints. It commonly causes red scaly patches to appear on the skin. The scaly patches caused by psoriasis, called psoriatic plaques, are areas of inflammation and excessive skin production. Skin rapidly accumulates at these sites and takes on a silvery-white appearance. Plaques frequently occur on the skin of the elbows and knees, but can affect any area including the scalp and genitals. In contrast to eczema, psoriasis is more likely to be found on the extensor aspect of the joint (the exterior part of the joint, such as the outside of the elbow).

In Ayurveda, this is Kapha Roga by location and structure (Rasa Dhatu). Functionally, it can be either Vataja or Pittaja or both together as the dry, red patches are characteristic of psoriasis. Usually both Doshas need to be treated for a cure.

The treatment begins by removing all agrochemicals from the diet by the use of fresh organic foods and by removing all animal products if possible. Some organic dairy products can be allowed if needed, however, dairy products are often linked to skin disorders and are best removed. Agni needs to be balanced and all Ama removed from the body – especially the digestive system. A Detoxifying Diet or Anti-Ama Diet is the best way to start treatment.

Use the Vataja herbs if Vata is predominant in the Vikriti (imbalance) with a Vata Vikriti diet / lifestyle.
Use the Pittaja herbs if Pitta is predominant in the Vikriti (imbalance) with a Pitta Vikriti diet / lifestyle.
Use the Kaphaja herbs if Kapha is predominant in the Vikriti (imbalance) with a Kapha Vikriti diet / lifestyle.

## Raynaud's disease

| Dosha | Code | Common Name | Latin Name |
|---|---|---|---|
| **Vataja** | 206 | Guduchi | Tinospora cordifolia |
| | 403 | Ginger | Zingiber officinale |
| | | Cumin | Cumimum cyminum |
| | | Fenugreek | Trigonella foenum-graecum |
| | 404 | Angelica | Angelica archangelica |
| | | Wild yam | Dioscorea villosa |
| | | Valerian | Valeriana officinalis |
| | 407 | Turmeric | Curcuma longa |
| | | Barberry | Berberis vulgaris |
| | | Dandelion | Taraxacum officinale |
| **Pittaja** | 206 | Guduchi | Tinospora cordifolia |
| | 403 | Ginger | Zingiber officinale |
| | | Cumin | Cumimum cyminum |
| | | Fenugreek | Trigonella foenum-graecum |
| | 405 | Burdock | Arctium lappa |
| | | Yellow dock | Rumex crispus |
| | | Milk Thistle | Silybum marianum |
| | 407 | Turmeric | Curcuma longa |
| | | Barberry | Berberis vulgaris |
| | | Dandelion | Taraxacum officinale |
| **Kaphaja** | 206 | Guduchi | Tinospora cordifolia |
| | 403 | Ginger | Zingiber officinale |
| | | Cumin | Cumimum cyminum |
| | | Fenugreek | Trigonella foenum-graecum |
| | 406 | Myrrh | Commiphora myrrha |
| | | Elecampane | Inula helenium |
| | | Yellow dock | Rumex crispus |
| | 407 | Turmeric | Curcuma longa |
| | | Barberry | Berberis vulgaris |
| | | Dandelion | Taraxacum officinale |

| Dosha | Low Dose | High Dose |
|---|---|---|
| **Vata** | 1 of each X2 per day before meals | 2 of each X2 per day before meals |
| **Pitta** | 1 of each X2 per day with meals | 2 of each X2 per day with meals |
| **Kapha** | 2 of each X2 per day after meals | 3 of each X2 per day after meals |

## Description:

Raynaud's disease, or Raynaud syndrome, is a medical condition in which spasm of arteries cause episodes of reduced blood flow to the peripheral members. Generally, the fingers, and less commonly the toes, are the main areas concerned. Rarely, the nose, ears, or lips are affected. The episodes result in the affected part turning white and then blue. Often there is numbness or pain. As blood flow returns, the area turns red and burns.

The cause of Primary Raynaud's is not known. For Ayurveda, it is a typical problem of Vyana Vayu and is thus a Vataja problem. As the blood circulation is the site of the problem it is Pitta Roga by location and Vataja by function.

Raynaud's phenomenon, or Secondary Raynaud's, is a symptom of another deeper disorder that causes vasoconstriction of the peripheral blood vessels. In this case, it remains up to the practitioner to correctly diagnose the disorder and so determine the treatment. For this type of disorder the cause needs to be treated rather than Raynaud's in order to heal the patient.

Treatment protocol is very clear and gives good results for Primary Raynaud's. Lifestyle should remove all forms of nicotine, stimulants, drugs, coffee and include daily exercise for thirty to sixty minutes per day. Diet should be based on whole foods as per Prakriti and be vegetarian or vegan during treatment. Daily practice of Nadishodhana pranayama is needed to control Vata Dosha.

Use the Vataja herbs if Vata is predominant in the Vikriti (imbalance) with a Vata Prakriti diet / lifestyle.

Use the Pittaja herbs if Pitta is predominant in the Vikriti (imbalance) with a Pitta Prakriti diet / lifestyle.

Use the Kaphaja herbs if Kapha is predominant in the Vikriti (imbalance) with a Kapha Prakriti diet / lifestyle.

## Reproductive disorders

| Dosha | Code | Common Name | Latin Name |
|---|---|---|---|
| Vataja | 203 | Ashwagandha | Withania somnifera |
| | 205 | Gokshura | Tribulus terrestris |
| | 211 | Shatavari | Asparagus racemosus |
| | 301 | Amalaki | Emblica officinalis |
| | | Bibhitaki | Terminalia belerica |
| | | Haritaki | Terminalia chebula |
| Pittaja | 203 | Ashwagandha | Withania somnifera |
| | 205 | Gokshura | Tribulus terrestris |
| | 211 | Shatavari | Asparagus racemosus |
| | 301 | Amalaki | Emblica officinalis |
| | | Bibhitaki | Terminalia belerica |
| | | Haritaki | Terminalia chebula |
| Kaphaja | 203 | Ashwagandha | Withania somnifera |
| | 205 | Gokshura | Tribulus terrestris |
| | 211 | Shatavari | Asparagus racemosus |
| | 301 | Amalaki | Emblica officinalis |
| | | Bibhitaki | Terminalia belerica |
| | | Haritaki | Terminalia chebula |

| Dosha | Low Dose | High Dose |
|---|---|---|
| Vata | 1 of each X2 per day before meals | 2 of each X2 per day before meals |
| Pitta | 1 of each X2 per day with meals | 2 of each X2 per day with meals |
| Kapha | 2 of each X2 per day after meals | 3 of each X2 per day after meals |

## Description:

See the description under Infertility. These are Rasayana herbal blends to support Shukra Dhatu and cover a broad range of general disorders in the reproductive system for men and women.

Use the Vataja herbs if Vata is predominant in the Vikriti (imbalance) with a Vata Vikriti diet / lifestyle.

Use the Pittaja herbs if Pitta is predominant in the Vikriti (imbalance) with a Pitta Vikriti diet / lifestyle.

Use the Kaphaja herbs if Kapha is predominant in the Vikriti (imbalance) with a Kapha Vikriti diet / lifestyle.

## Respiratory allergies

| Dosha | Code | Common Name | Latin Name |
|---|---|---|---|
| Vataja | 212 | Pau d'arco | Tabebuia impetiginosa |
| | 401 | Cumin | Cumimum cyminum |
| | | Fennel | Foeniculum vulgare |
| | | Cardamom | Elettaria cardamomum |
| | 409 | Marshmallow | Althaea officinalis |
| | | Gotu kola | Centella asiatica |
| | | Stinging nettles | Urtica dioica |
| Pittaja | 212 | Pau d'arco | Tabebuia impetiginosa |
| | 402 | Coriander | Coriandrum sativum |
| | | Cumin | Cumimum cyminum |
| | | Fennel | Foeniculum vulgare |
| | 409 | Marshmallow | Althaea officinalis |
| | | Gotu kola | Centella asiatica |
| | | Stinging nettles | Urtica dioica |
| Kaphaja | 212 | Pau d'arco | Tabebuia impetiginosa |
| | 403 | Ginger | Zingiber officinale |
| | | Cumin | Cumimum cyminum |
| | | Fenugreek | Trigonella foenum-graecum |
| | 409 | Marshmallow | Althaea officinalis |
| | | Gotu kola | Centella asiatica |
| | | Stinging nettles | Urtica dioica |

| Dosha | Low Dose | High Dose |
|---|---|---|
| Vata | 1 of each X2 per day before meals | 2 of each X2 per day before meals |
| Pitta | 1 of each X2 per day with meals | 2 of each X2 per day with meals |
| Kapha | 2 of each X2 per day after meals | 3 of each X2 per day after meals |

## Description:

Respiratory allergies show a reduction in the immune functions of the body. The immune system is becoming tired and fails to make the correct decisions for removing pathogens. Instead of removing pathological factors the immunity begins to confuse normal substances (hair, dust, pollen, etc.) as a pathogen. This is a precursor stage to autoimmune disorders. Allergies should be treated as soon as possible and corrected; a failure to do so will allow the immunity to continue to malfunction and eventually it will begin to attack the body itself (autoimmune disorder).

In Ayurveda, the main cause of respiratory allergies is due to having Ama in the system. The Ama needs to be removed and the body cleaned (Shodhana) and then the respiratory system should be rejuvenated (Rasayana). This is a Kapha Roga problem by location and a Vataja problem by function. Pitta can be a cause or implicated with there is inflammation in the lungs. All animal products, including dairy, should be removed from the diet. These herbal blends will clear and support correct immune function in the respiratory system. Treatment is best begun six months before Hay Fever season if the allergies are seasonal. Diet and lifestyle should follow Vikriti indications.

Use the Vataja herbs if Vata is predominant in the Vikriti (imbalance) with a Vata Vikriti diet / lifestyle.

Use the Pittaja herbs if Pitta is predominant in the Vikriti (imbalance) with a Pitta Vikriti diet / lifestyle.

Use the Kaphaja herbs if Kapha is predominant in the Vikriti (imbalance) with a Kapha Vikriti diet / lifestyle.

# Rheumatic pain

| Dosha | Code | Common Name | Latin Name |
|---|---|---|---|
| **Vataja** | 206 | Guduchi | Tinospora cordifolia |
| | 212 | Pau d'arco | Tabebuia impetiginosa |
| | 401 | Cumin | Cumimum cyminum |
| | | Fennel | Foeniculum vulgare |
| | | Cardamom | Elettaria cardamomum |
| | 404 | Angelica | Angelica archangelica |
| | | Wild yam | Dioscorea villosa |
| | | Valerian | Valeriana officinalis |
| | 407 | Turmeric | Curcuma longa |
| | | Barberry | Berberis vulgaris |
| | | Dandelion | Taraxacum officinale |
| **Pittaja** | 206 | Guduchi | Tinospora cordifolia |
| | 212 | Pau d'arco | Tabebuia impetiginosa |
| | 402 | Coriander | Coriandrum sativum |
| | | Cumin | Cumimum cyminum |
| | | Fennel | Foeniculum vulgare |
| | 405 | Burdock | Arctium lappa |
| | | Yellow dock | Rumex crispus |
| | | Milk Thistle | Silybum marianum |
| | 407 | Turmeric | Curcuma longa |
| | | Barberry | Berberis vulgaris |
| | | Dandelion | Taraxacum officinale |
| **Kaphaja** | 206 | Guduchi | Tinospora cordifolia |
| | 212 | Pau d'arco | Tabebuia impetiginosa |
| | 403 | Ginger | Zingiber officinale |
| | | Cumin | Cumimum cyminum |
| | | Fenugreek | Trigonella foenum-graecum |
| | 406 | Myrrh | Commiphora myrrha |
| | | Elecampane | Inula helenium |
| | | Yellow dock | Rumex crispus |
| | 407 | Turmeric | Curcuma longa |
| | | Barberry | Berberis vulgaris |
| | | Dandelion | Taraxacum officinale |

| Dosha | Low Dose | High Dose |
|---|---|---|
| **Vata** | 1 of each X2 per day before meals | 2 of each X2 per day before meals |
| **Pitta** | 1 of each X2 per day with meals | 2 of each X2 per day with meals |
| **Kapha** | 2 of each X2 per day after meals | 3 of each X2 per day after meals |

## Description:

See the description under Rheumatism.

Use the Vataja herbs if Vata is predominant in the Vikriti (imbalance) with a Vata Vikriti diet / lifestyle.

Use the Pittaja herbs if Pitta is predominant in the Vikriti (imbalance) with a Pitta Vikriti diet / lifestyle.

Use the Kaphaja herbs if Kapha is predominant in the Vikriti (imbalance) with a Kapha Vikriti diet / lifestyle.

## Rheumatism

| Dosha | Code | Common Name | Latin Name |
|---|---|---|---|
| **Vataja** | 206 | Guduchi | Tinospora cordifolia |
| | 212 | Pau d'arco | Tabebuia impetiginosa |
| | 401 | Cumin | Cumimum cyminum |
| | | Fennel | Foeniculum vulgare |
| | | Cardamom | Elettaria cardamomum |
| | 404 | Angelica | Angelica archangelica |
| | | Wild yam | Dioscorea villosa |
| | | Valerian | Valeriana officinalis |
| | 407 | Turmeric | Curcuma longa |
| | | Barberry | Berberis vulgaris |
| | | Dandelion | Taraxacum officinale |
| **Pittaja** | 206 | Guduchi | Tinospora cordifolia |
| | 212 | Pau d'arco | Tabebuia impetiginosa |
| | 402 | Coriander | Coriandrum sativum |
| | | Cumin | Cumimum cyminum |
| | | Fennel | Foeniculum vulgare |
| | 405 | Burdock | Arctium lappa |
| | | Yellow dock | Rumex crispus |
| | | Milk Thistle | Silybum marianum |
| | 407 | Turmeric | Curcuma longa |
| | | Barberry | Berberis vulgaris |
| | | Dandelion | Taraxacum officinale |
| **Kaphaja** | 206 | Guduchi | Tinospora cordifolia |
| | 212 | Pau d'arco | Tabebuia impetiginosa |
| | 403 | Ginger | Zingiber officinale |
| | | Cumin | Cumimum cyminum |
| | | Fenugreek | Trigonella foenum-graecum |
| | 406 | Myrrh | Commiphora myrrha |
| | | Elecampane | Inula helenium |
| | | Yellow dock | Rumex crispus |
| | 407 | Turmeric | Curcuma longa |
| | | Barberry | Berberis vulgaris |
| | | Dandelion | Taraxacum officinale |

| Dosha | Low Dose | High Dose |
|---|---|---|
| **Vata** | 1 of each X2 per day before meals | 2 of each X2 per day before meals |
| **Pitta** | 1 of each X2 per day with meals | 2 of each X2 per day with meals |
| **Kapha** | 2 of each X2 per day after meals | 3 of each X2 per day after meals |

## Description:

Rheumatism or rheumatic disorder is a non-specific term for medical problems affecting the joints, muscles and connective tissue. The study and therapeutic treatments for these disorders is called rheumatology. There are many reasons why a patient would manifest some form of Rheumatism. In Ayurveda, the main cause is Ama. Usually the main area of Ama accumulation is in Rasa Dhatu and Rakta Dhatu; in other words, the blood. Toxic blood is the main source of Ama building up in the joints, muscle and connective tissues. Hence the main treatment protocol is the removal of Ama from the body in general and from Rasa Dhatu and Rakta Dhatu specifically.

This is Pitta Roga by location (Rakta Dhatu) and can be caused by any of the three Doshas functionally. It is considered a Sama (with Ama) disorder and Agni is a main target in treatments. Following a diet to reduce Pitta is generally indicated, though it depends on which Dosha is causing the disorder.

Use the Vataja herbs if Vata is predominant in the Vikriti (imbalance) with a Vata Vikriti diet / lifestyle.

Use the Pittaja herbs if Pitta is predominant in the Vikriti (imbalance) with a Pitta Vikriti diet / lifestyle.

Use the Kaphaja herbs if Kapha is predominant in the Vikriti (imbalance) with a Kapha Vikriti diet / lifestyle.

## Rheumatoid arthritis

| Dosha | Code | Common Name | Latin Name |
|---|---|---|---|
| Vataja | 206 | Guduchi | Tinospora cordifolia |
| | 212 | Pau d'arco | Tabebuia impetiginosa |
| | 401 | Cumin | Cumimum cyminum |
| | | Fennel | Foeniculum vulgare |
| | | Cardamom | Elettaria cardamomum |
| | 404 | Angelica | Angelica archangelica |
| | | Wild yam | Dioscorea villosa |
| | | Valerian | Valeriana officinalis |
| | 407 | Turmeric | Curcuma longa |
| | | Barberry | Berberis vulgaris |
| | | Dandelion | Taraxacum officinale |
| Pittaja | 206 | Guduchi | Tinospora cordifolia |
| | 212 | Pau d'arco | Tabebuia impetiginosa |
| | 402 | Coriander | Coriandrum sativum |
| | | Cumin | Cumimum cyminum |
| | | Fennel | Foeniculum vulgare |
| | 405 | Burdock | Arctium lappa |
| | | Yellow dock | Rumex crispus |
| | | Milk Thistle | Silybum marianum |
| | 407 | Turmeric | Curcuma longa |
| | | Barberry | Berberis vulgaris |
| | | Dandelion | Taraxacum officinale |
| Kaphaja | 206 | Guduchi | Tinospora cordifolia |
| | 212 | Pau d'arco | Tabebuia impetiginosa |
| | 403 | Ginger | Zingiber officinale |
| | | Cumin | Cumimum cyminum |
| | | Fenugreek | Trigonella foenum-graecum |
| | 406 | Myrrh | Commiphora myrrha |
| | | Elecampane | Inula helenium |
| | | Yellow dock | Rumex crispus |
| | 407 | Turmeric | Curcuma longa |
| | | Barberry | Berberis vulgaris |
| | | Dandelion | Taraxacum officinale |

| Dosha | Low Dose | High Dose |
|---|---|---|
| Vata | 1 of each X2 per day before meals | 2 of each X2 per day before meals |
| Pitta | 1 of each X2 per day with meals | 2 of each X2 per day with meals |
| Kapha | 2 of each X2 per day after meals | 3 of each X2 per day after meals |

## Description:

Rheumatoid arthritis (RA) is considered to be an autoimmune form of Rheumatism and is a chronic, systemic inflammatory disorder that may affect many tissues and organs. Principally it attacks the joints producing an inflammatory synovitis that often progresses to destruction of the articular cartilage and ankylosis of the joints. Rheumatoid arthritis can also produce diffuse inflammation in the lungs, pericardium, pleura, and sclera, and also nodular lesions, most common in subcutaneous tissue under the skin. Although the cause of rheumatoid arthritis is unknown, autoimmunity plays a pivotal role in its chronicity and progression, hence its classification as an autoimmune disorder.

In Ayurveda, this is considered to be an Ama condition and the herbal blends work to remove Ama and increase immune function. The best treatment for RA in Ayurveda is Panchakarma. Diet and lifestyle are even more important than when treating normal Rheumatism because the disorder has now moved into the sixth stage of Kriya Kala (complications) and may be impossible to cure if the patient waits too long for treatment. With Panchakarma it is possible to stop the pathology, and depending when the patient starts treatment, cure the disorder.

Use the Vataja herbs if Vata is predominant in the Vikriti (imbalance) with a Vata Vikriti diet / lifestyle.

Use the Pittaja herbs if Pitta is predominant in the Vikriti (imbalance) with a Pitta Vikriti diet / lifestyle.

Use the Kaphaja herbs if Kapha is predominant in the Vikriti (imbalance) with a Kapha Vikriti diet / lifestyle.

## Sciatica

| Dosha | Code | Common Name | Latin Name |
|---|---|---|---|
| **Vataja** | 210 | Shankhpushpi | Convolvulus pluricaulis |
| | 410 | Passion flower | Passiflora incarnata |
| | | Skullcap | Scutellaria lateriflora |
| | | Gotu kola | Centella asiatica |
| | 301 | Amalaki | Emblica officinalis |
| | | Bibhitaki | Terminalia belerica |
| | | Haritaki | Terminalia chebula |
| **Pittaja** | 210 | Shankhpushpi | Convolvulus pluricaulis |
| | 410 | Passion flower | Passiflora incarnata |
| | | Skullcap | Scutellaria lateriflora |
| | | Gotu kola | Centella asiatica |
| | 301 | Amalaki | Emblica officinalis |
| | | Bibhitaki | Terminalia belerica |
| | | Haritaki | Terminalia chebula |
| **Kaphaja** | 210 | Shankhpushpi | Convolvulus pluricaulis |
| | 410 | Passion flower | Passiflora incarnata |
| | | Skullcap | Scutellaria lateriflora |
| | | Gotu kola | Centella asiatica |
| | 301 | Amalaki | Emblica officinalis |
| | | Bibhitaki | Terminalia belerica |
| | | Haritaki | Terminalia chebula |

| Dosha | Low Dose | High Dose |
|---|---|---|
| **Vata** | 1 of each X2 per day before meals | 2 of each X2 per day before meals |
| **Pitta** | 1 of each X2 per day with meals | 2 of each X2 per day with meals |
| **Kapha** | 2 of each X2 per day after meals | 3 of each X2 per day after meals |

## Description:

Sciatica is a term that describes symptoms of pain, numbness that radiate along the sciatic nerve from the lower back to the buttocks and leg. The vast majority of sciatica symptoms result from lower back disorders between the L4 and S1 levels that put pressure on, or cause irritation to, a lumbar nerve root.

In Ayurveda, this is a Kapha Roga disorder by structure (Majja Dhatu) and a Vataja problem by function (Majjavaha Srota). Vata can also be implicated structurally (Asthi Dhatu) if the cause is due to damage of the vertebra or intervertebral disks. When this occurs, the disorder can be classified as Vata Roga.

Treatment is mainly external with applications of oil and heat (Snehana and Svedhana). Mild Yoga asana are helpful once mobility has improved and to maintain the health of the lower back. These herbal blends help to support a normal function of Vata Dosha and restore correct movement in Majjavaha Srota. They will tend to accelerate healing of the nerve and bone tissues by balancing Vata. These blends do not work on the structure of Majja Dhatu.

Use the Vataja herbs if Vata is predominant in the Vikriti (imbalance) with a Vata Vikriti diet / lifestyle.

Use the Pittaja herbs if Pitta is predominant in the Vikriti (imbalance) with a Pitta Vikriti diet / lifestyle.

Use the Kaphaja herbs if Kapha is predominant in the Vikriti (imbalance) with a Kapha Vikriti diet / lifestyle.

## Senility (dementia)

| Dosha | Code | Common Name | Latin Name |
|---|---|---|---|
| **Vataja** | 203 | Ashwagandha | Withania somnifera |
| | 204 | Bramhi | Bacopa monnieri |
| | 211 | Shatavari | Asparagus racemosus |
| | 301 | Amalaki | Emblica officinalis |
| | | Bibhitaki | Terminalia belerica |
| | | Haritaki | Terminalia chebula |
| **Pittaja** | 203 | Ashwagandha | Withania somnifera |
| | 204 | Bramhi | Bacopa monnieri |
| | 211 | Shatavari | Asparagus racemosus |
| | 301 | Amalaki | Emblica officinalis |
| | | Bibhitaki | Terminalia belerica |
| | | Haritaki | Terminalia chebula |
| **Kaphaja** | 203 | Ashwagandha | Withania somnifera |
| | 204 | Bramhi | Bacopa monnieri |
| | 211 | Shatavari | Asparagus racemosus |
| | 301 | Amalaki | Emblica officinalis |
| | | Bibhitaki | Terminalia belerica |
| | | Haritaki | Terminalia chebula |

| Dosha | Low Dose | High Dose |
|---|---|---|
| **Vata** | 1 of each X2 per day before meals | 2 of each X2 per day before meals |
| **Pitta** | 1 of each X2 per day with meals | 2 of each X2 per day with meals |
| **Kapha** | 2 of each X2 per day after meals | 3 of each X2 per day after meals |

## Description:

Senility originally meant old age, and then became related with the physical decline associated with old age. Now the mental decline once associated with old age is known as dementia. This is a Vata Roga issue that is best treated years before old age. The Caraka Samhita says all humans should begin to take rejuvenating herbs from the age of forty onward to avoid problems in the seventies and eighties.

These herbal blends are classical Rasayana compounds to support Ojas and slow down the aging process. It is possible to start taking them at any age, however, once senility has started they work more to stabilize the decline rather than curing it. It is never too late to try. These herbs are Vata reducing and symptomatic in nature, therefore there is no difference between constitutional types. However, diet and lifestyle need to be modified accordingly, first by

Vikriti and then by age in order for these blends to help the patient. Remember that daily exercise is the single most important factor as we age. Daily practice of Pranayama is very important to support the mind and nervous system. Daily Abhyanga and Snehana Nasya treatments are also advised.

Use the Vataja herbs if Vata is predominant in the Vikriti (imbalance) with a Vata Vikriti diet / lifestyle.

Use the Pittaja herbs if Pitta is predominant in the Vikriti (imbalance) with a Pitta Vikriti diet / lifestyle.

Use the Kaphaja herbs if Kapha is predominant in the Vikriti (imbalance) with a Kapha Vikriti diet / lifestyle.

## Sexual debility

| Dosha | Code | Common Name | Latin Name |
|---|---|---|---|
| Vataja | 203 | Ashwagandha | Withania somnifera |
| | 207 | Haritaki | Terminalia chebula |
| | 211 | Shatavari | Asparagus racemosus |
| | 401 | Cumin | Cumimum cyminum |
| | | Fennel | Foeniculum vulgare |
| | | Cardamom | Elettaria cardamomum |
| Pittaja | 203 | Ashwagandha | Withania somnifera |
| | 207 | Haritaki | Terminalia chebula |
| | 211 | Shatavari | Asparagus racemosus |
| | 402 | Coriander | Coriandrum sativum |
| | | Cumin | Cumimum cyminum |
| | | Fennel | Foeniculum vulgare |
| Kaphaja | 203 | Ashwagandha | Withania somnifera |
| | 207 | Haritaki | Terminalia chebula |
| | 211 | Shatavari | Asparagus racemosus |
| | 403 | Ginger | Zingiber officinale |
| | | Cumin | Cumimum cyminum |
| | | Fenugreek | Trigonella foenum-graecum |

| Dosha | Low Dose | High Dose |
|---|---|---|
| Vata | 1 of each X2 per day before meals | 2 of each X2 per day before meals |
| Pitta | 1 of each X2 per day with meals | 2 of each X2 per day with meals |
| Kapha | 2 of each X2 per day after meals | 3 of each X2 per day after meals |

## Description:
These are herbal blends that support Shukra Dhatu and are classified as Vajikarana in Ayurveda. See the description under infertility for more information.

Use the Vataja herbs if Vata is predominant in the Vikriti (imbalance) with a Vata Vikriti diet / lifestyle.

Use the Pittaja herbs if Pitta is predominant in the Vikriti (imbalance) with a Pitta Vikriti diet / lifestyle.

Use the Kaphaja herbs if Kapha is predominant in the Vikriti (imbalance) with a Kapha Vikriti diet / lifestyle.

## Shingles (herpes zoster)

| Dosha | Code | Common Name | Latin Name |
|-------|------|-------------|------------|
| Vataja | 207 | Haritaki | Terminalia chebula |
| | 208 | Manjishta | Rubia cordifolia |
| | 212 | Pau d'arco | Tabebuia impetiginosa |
| | 401 | Cumin | Cumimum cyminum |
| | | Fennel | Foeniculum vulgare |
| | | Cardamom | Elettaria cardamomum |
| Pittaja | 207 | Haritaki | Terminalia chebula |
| | 208 | Manjishta | Rubia cordifolia |
| | 212 | Pau d'arco | Tabebuia impetiginosa |
| | 402 | Coriander | Coriandrum sativum |
| | | Cumin | Cumimum cyminum |
| | | Fennel | Foeniculum vulgare |
| Kaphaja | 207 | Haritaki | Terminalia chebula |
| | 208 | Manjishta | Rubia cordifolia |
| | 212 | Pau d'arco | Tabebuia impetiginosa |
| | 403 | Ginger | Zingiber officinale |
| | | Cumin | Cumimum cyminum |
| | | Fenugreek | Trigonella foenum-graecum |

| Dosha | Low Dose | High Dose |
|-------|----------|-----------|
| Vata | 1 of each X2 per day before meals | 2 of each X2 per day before meals |
| Pitta | 1 of each X2 per day with meals | 2 of each X2 per day with meals |
| Kapha | 2 of each X2 per day after meals | 3 of each X2 per day after meals |

## Description:

Shingles is a painful skin rash. It is caused by the Varicella Zoster Virus. It is also called herpes zoster. Shingles usually appears in a band, a strip, or a small area on one side of the face or body. The rash usually heals within two to four weeks although some people develop nerve pain that last much longer. It is common for Shingles to reoccur. This is a Pitta Roga problem cause by a viral pathogen. These herbal blends work to reduce inflammation and to support the immune system that will fight off the viral infection.

For an external treatment use *Melissa officinalis* (Lemon balm) directly on sores or the rashes. Make a strong infusion (4 g per 260 ml, or 1 cup of water) and apply directly on the skin as needed during the day, usually five to ten times a day is needed. Aloe Vera gel can also be used externally to sooth Shingles.

Diet and lifestyle should follow Vikriti indications. Stress is often a factor to trigger episodes of Shingles, so anti-stress therapies (Vata reducing therapies) may be needed in addition to normal lifestyle.

Use the Vataja herbs if Vata is predominant in the Vikriti (imbalance) with a Vata Vikriti diet / lifestyle.

Use the Pittaja herbs if Pitta is predominant in the Vikriti (imbalance) with a Pitta Vikriti diet / lifestyle.

Use the Kaphaja herbs if Kapha is predominant in the Vikriti (imbalance) with a Kapha Vikriti diet / lifestyle.

## Sinus congestion

| Dosha | Code | Common Name | Latin Name |
|---|---|---|---|
| **Vataja** | 405 | Burdock | Arctium lappa |
| | | Yellow dock | Rumex crispus |
| | | Milk Thistle | Silybum marianum |
| | 406 | Myrrh | Commiphora myrrha |
| | | Elecampane | Inula helenium |
| | | Yellow dock | Rumex crispus |
| | 401 | Cumin | Cumimum cyminum |
| | | Fennel | Foeniculum vulgare |
| | | Cardamom | Elettaria cardamomum |
| **Pittaja** | 405 | Burdock | Arctium lappa |
| | | Yellow dock | Rumex crispus |
| | | Milk Thistle | Silybum marianum |
| | 406 | Myrrh | Commiphora myrrha |
| | | Elecampane | Inula helenium |
| | | Yellow dock | Rumex crispus |
| | 402 | Coriander | Coriandrum sativum |
| | | Cumin | Cumimum cyminum |
| | | Fennel | Foeniculum vulgare |
| **Kaphaja** | 405 | Burdock | Arctium lappa |
| | | Yellow dock | Rumex crispus |
| | | Milk Thistle | Silybum marianum |
| | 406 | Myrrh | Commiphora myrrha |
| | | Elecampane | Inula helenium |
| | | Yellow dock | Rumex crispus |
| | 403 | Ginger | Zingiber officinale |
| | | Cumin | Cumimum cyminum |
| | | Fenugreek | Trigonella foenum-graecum |

| Dosha | Low Dose | High Dose |
|---|---|---|
| **Vata** | 1 of each X2 per day before meals | 2 of each X2 per day before meals |
| **Pitta** | 1 of each X2 per day with meals | 2 of each X2 per day with meals |
| **Kapha** | 2 of each X2 per day after meals | 3 of each X2 per day after meals |

## Description:

See the description for 'Colds'. Sinus congestion is a problem of Bodhaka Kapha and Rasa Dhatu so is classified as Kapha Roga. Sinus congestion may or may not be related to a Cold and usually does not include inflammation or infections (Pittaja issues); for inflammation see 'Sinusitis'. Diet and lifestyle should follow Vikriti.

These blends are very effective to reduce Ama and Kapha in both Rasa Dhatu and specifically the respiratory system. Both Avalambaka and Bodhaka Kapha are reduced and controlled by these blends which combine well with all of the other treatments of the respiratory system. This treatment can be followed by several months the "Low immunity" blends to strengthen the person.

Use the Vataja herbs if Vata is predominant in the Vikriti (imbalance) with a Vata Vikriti diet / lifestyle.

Use the Pittaja herbs if Pitta is predominant in the Vikriti (imbalance) with a Pitta Vikriti diet / lifestyle.

Use the Kaphaja herbs if Kapha is predominant in the Vikriti (imbalance) with a Kapha Vikriti diet / lifestyle.

## Sinusitis

| Dosha | Code | Common Name | Latin Name |
|---|---|---|---|
| **Vataja** | 405 | Burdock | Arctium lappa |
| | | Yellow dock | Rumex crispus |
| | | Milk Thistle | Silybum marianum |
| | 406 | Myrrh | Commiphora myrrha |
| | | Elecampane | Inula helenium |
| | | Yellow dock | Rumex crispus |
| | 401 | Cumin | Cumimum cyminum |
| | | Fennel | Foeniculum vulgare |
| | | Cardamom | Elettaria cardamomum |
| **Pittaja** | 405 | Burdock | Arctium lappa |
| | | Yellow dock | Rumex crispus |
| | | Milk Thistle | Silybum marianum |
| | 406 | Myrrh | Commiphora myrrha |
| | | Elecampane | Inula helenium |
| | | Yellow dock | Rumex crispus |
| | 402 | Coriander | Coriandrum sativum |
| | | Cumin | Cumimum cyminum |
| | | Fennel | Foeniculum vulgare |
| **Kaphaja** | 405 | Burdock | Arctium lappa |
| | | Yellow dock | Rumex crispus |
| | | Milk Thistle | Silybum marianum |
| | 406 | Myrrh | Commiphora myrrha |
| | | Elecampane | Inula helenium |
| | | Yellow dock | Rumex crispus |
| | 403 | Ginger | Zingiber officinale |
| | | Cumin | Cumimum cyminum |
| | | Fenugreek | Trigonella foenum-graecum |

| Dosha | Low Dose | High Dose |
|---|---|---|
| **Vata** | 1 of each X2 per day before meals | 2 of each X2 per day before meals |
| **Pitta** | 1 of each X2 per day with meals | 2 of each X2 per day with meals |
| **Kapha** | 2 of each X2 per day after meals | 3 of each X2 per day after meals |

## Description:

Ayurveda classifies Sinusitis as Kapha Roga by both location and function as it is an increase of Avalambaka and Bodhaka Kapha in Rasa Dhatu. Sinusitis is different than a cold because it is mixed with Pitta and manifests inflammation and irritation in the mucus membranes. There are a number of reasons behind Kapha increasing and becoming mixed with Pitta to provoke chronic sinus inflammation. Diet and lifestyle are the main causes. The excessive use of salt water to clean the sinus (*Jala Neti*) can also cause this condition. This method is safe when used correctly, but salt is drying and irritating to the mucus membranes and increases both Vata and Pitta in the sinus. It is done in Ayurveda specifically for Kapha problems, e.g., colds, congestion, mucus; or for Kapha Prakriti.

Rest with lots of fluids and avoiding Kapha increasing foods is the main treatment. Thyme (*Thymus vulgaris*) is the best single herb to use as it is antiviral and works to reduce both Vata and Kapha strongly. Thyme can be used as an infusion, inhalation, or both together. The inhalation of Thyme is an excellent treatment X2 to X3 per day when possible. If it is not available, then Eucalyptus leaves can be used instead for inhalations.

These blends are very effective to reduce Ama and Kapha in both Rasa Dhatu and specifically the respiratory system. Both Avalambaka and Bodhaka Kapha are reduced and controlled by these blends which combine well with all of the other treatments suggested above. This treatment can be followed by several months the 'Low immunity' blends to strengthen the person.

Use the Vataja herbs if Vata is predominant in the Vikriti (imbalance) with a Vata Vikriti diet / lifestyle.

Use the Pittaja herbs if Pitta is predominant in the Vikriti (imbalance) with a Pitta Vikriti diet / lifestyle.

Use the Kaphaja herbs if Kapha is predominant in the Vikriti (imbalance) with a Kapha Vikriti diet / lifestyle.

## Skin disorders

| Dosha | Code | Common Name | Latin Name |
|---|---|---|---|
| **Vataja** | 401 | Cumin | Cumimum cyminum |
| | | Fennel | Foeniculum vulgare |
| | | Cardamom | Elettaria cardamomum |
| | 404 | Angelica | Angelica archangelica |
| | | Wild yam | Dioscorea villosa |
| | | Valerian | Valeriana officinalis |
| | 407 | Turmeric | Curcuma longa |
| | | Barberry | Berberis vulgaris |
| | | Dandelion | Taraxacum officinale |
| | 410 | Passion flower | Passiflora incarnata |
| | | Skullcap | Scutellaria lateriflora |
| | | Gotu kola | Centella asiatica |
| **Pittaja** | 402 | Coriander | Coriandrum sativum |
| | | Cumin | Cumimum cyminum |
| | | Fennel | Foeniculum vulgare |
| | 405 | Burdock | Arctium lappa |
| | | Yellow dock | Rumex crispus |
| | | Milk Thistle | Silybum marianum |
| | 407 | Turmeric | Curcuma longa |
| | | Barberry | Berberis vulgaris |
| | | Dandelion | Taraxacum officinale |
| | 410 | Passion flower | Passiflora incarnata |
| | | Skullcap | Scutellaria lateriflora |
| | | Gotu kola | Centella asiatica |
| **Kaphaja** | 403 | Ginger | Zingiber officinale |
| | | Cumin | Cumimum cyminum |
| | | Fenugreek | Trigonella foenum-graecum |
| | 405 | Burdock | Arctium lappa |
| | | Yellow dock | Rumex crispus |
| | | Milk Thistle | Silybum marianum |
| | 407 | Turmeric | Curcuma longa |
| | | Barberry | Berberis vulgaris |
| | | Dandelion | Taraxacum officinale |
| | 410 | Passion flower | Passiflora incarnata |
| | | Skullcap | Scutellaria lateriflora |
| | | Gotu kola | Centella asiatica |

| Dosha | Low Dose | High Dose |
|-------|----------|-----------|
| Vata | 1 of each X2 per day before meals | 2 of each X2 per day before meals |
| Pitta | 1 of each X2 per day with meals | 2 of each X2 per day with meals |
| Kapha | 2 of each X2 per day after meals | 3 of each X2 per day after meals |

## Description:

Rasadhatu has a special relationship to the skin (*Tvaca*) and controls the top layer of the seven layers of the skin, called *Avabhasini* in Sanskrit; the other six layers are controlled by Mamsa Dhatu. Remembering that Rasa Dhatu includes blood plasma indicates that a poorly formed, or toxic Rasa Dhatu will cause the blood to become disturbed in some manner.

Through the same mechanism Rakta Dhatu is able to create a toxic or heat condition in the blood through hemoglobin. When this happens Rasa Dhatu, or blood plasma, gets affected and takes on the disorder of Rakta Dhatu. Hence, both Rasa and Rakta have the ability to affect each other and cause skin disorders because skin is part of Rasa. The skin is one of the first areas to become affected by any Dosha Vriddhi or Ama condition manifesting in either Rasa Dhatu or Rakta Dhatu.

Skin problems are often classified as Kapha Roga because of Rasa and Mamsa Dhatus. Inflammatory skin problems are usually classified as Pitta Roga and dry, flaky skin disorders are often classified as Vata Roga. Hence, classification tends to follow the functional causal Dosha as any Dosha can cause these types of disorders on the skin.

Treatment begins with diet and lifestyle as per Vikriti and then uses these herbal blends to control the causal Dosha and remove Ama.

Use the Vataja herbs if Vata is predominant in the Vikriti (imbalance) with a Vata Vikriti diet / lifestyle.

Use the Pittaja herbs if Pitta is predominant in the Vikriti (imbalance) with a Pitta Vikriti diet / lifestyle.

Use the Kaphaja herbs if Kapha is predominant in the Vikriti (imbalance) with a Kapha Vikriti diet / lifestyle.

## Skin inflammations

| Dosha | Code | Common Name | Latin Name |
|---|---|---|---|
| **Vataja** | 401 | Cumin | Cumimum cyminum |
| | | Fennel | Foeniculum vulgare |
| | | Cardamom | Elettaria cardamomum |
| | 404 | Angelica | Angelica archangelica |
| | | Wild yam | Dioscorea villosa |
| | | Valerian | Valeriana officinalis |
| | 407 | Turmeric | Curcuma longa |
| | | Barberry | Berberis vulgaris |
| | | Dandelion | Taraxacum officinale |
| | 410 | Passion flower | Passiflora incarnata |
| | | Skullcap | Scutellaria lateriflora |
| | | Gotu kola | Centella asiatica |
| **Pittaja** | 402 | Coriander | Coriandrum sativum |
| | | Cumin | Cumimum cyminum |
| | | Fennel | Foeniculum vulgare |
| | 405 | Burdock | Arctium lappa |
| | | Yellow dock | Rumex crispus |
| | | Milk Thistle | Silybum marianum |
| | 407 | Turmeric | Curcuma longa |
| | | Barberry | Berberis vulgaris |
| | | Dandelion | Taraxacum officinale |
| | 410 | Passion flower | Passiflora incarnata |
| | | Skullcap | Scutellaria lateriflora |
| | | Gotu kola | Centella asiatica |
| **Kaphaja** | 403 | Ginger | Zingiber officinale |
| | | Cumin | Cumimum cyminum |
| | | Fenugreek | Trigonella foenum-graecum |
| | 405 | Burdock | Arctium lappa |
| | | Yellow dock | Rumex crispus |
| | | Milk Thistle | Silybum marianum |
| | 407 | Turmeric | Curcuma longa |
| | | Barberry | Berberis vulgaris |
| | | Dandelion | Taraxacum officinale |
| | 410 | Passion flower | Passiflora incarnata |
| | | Skullcap | Scutellaria lateriflora |
| | | Gotu kola | Centella asiatica |

| Dosha | Low Dose | High Dose |
|-------|----------|-----------|
| **Vata** | 1 of each X2 per day before meals | 2 of each X2 per day before meals |
| **Pitta** | 1 of each X2 per day with meals | 2 of each X2 per day with meals |
| **Kapha** | 2 of each X2 per day after meals | 3 of each X2 per day after meals |

## Description:

These are Pitta Roga problems, see the description under 'Skin Disorders'.

Use the Vataja herbs if Vata is predominant in the Vikriti (imbalance) with a Vata Vikriti diet / lifestyle.

Use the Pittaja herbs if Pitta is predominant in the Vikriti (imbalance) with a Pitta Vikriti diet / lifestyle.

Use the Kaphaja herbs if Kapha is predominant in the Vikriti (imbalance) with a Kapha Vikriti diet / lifestyle.

## Sore breasts

| Dosha | Code | Common Name | Latin Name |
|---|---|---|---|
| **Vataja** | 211 | Shatavari | Asparagus racemosus |
| | 401 | Cumin | Cumimum cyminum |
| | | Fennel | Foeniculum vulgare |
| | | Cardamom | Elettaria cardamomum |
| | 404 | Angelica | Angelica archangelica |
| | | Wild yam | Dioscorea villosa |
| | | Valerian | Valeriana officinalis |
| | 408 | Vitex | Vitex agnus-castus |
| | | Black cohosh | Cimicifuga racemosa |
| | | Cramp bark | Viburnum opulus |
| **Pittaja** | 211 | Shatavari | Asparagus racemosus |
| | 402 | Coriander | Coriandrum sativum |
| | | Cumin | Cumimum cyminum |
| | | Fennel | Foeniculum vulgare |
| | 404 | Angelica | Angelica archangelica |
| | | Wild yam | Dioscorea villosa |
| | | Valerian | Valeriana officinalis |
| | 408 | Vitex | Vitex agnus-castus |
| | | Black cohosh | Cimicifuga racemosa |
| | | Cramp bark | Viburnum opulus |
| **Kaphaja** | 211 | Shatavari | Asparagus racemosus |
| | 403 | Ginger | Zingiber officinale |
| | | Cumin | Cumimum cyminum |
| | | Fenugreek | Trigonella foenum-graecum |
| | 404 | Angelica | Angelica archangelica |
| | | Wild yam | Dioscorea villosa |
| | | Valerian | Valeriana officinalis |
| | 408 | Vitex | Vitex agnus-castus |
| | | Black cohosh | Cimicifuga racemosa |
| | | Cramp bark | Viburnum opulus |

| Dosha | Low Dose | High Dose |
|---|---|---|
| **Vata** | 1 of each X2 per day before meals | 2 of each X2 per day before meals |
| **Pitta** | 1 of each X2 per day with meals | 2 of each X2 per day with meals |
| **Kapha** | 2 of each X2 per day after meals | 3 of each X2 per day after meals |

## Description:

Sore breasts are a common issue related to hormone cycles. In Ayurveda, this problem is usually associated with Kapha Prakriti women although it can happen to any type of person. Vata Dosha controls the functioning of the endocrine system and hormone levels. These herbal blends work to balance Vata and restore normal balance in the endocrine functions. It is a symptomatic approach using the same blend for each type of person. Other individual blends could also be used, for example, PMS blends. If the sore breasts occur during ovulation I suggest using the above blends. Diet and lifestyle should follow Vikriti indications.

Use the Vataja herbs if Vata is predominant in the Vikriti (imbalance) with a Vata Vikriti diet / lifestyle.
Use the Pittaja herbs if Pitta is predominant in the Vikriti (imbalance) with a Pitta Vikriti diet / lifestyle.
Use the Kaphaja herbs if Kapha is predominant in the Vikriti (imbalance) with a Kapha Vikriti diet / lifestyle.

## Spermatorrhea

| Dosha | Code | Common Name | Latin Name |
|---|---|---|---|
| **Vataja** | 203 | Ashwagandha | Withania somnifera |
| | 204 | Bramhi | Bacopa monnieri |
| | 205 | Gokshura | Tribulus terrestris |
| | 301 | Amalaki | Emblica officinalis |
| | | Bibhitaki | Terminalia belerica |
| | | Haritaki | Terminalia chebula |
| **Pittaja** | 203 | Ashwagandha | Withania somnifera |
| | 204 | Bramhi | Bacopa monnieri |
| | 205 | Gokshura | Tribulus terrestris |
| | 301 | Amalaki | Emblica officinalis |
| | | Bibhitaki | Terminalia belerica |
| | | Haritaki | Terminalia chebula |
| **Kaphaja** | 203 | Ashwagandha | Withania somnifera |
| | 204 | Bramhi | Bacopa monnieri |
| | 205 | Gokshura | Tribulus terrestris |
| | 301 | Amalaki | Emblica officinalis |
| | | Bibhitaki | Terminalia belerica |
| | | Haritaki | Terminalia chebula |

| Dosha | Low Dose | High Dose |
|---|---|---|
| **Vata** | 1 of each X2 per day before meals | 2 of each X2 per day before meals |
| **Pitta** | 1 of each X2 per day with meals | 2 of each X2 per day with meals |
| **Kapha** | 2 of each X2 per day after meals | 3 of each X2 per day after meals |

## Description:

Spermatorrhea is a condition of excessive, involuntary ejaculation caused by Vata Dosha (Apana and Prana Vayus). This herbal treatment is symptomatic for Apana Vayu and supports Shukra Dhatu.

Use the Vataja herbs if Vata is predominant in the Vikriti (imbalance) with a Vata Vikriti diet / lifestyle.

Use the Pittaja herbs if Pitta is predominant in the Vikriti (imbalance) with a Pitta Vikriti diet / lifestyle.

Use the Kaphaja herbs if Kapha is predominant in the Vikriti (imbalance) with a Kapha Vikriti diet / lifestyle.

## Staphylococcus (staph)

| Dosha | Code | Common Name | Latin Name |
|---|---|---|---|
| **Vataja** | 207 | Haritaki | Terminalia chebula |
| | 212 | Pau d'arco | Tabebuia impetiginosa |
| | 401 | Cumin | Cumimum cyminum |
| | | Fennel | Foeniculum vulgare |
| | | Cardamom | Elettaria cardamomum |
| | 407 | Turmeric | Curcuma longa |
| | | Barberry | Berberis vulgaris |
| | | Dandelion | Taraxacum officinale |
| **Pittaja** | 207 | Haritaki | Terminalia chebula |
| | 212 | Pau d'arco | Tabebuia impetiginosa |
| | 401 | Coriander | Coriandrum sativum |
| | | Cumin | Cumimum cyminum |
| | | Fennel | Foeniculum vulgare |
| | 407 | Turmeric | Curcuma longa |
| | | Barberry | Berberis vulgaris |
| | | Dandelion | Taraxacum officinale |
| **Kaphaja** | 207 | Haritaki | Terminalia chebula |
| | 212 | Pau d'arco | Tabebuia impetiginosa |
| | 401 | Ginger | Zingiber officinale |
| | | Cumin | Cumimum cyminum |
| | | Fenugreek | Trigonella foenum-graecum |
| | 407 | Turmeric | Curcuma longa |
| | | Barberry | Berberis vulgaris |
| | | Dandelion | Taraxacum officinale |

| Dosha | Low Dose | High Dose |
|---|---|---|
| **Vata** | 1 of each X2 per day before meals | 2 of each X2 per day before meals |
| **Pitta** | 1 of each X2 per day with meals | 2 of each X2 per day with meals |
| **Kapha** | 2 of each X2 per day after meals | 3 of each X2 per day after meals |

## Description:

Staphylococcus (also called 'staph') is a group of bacteria that can cause a multitude of diseases. Staph infections may cause disease due to direct infection or due to the production of toxins by the bacteria. Boils, impetigo, food poisoning, and toxic shock syndrome are all examples of diseases that can be caused by Staphylococcus.

Pathogenic infections tend to be classified by the Dhatu affected. Therefore, the Dosha controlling the Dhatu gets the name, e.g., Pitta Roga if Rakta Dhatu is implicated, Kapha Roga if Rasa Dhatu is implicated, etc. These herbal blends are a symptomatic treatment to reduce the staph infection and increase immune response to remove the bacteria. Diet and lifestyle should follow Vikriti.

Use the Vataja herbs if Vata is predominant in the Vikriti (imbalance) with a Vata Vikriti diet / lifestyle.

Use the Pittaja herbs if Pitta is predominant in the Vikriti (imbalance) with a Pitta Vikriti diet / lifestyle.

Use the Kaphaja herbs if Kapha is predominant in the Vikriti (imbalance) with a Kapha Vikriti diet / lifestyle.

## Stomach cramps

| Dosha | Code | Common Name | Latin Name |
|-------|------|-------------|------------|
| Vataja | 207 | Haritaki | Terminalia chebula |
| | 401 | Cumin | Cumimum cyminum |
| | | Fennel | Foeniculum vulgare |
| | | Cardamom | Elettaria cardamomum |
| | 404 | Angelica | Angelica archangelica |
| | | Wild yam | Dioscorea villosa |
| | | Valerian | Valeriana officinalis |
| Pittaja | 201 | Amalaki | Emblica officinalis |
| | 402 | Coriander | Coriandrum sativum |
| | | Cumin | Cumimum cyminum |
| | | Fennel | Foeniculum vulgare |
| | 407 | Turmeric | Curcuma longa |
| | | Barberry | Berberis vulgaris |
| | | Dandelion | Taraxacum officinale |
| Kaphaja | 207 | Haritaki | Terminalia chebula |
| | 403 | Ginger | Zingiber officinale |
| | | Cumin | Cumimum cyminum |
| | | Fenugreek | Trigonella foenum-graecum |
| | 407 | Turmeric | Curcuma longa |
| | | Barberry | Berberis vulgaris |
| | | Dandelion | Taraxacum officinale |

| Dosha | Low Dose | High Dose |
|-------|----------|-----------|
| Vata | 1 of each X2 per day before meals | 2 of each X2 per day before meals |
| Pitta | 1 of each X2 per day with meals | 2 of each X2 per day with meals |
| Kapha | 2 of each X2 per day after meals | 3 of each X2 per day after meals |

## Description:

Stomach cramps are the symptom of some underlying problem. The cause should be diagnosed and corrected. Cramping and abdominal pain are Vataja and can be triggered by typical causes such as: food poisoning, intestinal gas, indigestion, infections, and inflammatory type bowel disease. For mild, occasional cramping or abdominal pain these herbal blends can be used. Any Dosha is able to aggravate Agni and Samana Vayu causing cramping and distention in the stomach and intestines. Treatment should target the causal Dosha and just Vata. Diet and lifestyle should follow the Vikriti indications in the test as well.

Use the Vataja herbs if Vata is predominant in the Vikriti (imbalance) with a Vata Vikriti diet / lifestyle.

Use the Pittaja herbs if Pitta is predominant in the Vikriti (imbalance) with a Pitta Vikriti diet / lifestyle.

Use the Kaphaja herbs if Kapha is predominant in the Vikriti (imbalance) with a Kapha Vikriti diet / lifestyle.

## Stress

| Dosha | Code | Common Name | Latin Name |
|---|---|---|---|
| **Vataja** | 204 | Bramhi | Bacopa monnieri |
| | 210 | Shankhpushpi | Convolvulus pluricaulis |
| | 401 | Cumin | Cumimum cyminum |
| | | Fennel | Foeniculum vulgare |
| | | Cardamom | Elettaria cardamomum |
| | 410 | Passion flower | Passiflora incarnata |
| | | Skullcap | Scutellaria lateriflora |
| | | Gotu kola | Centella asiatica |
| **Pittaja** | 204 | Bramhi | Bacopa monnieri |
| | 210 | Shankhpushpi | Convolvulus pluricaulis |
| | 402 | Coriander | Coriandrum sativum |
| | | Cumin | Cumimum cyminum |
| | | Fennel | Foeniculum vulgare |
| | 410 | Passion flower | Passiflora incarnata |
| | | Skullcap | Scutellaria lateriflora |
| | | Gotu kola | Centella asiatica |
| **Kaphaja** | 204 | Bramhi | Bacopa monnieri |
| | 210 | Shankhpushpi | Convolvulus pluricaulis |
| | 403 | Ginger | Zingiber officinale |
| | | Cumin | Cumimum cyminum |
| | | Fenugreek | Trigonella foenum-graecum |
| | 410 | Passion flower | Passiflora incarnata |
| | | Skullcap | Scutellaria lateriflora |
| | | Gotu kola | Centella asiatica |

| Dosha | Low Dose | High Dose |
|---|---|---|
| **Vata** | 1 of each X2 per day before meals | 2 of each X2 per day before meals |
| **Pitta** | 1 of each X2 per day with meals | 2 of each X2 per day with meals |
| **Kapha** | 2 of each X2 per day after meals | 3 of each X2 per day after meals |

## Description:

The death rate due to stress-related illness is alarming today. Emotional stress is considered to be a major contributing factor to the six leading causes of death in the United States: cancer, coronary heart disease, accidental injuries, respiratory disorders, cirrhosis of the liver and suicide (National Institutes of Health, 2008, USA).

Stress can be classified as Vata Roga by function. These herbal blends work mainly on the movement of Vata in the mind with the nervous system as a secondary target (Majja Dhatu). If the nervous system is the main problem due to weak Majja Dhatu or Ama in the Majjavahasrota use the description under 'Nervous disorders' instead of these blends. Anxiety is the result of stress factors and is a normal human response. When stress becomes chronic it needs to be treated and the cause removed. Prolonged stress weakens Majja Dhatu and Majjavaha Srota. These blends should be used for a minimum of two months and up to twelve months.

If there is no clear pathology or symptomology for the patient, then use these blends according to Prakriti. Lifestyle therapies are extremely important. Ayurvedic therapies such as Nadishodhana pranayama, yoga asana, mild exercise and relaxation are needed daily.

NOTE: These blends are CONTRAINDICATED with anti-depressant or antianxiety medications as they may reduce the effectiveness of the treatment.

Use the Vataja herbs if Vata is predominant in the Prakriti with a Vata Prakriti diet / lifestyle.

Use the Pittaja herbs if Pitta is predominant in the Prakriti with a Pitta Prakriti diet / lifestyle.

Use the Kaphaja herbs if Kapha is predominant in the Prakriti with a Kapha Prakriti diet / lifestyle.

## Thrombosis

| Dosha | Code | Common Name | Latin Name |
|-------|------|-------------|------------|
| **Vataja** | 208 | Manjishta | Rubia cordifolia |
| | 401 | Cumin | Cumimum cyminum |
| | | Fennel | Foeniculum vulgare |
| | | Cardamom | Elettaria cardamomum |
| | 404 | Angelica | Angelica archangelica |
| | | Wild yam | Dioscorea villosa |
| | | Valerian | Valeriana officinalis |
| | 407 | Turmeric | Curcuma longa |
| | | Barberry | Berberis vulgaris |
| | | Dandelion | Taraxacum officinale |
| **Pittaja** | 208 | Manjishta | Rubia cordifolia |
| | 402 | Coriander | Coriandrum sativum |
| | | Cumin | Cumimum cyminum |
| | | Fennel | Foeniculum vulgare |
| | 405 | Burdock | Arctium lappa |
| | | Yellow dock | Rumex crispus |
| | | Milk Thistle | Silybum marianum |
| | 407 | Turmeric | Curcuma longa |
| | | Barberry | Berberis vulgaris |
| | | Dandelion | Taraxacum officinale |
| **Kaphaja** | 208 | Manjishta | Rubia cordifolia |
| | 403 | Ginger | Zingiber officinale |
| | | Cumin | Cumimum cyminum |
| | | Fenugreek | Trigonella foenum-graecum |
| | 407 | Turmeric | Curcuma longa |
| | | Barberry | Berberis vulgaris |
| | | Dandelion | Taraxacum officinale |

| Dosha | Low Dose | High Dose |
|-------|----------|-----------|
| **Vata** | 1 of each X2 per day before meals | 2 of each X2 per day before meals |
| **Pitta** | 1 of each X2 per day with meals | 2 of each X2 per day with meals |
| **Kapha** | 2 of each X2 per day after meals | 3 of each X2 per day after meals |

## Description:

Thrombosis is the formation of a blood clot inside a blood vessel, obstructing the flow of blood through the circulatory system. Thrombosis is a serious condition because blood clots in the veins can break loose, travel through the bloodstream and lodge in the lungs, blocking blood flow and cause pulmonary embolism, heart attacks and strokes, all of which are life threatening.

Thrombosis is a combination of Vata and Pitta. I have written out a full explanation of this disorder and the various sub-types in Vol. 5 of my textbooks for those practitioners who need more information. According to the sub-type either Vata or Pitta can be the casual factor behind the disorder. These herbal blends are for Deep Vein Thrombosis (DVT). As this can be a life-threating disorder it is important to know what the cause is and remove it. DVT is typically a Vata Roga problem due to excess dryness in the blood – Vata moving into Raktavaha Srota and causing dryness. Vata can also move in the wrong way in this Srota causing further complications.

Diet is very important and should follow Vikriti diets as per the test or diagnosis. Lifestyle should follow a Vata Vikriti plan for everyone in order to control the movement of Vata Dosha. This would include mild exercise, daily Nadishodhana pranayama, regularity in meals and sleeping, and finally, reduced or eliminated travel by airplanes.

NOTE: These blends are CONTRAINDICATED with blood thinners or anticoagulants such as warfarin (e.g., Coumadin, Jantoven, Marevan, Uniwarfin) and fluindione (Previscan).

Use the Vataja herbs if Vata is predominant in the Vikriti (imbalance) with a Vata Vikriti diet and lifestyle.

Use the Pittaja herbs if Pitta is predominant in the Vikriti (imbalance) with a Pitta Vikriti diet and Vata Vikriti lifestyle.

Use the Kaphaja herbs if Kapha is predominant in the Vikriti (imbalance) with a Kapha Vikriti diet and Vata Vikriti lifestyle.

For more information on Thrombosis disorders refer to: *Ayurvedic Medicine for Westerners, Application of Ayurvedic Treatments Throughout Life* (Volume 5), chapter 15

## Thyroid

| Dosha | Code | Common Name | Latin Name |
|-------|------|-------------|------------|
| **Vataja** | 203 | Ashwagandha | Withania somnifera |
| | 401 | Cumin | Cumimum cyminum |
| | | Fennel | Foeniculum vulgare |
| | | Cardamom | Elettaria cardamomum |
| | 407 | Turmeric | Curcuma longa |
| | | Barberry | Berberis vulgaris |
| | | Dandelion | Taraxacum officinale |
| | 410 | Passion flower | Passiflora incarnata |
| | | Skullcap | Scutellaria lateriflora |
| | | Gotu kola | Centella asiatica |
| **Pittaja** | 203 | Ashwagandha | Withania somnifera |
| | 402 | Coriander | Coriandrum sativum |
| | | Cumin | Cumimum cyminum |
| | | Fennel | Foeniculum vulgare |
| | 407 | Turmeric | Curcuma longa |
| | | Barberry | Berberis vulgaris |
| | | Dandelion | Taraxacum officinale |
| | 410 | Passion flower | Passiflora incarnata |
| | | Skullcap | Scutellaria lateriflora |
| | | Gotu kola | Centella asiatica |
| **Kaphaja** | 203 | Ashwagandha | Withania somnifera |
| | 403 | Ginger | Zingiber officinale |
| | | Cumin | Cumimum cyminum |
| | | Fenugreek | Trigonella foenum-graecum |
| | 407 | Turmeric | Curcuma longa |
| | | Barberry | Berberis vulgaris |
| | | Dandelion | Taraxacum officinale |
| | 410 | Passion flower | Passiflora incarnata |
| | | Skullcap | Scutellaria lateriflora |
| | | Gotu kola | Centella asiatica |

| Dosha | Low Dose | High Dose |
|-------|----------|-----------|
| **Vata** | 1 of each X2 per day before meals | 2 of each X2 per day before meals |
| **Pitta** | 1 of each X2 per day with meals | 2 of each X2 per day with meals |
| **Kapha** | 2 of each X2 per day after meals | 3 of each X2 per day after meals |

## Description:

According to Ayurveda the thyroid is located in the sixth tissue level or Majja Dhatu. Majja is controlled by Kapha Dosha. Additionally, in

Ayurveda the thyroid function is controlled by Pitta Dosha. Pitta is responsible for all of the metabolic actions carried out by the thyroid gland. Vata Dosha allows the movement and functioning of both Kapha and Pitta. Therefore, all three Doshas can cause thyroid diseases; Kapha by controlling the structure, Pitta by controlling the function, and Vata by controlling both Kapha and Pitta. Hypothyroidism is considered to be a Munda Agni problem of the Majja Dhatu Agni and Hyperthyroidism is considered to a Tikshna Agni problem of Majja Dhatu. Obviously Kapha would cause Munda Agni and Hypothyroidism and Pitta would cause Tikshna Agni and Hyperthyroidism. Vata Vriddhi could cause either of these by disrupting the function of Kapha or Pitta and fluctuating between hypo and hyper conditions as in Hashimoto's disease.

These herbal blends and advice are to regulate thyroid function in the beginning stages of thyroid imbalance. The main problem with all thyroid disorders is the Dhatu Agni. Therefore, diet should be controlled and the main digestive Agni stabilized. This will stabilize the Dhatu Agni and help all thyroid conditions. Lifestyle should support the diet as per Vikriti. For a full explanation and treatment options of all thyroid problems see the note below.

Use the Vataja herbs if Vata is predominant in the Vikriti (imbalance) with a Vata Vikriti diet / lifestyle.

Use the Pittaja herbs if Pitta is predominant in the Vikriti (imbalance) with a Pitta Vikriti diet / lifestyle.

Use the Kaphaja herbs if Kapha is predominant in the Vikriti (imbalance) with a Kapha Vikriti diet / lifestyle.

For more information on Thyroid disorders and more specific herbal formulas refer to: *Ayurvedic Medicine for Westerners, Application of Ayurvedic Treatments Throughout Life* (Volume 5), chapter 10

## Tinnitus

| Dosha | Code | Common Name | Latin Name |
|-------|------|-------------|------------|
| Vataja | 203 | Ashwagandha | Withania somnifera |
| | 204 | Bramhi | Bacopa monnieri |
| | 401 | Cumin | Cumimum cyminum |
| | | Fennel | Foeniculum vulgare |
| | | Cardamom | Elettaria cardamomum |
| Pittaja | 203 | Ashwagandha | Withania somnifera |
| | 204 | Bramhi | Bacopa monnieri |
| | 402 | Coriander | Coriandrum sativum |
| | | Cumin | Cumimum cyminum |
| | | Fennel | Foeniculum vulgare |
| Kaphaja | 203 | Ashwagandha | Withania somnifera |
| | 204 | Bramhi | Bacopa monnieri |
| | 403 | Ginger | Zingiber officinale |
| | | Cumin | Cumimum cyminum |
| | | Fenugreek | Trigonella foenum-graecum |

| Dosha | Low Dose | High Dose |
|-------|----------|-----------|
| Vata | 1 of each X2 per day before meals | 2 of each X2 per day before meals |
| Pitta | 1 of each X2 per day with meals | 2 of each X2 per day with meals |
| Kapha | 2 of each X2 per day after meals | 3 of each X2 per day after meals |

## Description:

Tinnitus is the perception of noise or ringing in the ears. It is a common problem and affects about one in five people. Tinnitus isn't considered to be a condition itself, rather it's a symptom of an underlying condition, such as age-related hearing loss, ear injury or a circulatory system disorder.

Ayurveda considers tinnitus to be a Vata Roga disorder, specifically of Prana Vayu. Treatment revolves around controlling the movement of Vata Dosha and Prana Vayu. Nadishodhana pranayama is the main treatment for the five sense organs and Prana Vayu. These herbal blends help both Vata and the brain (Majja Dhatu). Traditionally, Ayurveda treats the ears through the nose. These therapies are collectively called *Nasya* therapies and can range from simple to complex depending on the method and therapeutic goal. For this disorder Snehana Nasya is indicated. Take one or two drops of sesame oil (Vata or Kapha Vikriti) or Ghee (Pitta Vikriti) and put them in each nostril. Take several deep breaths to allow the oil to penetrate deeper into the sinus. For acute tinnitus, this Nasya should be done twice per day in the morning and evening.

These herbal blends work on controlling the movement of Prana Vayu and Vata Dosha in general. Diet should be followed as per Vikriti and lifestyle should follow a Vata reducing regime for all types to help control Prana Vayu.

Use the Vataja herbs if Vata is predominant in the Vikriti (imbalance) with a Vata Vikriti diet and Vata lifestyle.

Use the Pittaja herbs if Pitta is predominant in the Vikriti (imbalance) with a Pitta Vikriti diet and Vata lifestyle.

Use the Kaphaja herbs if Kapha is predominant in the Vikriti (imbalance) with a Kapha Vikriti diet and Vata lifestyle.

## Toxic blood

| Dosha | Code | Common Name | Latin Name |
|---|---|---|---|
| **Vataja** | 207 | Haritaki | Terminalia chebula |
| | 208 | Manjishta | Rubia cordifolia |
| | 403 | Ginger | Zingiber officinale |
| | | Cumin | Cumimum cyminum |
| | | Fenugreek | Trigonella foenum-graecum |
| **Pittaja** | 207 | Haritaki | Terminalia chebula |
| | 208 | Manjishta | Rubia cordifolia |
| | 402 | Coriander | Coriandrum sativum |
| | | Cumin | Cumimum cyminum |
| | | Fennel | Foeniculum vulgare |
| | 405 | Burdock | Arctium lappa |
| | | Yellow dock | Rumex crispus |
| | | Milk Thistle | Silybum marianum |
| **Kaphaja** | 207 | Haritaki | Terminalia chebula |
| | 208 | Manjishta | Rubia cordifolia |
| | 403 | Ginger | Zingiber officinale |
| | | Cumin | Cumimum cyminum |
| | | Fenugreek | Trigonella foenum-graecum |
| | 405 | Burdock | Arctium lappa |
| | | Yellow dock | Rumex crispus |
| | | Milk Thistle | Silybum marianum |

| Dosha | Low Dose | High Dose |
|---|---|---|
| **Vata** | 1 of each X2 per day before meals | 2 of each X2 per day before meals |
| **Pitta** | 1 of each X2 per day with meals | 2 of each X2 per day with meals |
| **Kapha** | 2 of each X2 per day after meals | 3 of each X2 per day after meals |

## Description:

Toxic blood means that Ama is in Raktavaha Srota. When Ama is in the blood it can cause many different kinds of disorders, such as skin problems, fatigue, headaches, etc. This is a Pitta Roga problem and the diet should be adjusted to reduce Pitta and Ama; this means following a Pitta reducing diet. These herbal blends work on gently removing Ama from Rasa and Rakta Dhatus. Because the liver is the Mulasthana of Rakta Dhatu these herbs also help to detoxify the liver and thereby assisting to clean the blood. Lifestyle should follow Vikriti dominance including regular exercise to help the body remove impurities in the blood.

Use the Vataja herbs if Vata is predominant in the Vikriti (imbalance) with a Pitta Vikriti diet and Vata lifestyle.

Use the Pittaja herbs if Pitta is predominant in the Vikriti (imbalance) with a Pitta Vikriti diet and lifestyle.

Use the Kaphaja herbs if Kapha is predominant in the Vikriti (imbalance) with a Pitta Vikriti diet and Kapha lifestyle.

## Tuberculosis

| Dosha | Code | Common Name | Latin Name |
|-------|------|-------------|------------|
| **Vataja** | 211 | Shatavari | Asparagus racemosus |
| | 212 | Pau d'arco | Tabebuia impetiginosa |
| | 401 | Cumin | Cumimum cyminum |
| | | Fennel | Foeniculum vulgare |
| | | Cardamom | Elettaria cardamomum |
| | 406 | Myrrh | Commiphora myrrha |
| | | Elecampane | Inula helenium |
| | | Yellow dock | Rumex crispus |
| **Pittaja** | 211 | Shatavari | Asparagus racemosus |
| | 212 | Pau d'arco | Tabebuia impetiginosa |
| | 402 | Coriander | Coriandrum sativum |
| | | Cumin | Cumimum cyminum |
| | | Fennel | Foeniculum vulgare |
| | 406 | Myrrh | Commiphora myrrha |
| | | Elecampane | Inula helenium |
| | | Yellow dock | Rumex crispus |
| **Kaphaja** | 212 | Pau d'arco | Tabebuia impetiginosa |
| | 403 | Ginger | Zingiber officinale |
| | | Cumin | Cumimum cyminum |
| | | Fenugreek | Trigonella foenum-graecum |
| | 406 | Myrrh | Commiphora myrrha |
| | | Elecampane | Inula helenium |
| | | Yellow dock | Rumex crispus |

| Dosha | Low Dose | High Dose |
|-------|----------|-----------|
| **Vata** | 1 of each X2 per day before meals | 2 of each X2 per day before meals |
| **Pitta** | 1 of each X2 per day with meals | 2 of each X2 per day with meals |
| **Kapha** | 2 of each X2 per day after meals | 3 of each X2 per day after meals |

## Description:

Tuberculosis (TB) is a widespread, and in many cases fatal, infectious disease caused by various strains of mycobacteria, usually *Mycobacterium tuberculosis*. Tuberculosis typically attacks the lungs, but can also affect other parts of the body. It is spread through the air when people who have an active TB infection cough, sneeze, or otherwise transmit respiratory fluids through the air. If left untreated it kills more than fifty percent of those infected. These kinds of infectious diseases are causing both inflammation (Pitta) and tissue depletion (Vata) symptoms. Any Dosha can create an Ama environment favorable for these mycobacteria to take hold in the body. Main causes can be dietary, bad food combinations, low immunity, or chronic fatigue. The treatment for Tuberculosis is a bit different than most lung disorders as it is a life-threatening disease. Also, it is strongly reducing the tissues and literally consumes the Dhatus (hence the old name 'consumption').

These herbal blends will work in mild cases of TB, or will help patients to recover after TB has been treated with antibiotics. When treated early these herbs may be enough to stop the pathology. Diet and lifestyle should follow Vikriti.

Use the Vataja herbs if Vata is predominant in the Vikriti (imbalance) with a Vata Vikriti diet / lifestyle.

Use the Pittaja herbs if Pitta is predominant in the Vikriti (imbalance) with a Pitta Vikriti diet / lifestyle.

Use the Kaphaja herbs if Kapha is predominant in the Vikriti (imbalance) with a Kapha Vikriti diet / lifestyle.

## Tumors

| Dosha | Code | Common Name | Latin Name |
|---|---|---|---|
| Vataja | 204 | Bramhi | Bacopa monnieri |
| | 208 | Manjishta | Rubia cordifolia |
| | 212 | Pau d'arco | Tabebuia impetiginosa |
| | 401 | Cumin | Cumimum cyminum |
| | | Fennel | Foeniculum vulgare |
| | | Cardamom | Elettaria cardamomum |
| Pittaja | 204 | Bramhi | Bacopa monnieri |
| | 208 | Manjishta | Rubia cordifolia |
| | 212 | Pau d'arco | Tabebuia impetiginosa |
| | 402 | Coriander | Coriandrum sativum |
| | | Cumin | Cumimum cyminum |
| | | Fennel | Foeniculum vulgare |
| Kaphaja | 204 | Bramhi | Bacopa monnieri |
| | 208 | Manjishta | Rubia cordifolia |
| | 212 | Pau d'arco | Tabebuia impetiginosa |
| | 403 | Ginger | Zingiber officinale |
| | | Cumin | Cumimum cyminum |
| | | Fenugreek | Trigonella foenum-graecum |
| | 406 | Myrrh | Commiphora myrrha |
| | | Elecampane | Inula helenium |
| | | Yellow dock | Rumex crispus |

| Dosha | Low Dose | High Dose |
|---|---|---|
| Vata | 1 of each X2 per day before meals | 2 of each X2 per day before meals |
| Pitta | 1 of each X2 per day with meals | 2 of each X2 per day with meals |
| Kapha | 2 of each X2 per day after meals | 3 of each X2 per day after meals |

## Description:

In general, benign tumors should be treated like cysts, as there is little difference from the Ayurvedic point of view. Accumulation or congestion is Kapha in nature and can be caused by Kapha itself or by a constriction of Vata or Pitta. Thus, tumors are classified as Kapha Roga disorders.

What determines the treatment is the location (Dhatu) and system (Srota) involved. If the system is related to Vata treat Vata primarily. If the system is a Kapha system, treat Kapha first. Pitta must always be considered because of the digestive relationship and the control it exerts on Agni.

Remember that in Ayurvedic pathology cysts and tumors start forming in the fourth stage of 'relocation' or *Sthana Samsraya*. The progression of disease is called *Kriyakala*, or the six stages of disease manifestation (see Chapter Two, *Ayurvedic Medicine for Westerners, Vol. 2, Pathology and Diagnosis in Ayurveda*). The Srotamsi, as the systems of communication and transportation, are greatly affected in this stage of the disease process. They are transporting the excess Dosha, Ama and Mala and so become weakened and abnormal in their function.

Reducing or balancing Kapha is the most important factor in treatment after understanding the cause and the location (Dhatu). Perhaps the next most important step is to eliminate all processed and manufactured foods from the diet. This includes all forms of pre-made drinks such as colas. All dairy products are laced with estrogenic hormones, antibiotics and are contraindicated for functional cysts and tumors. All meats are also contraindicated for the same reasons. A Vegan diet that balances Kapha and Pitta is the right approach according to Ayurveda. A low protein diet will also help. Lifestyle should follow Vikriti of the patient.

Use the Vataja herbs if Vata is predominant in the Vikriti (imbalance) with a Vata Vikriti diet / lifestyle.

Use the Pittaja herbs if Pitta is predominant in the Vikriti (imbalance) with a Pitta Vikriti diet / lifestyle.

Use the Kaphaja herbs if Kapha is predominant in the Vikriti (imbalance) with a Kapha Vikriti diet / lifestyle.

## Ulcers

| Dosha | Code | Common Name | Latin Name |
|-------|------|-------------|------------|
| **Vataja** | 201 | Amalaki | Emblica officinalis |
|  | 211 | Shatavari | Asparagus racemosus |
|  | 401 | Cumin | Cumimum cyminum |
|  |  | Fennel | Foeniculum vulgare |
|  |  | Cardamom | Elettaria cardamomum |
|  | 404 | Angelica | Angelica archangelica |
|  |  | Wild yam | Dioscorea villosa |
|  |  | Valerian | Valeriana officinalis |
| **Pittaja** | 201 | Amalaki | Emblica officinalis |
|  | 211 | Shatavari | Asparagus racemosus |
|  | 402 | Coriander | Coriandrum sativum |
|  |  | Cumin | Cumimum cyminum |
|  |  | Fennel | Foeniculum vulgare |
|  | 405 | Burdock | Arctium lappa |
|  |  | Yellow dock | Rumex crispus |
|  |  | Milk Thistle | Silybum marianum |
| **Kaphaja** | 201 | Amalaki | Emblica officinalis |
|  | 211 | Shatavari | Asparagus racemosus |
|  | 402 | Coriander | Coriandrum sativum |
|  |  | Cumin | Cumimum cyminum |
|  |  | Fennel | Foeniculum vulgare |
|  | 404 | Angelica | Angelica archangelica |
|  |  | Wild yam | Dioscorea villosa |
|  |  | Valerian | Valeriana officinalis |

| Dosha | Low Dose | High Dose |
|-------|----------|-----------|
| **Vata** | 1 of each X2 per day before meals | 2 of each X2 per day before meals |
| **Pitta** | 1 of each X2 per day with meals | 2 of each X2 per day with meals |
| **Kapha** | 2 of each X2 per day after meals | 3 of each X2 per day after meals |

## Description:

These herbal blends can be used for the treatment of peptic ulcers or oral ulcers; e.g., aphthous ulcers (canker sores), and cold sores (fever blisters). This is a Pitta Roga condition that can be caused from stress (Vata), emotions (Kapha) or Pitta (frustration) Vriddhi. Thus, it is important to diagnose correctly which Dosha is causing the problem. These blends reduce Pitta and heal the mucous membrane. See the description under 'Peptic ulcer'.

Use the Vataja herbs if Vata is predominant in the Vikriti (imbalance) with a Vata Vikriti diet / lifestyle.

Use the Pittaja herbs if Pitta is predominant in the Vikriti (imbalance) with a Pitta Vikriti diet / lifestyle.

Use the Kaphaja herbs if Kapha is predominant in the Vikriti (imbalance) with a Kapha Vikriti diet / lifestyle.

## Ulcers of the mouth

| Dosha | Code | Common Name | Latin Name |
|---|---|---|---|
| Vataja | 201 | Amalaki | Emblica officinalis |
| | 208 | Manjishta | Rubia cordifolia |
| | 401 | Cumin | Cumimum cyminum |
| | | Fennel | Foeniculum vulgare |
| | | Cardamom | Elettaria cardamomum |
| Pittaja | 201 | Amalaki | Emblica officinalis |
| | 208 | Manjishta | Rubia cordifolia |
| | 402 | Coriander | Coriandrum sativum |
| | | Cumin | Cumimum cyminum |
| | | Fennel | Foeniculum vulgare |
| | 405 | Burdock | Arctium lappa |
| | | Yellow dock | Rumex crispus |
| | | Milk Thistle | Silybum marianum |
| Kaphaja | 201 | Amalaki | Emblica officinalis |
| | 208 | Manjishta | Rubia cordifolia |
| | 403 | Ginger | Zingiber officinale |
| | | Cumin | Cumimum cyminum |
| | | Fenugreek | Trigonella foenum-graecum |

| Dosha | Low Dose | High Dose |
|---|---|---|
| Vata | 1 of each X2 per day before meals | 2 of each X2 per day before meals |
| Pitta | 1 of each X2 per day with meals | 2 of each X2 per day with meals |
| Kapha | 2 of each X2 per day after meals | 3 of each X2 per day after meals |

## Description:

See the description under 'Ulcer'. These blends are specific for oral ulcers; e.g., aphthous ulcers (canker sores), and cold sores (fever blisters).

Use the Vataja herbs if Vata is predominant in the Vikriti (imbalance) with a Vata Vikriti diet / lifestyle.

Use the Pittaja herbs if Pitta is predominant in the Vikriti (imbalance) with a Pitta Vikriti diet / lifestyle.

Use the Kaphaja herbs if Kapha is predominant in the Vikriti (imbalance) with a Kapha Vikriti diet / lifestyle.

## Urinary disorders

| Dosha | Code | Common Name | Latin Name |
|---|---|---|---|
| **Vataja** | 205 | Gokshura | Tribulus terrestris |
| | 402 | Coriander | Coriandrum sativum |
| | | Cumin | Cumimum cyminum |
| | | Fennel | Foeniculum vulgare |
| | 405 | Burdock | Arctium lappa |
| | | Yellow dock | Rumex crispus |
| | | Milk Thistle | Silybum marianum |
| | 409 | Marshmallow | Althaea officinalis |
| | | Gotu kola | Centella asiatica |
| | | Stinging nettles | Urtica dioica |
| **Pittaja** | 205 | Gokshura | Tribulus terrestris |
| | 402 | Coriander | Coriandrum sativum |
| | | Cumin | Cumimum cyminum |
| | | Fennel | Foeniculum vulgare |
| | 405 | Burdock | Arctium lappa |
| | | Yellow dock | Rumex crispus |
| | | Milk Thistle | Silybum marianum |
| | 409 | Marshmallow | Althaea officinalis |
| | | Gotu kola | Centella asiatica |
| | | Stinging nettles | Urtica dioica |
| **Kaphaja** | 205 | Gokshura | Tribulus terrestris |
| | 209 | Punarnava | Boerhaavia diffusa |
| | 402 | Coriander | Coriandrum sativum |
| | | Cumin | Cumimum cyminum |
| | | Fennel | Foeniculum vulgare |
| | 405 | Burdock | Arctium lappa |
| | | Yellow dock | Rumex crispus |
| | | Milk Thistle | Silybum marianum |

| Dosha | Low Dose | High Dose |
|---|---|---|
| **Vata** | 1 of each X2 per day before meals | 2 of each X2 per day before meals |
| **Pitta** | 1 of each X2 per day with meals | 2 of each X2 per day with meals |
| **Kapha** | 2 of each X2 per day after meals | 3 of each X2 per day after meals |

## Description:

These herbal blends can be used as a tonic for the whole urinary system including urethra, bladder and kidneys (Mutravaha Srota). One of the main reasons why the urinary system becomes weak is due to inflammatory conditions. Very often inflammation is caused from an imbalance in the colon or an excessive amount of Ama in the colon. Either one will create a bacterial imbalance in the flora that will affect the bladder by proximity. Other causes are poor hygiene, excessive sex, not drinking enough liquids or drinking too much alcohol. For women, vaginal flora should also be monitored. This is a classic Pitta Roga problem that often plagues Pitta Prakriti people.

Functionally any Dosha can cause this problem as the Dosha disrupts the function of Agni and then Ama is created. The main cause of urinary tract weakness is Ama or Mala according to Ayurveda. One common form of Mala in the body is uric acid; it is known to weaken the urinary system in excess. Structurally the whole urinary system is under the control of Kapha Dosha. Thus, we often see Kapha implicated in the disorders of this system.

If this system is weak it is best to stop eating all animal products for some months to clear and remove uric acid from the tissues. A vegan diet is best to use for this purpose. Drinking water and herbal teas instead of chemical drinks such as sodas is important. It is advised to stop drinking coffee and black or green tea as well during treatment.

Use the Vataja herbs if Vata is predominant in the Vikriti (imbalance) with a Vata Vikriti diet / lifestyle.

Use the Pittaja herbs if Pitta is predominant in the Vikriti (imbalance) with a Pitta Vikriti diet / lifestyle.

Use the Kaphaja herbs if Kapha is predominant in the Vikriti (imbalance) with a Kapha Vikriti diet / lifestyle.

## Uterine fibroids

| Dosha | Code | Common Name | Latin Name |
|---|---|---|---|
| **Vataja** | 401 | Cumin | Cumimum cyminum |
| | | Fennel | Foeniculum vulgare |
| | | Cardamom | Elettaria cardamomum |
| | 404 | Angelica | Angelica archangelica |
| | | Wild yam | Dioscorea villosa |
| | | Valerian | Valeriana officinalis |
| | 406 | Myrrh | Commiphora myrrha |
| | | Elecampane | Inula helenium |
| | | Yellow dock | Rumex crispus |
| | 407 | Turmeric | Curcuma longa |
| | | Barberry | Berberis vulgaris |
| | | Dandelion | Taraxacum officinale |
| | 408 | Vitex | Vitex agnus-castus |
| | | Black cohosh | Cimicifuga racemosa |
| | | Cramp bark | Viburnum opulus |
| **Pittaja** | 402 | Coriander | Coriandrum sativum |
| | | Cumin | Cumimum cyminum |
| | | Fennel | Foeniculum vulgare |
| | 405 | Burdock | Arctium lappa |
| | | Yellow dock | Rumex crispus |
| | | Milk Thistle | Silybum marianum |
| | 406 | Myrrh | Commiphora myrrha |
| | | Elecampane | Inula helenium |
| | | Yellow dock | Rumex crispus |
| | 407 | Turmeric | Curcuma longa |
| | | Barberry | Berberis vulgaris |
| | | Dandelion | Taraxacum officinale |
| | 408 | Vitex | Vitex agnus-castus |
| | | Black cohosh | Cimicifuga racemosa |
| | | Cramp bark | Viburnum opulus |
| **Kaphaja** | 403 | Ginger | Zingiber officinale |
| | | Cumin | Cumimum cyminum |
| | | Fenugreek | Trigonella foenum-graecum |
| | 406 | Myrrh | Commiphora myrrha |
| | | Elecampane | Inula helenium |
| | | Yellow dock | Rumex crispus |
| | 407 | Turmeric | Curcuma longa |
| | | Barberry | Berberis vulgaris |
| | | Dandelion | Taraxacum officinale |
| | 408 | Vitex | Vitex agnus-castus |

| | | Black cohosh | Cimicifuga racemosa |
|---|---|---|---|
| | | Cramp bark | Viburnum opulus |

| Dosha | Low Dose | High Dose |
|---|---|---|
| Vata | 1 of each X2 per day before meals | 2 of each X2 per day before meals |
| Pitta | 1 of each X2 per day with meals | 2 of each X2 per day with meals |
| Kapha | 2 of each X2 per day after meals | 3 of each X2 per day after meals |

## Description:

Fibroids are muscular tumors that grow in the wall of the uterus (womb). Another medical term for fibroids is leiomyoma or just myoma. Fibroids are almost always benign (non-cancerous). Fibroids can grow as a single tumor, or there can be many of them in the uterus. Fibroids are known to grow with increased estrogen and decrease with an increase of progesterone and are therefore called 'functional'. There is an obvious relation to endocrine function and external factors such as estrogenic chemicals in the food chain.

Fibroids are mainly classified as Pitta Roga because Pitta controls the uterus as part of Rakta Dhatu. Fibroids are usually associated with Vata Vriddhi, specifically Apana Vayu which causes the accumulation of Pitta or Kapha in the uterus. There is always a Kapha aspect to fibroids because of the increased growth due to estrogen. Functionally it is possible to say that fibroids are Kapha Roga because Kapha controls growth.

Reducing or balancing Vata is the most important factor in treatment after understanding the cause. Perhaps the next most important step is to eliminate all processed and manufactured foods from the diet. This includes all forms of pre-made drinks such as colas. All dairy products are laced with estrogenic hormones, antibiotics and are contraindicated for fibroids and tumors. All meats are also contraindicated for the same reasons. A Vegan diet that balances Kapha and Pitta is the right approach according to Ayurveda. A low protein diet will also help.

Use the Vataja herbs if Vata is predominant in the Vikriti (imbalance) with a Vata Vikriti diet / lifestyle.

Use the Pittaja herbs if Pitta is predominant in the Vikriti (imbalance) with a Pitta Vikriti diet / lifestyle.

Use the Kaphaja herbs if Kapha is predominant in the Vikriti (imbalance) with a Kapha Vikriti diet / lifestyle.

## Vaginitis

| Dosha | Code | Common Name | Latin Name |
|---|---|---|---|
| Vataja | 206 | Guduchi | Tinospora cordifolia |
| | 211 | Shatavari | Asparagus racemosus |
| | 301 | Amalaki | Emblica officinalis |
| | | Bibhitaki | Terminalia belerica |
| | | Haritaki | Terminalia chebula |
| | 401 | Cumin | Cumimum cyminum |
| | | Fennel | Foeniculum vulgare |
| | | Cardamom | Elettaria cardamomum |
| Pittaja | 206 | Guduchi | Tinospora cordifolia |
| | 211 | Shatavari | Asparagus racemosus |
| | 301 | Amalaki | Emblica officinalis |
| | | Bibhitaki | Terminalia belerica |
| | | Haritaki | Terminalia chebula |
| | 402 | Coriander | Coriandrum sativum |
| | | Cumin | Cumimum cyminum |
| | | Fennel | Foeniculum vulgare |
| Kaphaja | 206 | Guduchi | Tinospora cordifolia |
| | 211 | Shatavari | Asparagus racemosus |
| | 301 | Amalaki | Emblica officinalis |
| | | Bibhitaki | Terminalia belerica |
| | | Haritaki | Terminalia chebula |
| | 403 | Ginger | Zingiber officinale |
| | | Cumin | Cumimum cyminum |
| | | Fenugreek | Trigonella foenum-graecum |

| Dosha | Low Dose | High Dose |
|---|---|---|
| Vata | 1 of each X2 per day before meals | 2 of each X2 per day before meals |
| Pitta | 1 of each X2 per day with meals | 2 of each X2 per day with meals |
| Kapha | 2 of each X2 per day after meals | 3 of each X2 per day after meals |

## Description:

This is primarily a Vata Roga disturbance which can come from mental aggravation of the mind or any chronic Vata disturbance which moves into the uterus / vagina through Artavavaha Srota or Raktavaha Srota. It is important to address diet and lifestyle to lower Vata in general and to balance the digestion. As with all forms of Vata disorders it is highly advised to do Nadishodhana pranayama, oil Nasya and Abhyanga treatments daily or even twice a day to reduce and control Vata Dosha.

Creams are useful symptomatically and can be used alike for all constitutions. Use either Marigold / Calendula creams (*Calendula officinalis*) which are available from your herbalist or health food store. The Calendula cream can be used alone or it is possible to add 5 drops (each) of Golden Seal (*Hydrastis canadensis*) and Chamomile (*Chamaemelum nobile*) mother tinctures (MT) per teaspoon of cream. Mix and apply as needed. Never use essential oils on the skin or genitals, even diluted in oil bases.

Diet and stress are key factors. Often a change in diet will bring relief from reoccurring vaginitis. If burning is involved it means Bhrajaka and Ranjaka Pitta are involved. Also, stimulants such as coffee, tea, white sugar, alcohol and smoking should be stopped to aid the healing process. In general, a Vata reducing diet is usually helpful.

Use the Vataja herbs if Vata is predominant in the Vikriti (imbalance) with a Vata Vikriti diet / lifestyle.

Use the Pittaja herbs if Pitta is predominant in the Vikriti (imbalance) with a Pitta Vikriti diet / lifestyle.

Use the Kaphaja herbs if Kapha is predominant in the Vikriti (imbalance) with a Kapha Vikriti diet / lifestyle.

## Varicose veins

| Dosha | Code | Common Name | Latin Name |
|---|---|---|---|
| **Vataja** | 208 | Manjishta | Rubia cordifolia |
| | 401 | Cumin | Cumimum cyminum |
| | | Fennel | Foeniculum vulgare |
| | | Cardamom | Elettaria cardamomum |
| | 407 | Turmeric | Curcuma longa |
| | | Barberry | Berberis vulgaris |
| | | Dandelion | Taraxacum officinale |
| **Pittaja** | 208 | Manjishta | Rubia cordifolia |
| | 402 | Coriander | Coriandrum sativum |
| | | Cumin | Cumimum cyminum |
| | | Fennel | Foeniculum vulgare |
| | 405 | Burdock | Arctium lappa |
| | | Yellow dock | Rumex crispus |
| | | Milk Thistle | Silybum marianum |
| | 407 | Turmeric | Curcuma longa |
| | | Barberry | Berberis vulgaris |
| | | Dandelion | Taraxacum officinale |
| **Kaphaja** | 208 | Manjishta | Rubia cordifolia |
| | 403 | Ginger | Zingiber officinale |
| | | Cumin | Cumimum cyminum |
| | | Fenugreek | Trigonella foenum-graecum |
| | 406 | Myrrh | Commiphora myrrha |
| | | Elecampane | Inula helenium |
| | | Yellow dock | Rumex crispus |
| | 407 | Turmeric | Curcuma longa |
| | | Barberry | Berberis vulgaris |
| | | Dandelion | Taraxacum officinale |

| Dosha | Low Dose | High Dose |
|---|---|---|
| **Vata** | 1 of each X2 per day before meals | 2 of each X2 per day before meals |
| **Pitta** | 1 of each X2 per day with meals | 2 of each X2 per day with meals |
| **Kapha** | 2 of each X2 per day after meals | 3 of each X2 per day after meals |

## Description:

Varicose veins are gnarled, enlarged veins. Any vein may become varicose, but the veins most commonly affected are those in the legs and feet. That's because standing and walking upright increases the pressure in the veins of your lower body.

In Ayurveda, this problem is linked with Ama accumulation in blood and veins. As the veins become congested the veins move towards the surface of the body provoking Varicose veins. This process continues until the cause is removed. Agni should be balanced and Ama removed as well as reducing the causal Dosha. Diet and lifestyle are both important and should follow the Vikriti indications.

Use the Vataja herbs if Vata is predominant in the Vikriti (imbalance) with a Vata Vikriti diet / lifestyle.

Use the Pittaja herbs if Pitta is predominant in the Vikriti (imbalance) with a Pitta Vikriti diet / lifestyle.

Use the Kaphaja herbs if Kapha is predominant in the Vikriti (imbalance) with a Kapha Vikriti diet / lifestyle.

## Wasting diseases (cachexia)

| Dosha | Code | Common Name | Latin Name |
|---|---|---|---|
| Vataja | 203 | Ashwagandha | Withania somnifera |
| | 206 | Guduchi | Tinospora cordifolia |
| | 211 | Shatavari | Asparagus racemosus |
| | 301 | Amalaki | Emblica officinalis |
| | | Bibhitaki | Terminalia belerica |
| | | Haritaki | Terminalia chebula |
| Pittaja | 201 | Amalaki | Emblica officinalis |
| | 206 | Guduchi | Tinospora cordifolia |
| | 211 | Shatavari | Asparagus racemosus |
| | 301 | Amalaki | Emblica officinalis |
| | | Bibhitaki | Terminalia belerica |
| | | Haritaki | Terminalia chebula |
| Kaphaja | 203 | Ashwagandha | Withania somnifera |
| | 206 | Guduchi | Tinospora cordifolia |
| | 209 | Punarnava | Boerhaavia diffusa |
| | 301 | Amalaki | Emblica officinalis |
| | | Bibhitaki | Terminalia belerica |
| | | Haritaki | Terminalia chebula |

| Dosha | Low Dose | High Dose |
|---|---|---|
| Vata | 1 of each X2 per day before meals | 2 of each X2 per day before meals |
| Pitta | 1 of each X2 per day with meals | 2 of each X2 per day with meals |
| Kapha | 2 of each X2 per day after meals | 3 of each X2 per day after meals |

## Description:

Wasting syndrome is loss of weight, muscle atrophy, fatigue, weakness, and significant loss of appetite in someone who is not actively trying to lose weight. The formal definition of cachexia is the loss of body mass that cannot be reversed nutritionally. Even if the affected patient eats more calories, lean body mass will be lost, indicating a primary pathology is in place. Cachexia can be seen in patients with cancer, AIDS, chronic obstructive lung disease, multiple sclerosis, congestive heart failure, tuberculosis, familial amyloid polyneuropathy, mercury poisoning, heavy metal poisoning and hormonal deficiency.

In Ayurvedic medicine these kinds of disorders are related to poor lifestyle choices, poor diets and low immunity, or Ojas. Usually all Doshas are implicated in this kind of pathology, therefore it is advised to follow the Prakriti of the patient; if this is not known treat the dominate Dosha of Vikriti. These formulas can be used as a starting point for building immunity and increasing nutrient absorption in the intestines. These formulas build Ojas and Shukra Dhatu as per Prakriti.

Care needs to be given regarding Agni and Ama formation when using these formulas as they are Rasayana blends. It is best to begin with a low dose and work up to the higher dose over one month. These blends can be used when there is a small amount of Ama present on the tongue as there are enough digestives to help remove Ama. These blends are safe to use for several years, the minimum time for treatment would be three months.

Use the Vataja herbs if Vata is predominant in the Prakriti with a Vata Prakriti diet / lifestyle.

Use the Pittaja herbs if Pitta is predominant in the Prakriti with a Pitta Prakriti diet / lifestyle.

Use the Kaphaja herbs if Kapha is predominant in the Prakriti with a Kapha Prakriti diet / lifestyle.

## Water retention

| Dosha | Code | Common Name | Latin Name |
|---|---|---|---|
| **Vataja** | 204 | Bramhi | Bacopa monnieri |
| | 209 | Punarnava | Boerhaavia diffusa |
| | 403 | Ginger | Zingiber officinale |
| | | Cumin | Cumimum cyminum |
| | | Fenugreek | Trigonella foenum-graecum |
| | 409 | Marshmallow | Althaea officinalis |
| | | Gotu kola | Centella asiatica |
| | | Stinging nettles | Urtica dioica |
| **Pittaja** | 204 | Bramhi | Bacopa monnieri |
| | 209 | Punarnava | Boerhaavia diffusa |
| | 402 | Coriander | Coriandrum sativum |
| | | Cumin | Cumimum cyminum |
| | | Fennel | Foeniculum vulgare |
| | 409 | Marshmallow | Althaea officinalis |
| | | Gotu kola | Centella asiatica |
| | | Stinging nettles | Urtica dioica |
| **Kaphaja** | 204 | Bramhi | Bacopa monnieri |
| | 209 | Punarnava | Boerhaavia diffusa |
| | 403 | Ginger | Zingiber officinale |
| | | Cumin | Cumimum cyminum |
| | | Fenugreek | Trigonella foenum-graecum |
| | 409 | Marshmallow | Althaea officinalis |
| | | Gotu kola | Centella asiatica |
| | | Stinging nettles | Urtica dioica |

| Dosha | Low Dose | High Dose |
|---|---|---|
| **Vata** | 1 of each X2 per day before meals | 2 of each X2 per day before meals |
| **Pitta** | 1 of each X2 per day with meals | 2 of each X2 per day with meals |
| **Kapha** | 2 of each X2 per day after meals | 3 of each X2 per day after meals |

## Description:
See the description under Edema.

Use the Vataja herbs if Vata is predominant in the Vikriti (imbalance) with a Vata Vikriti diet / lifestyle.

Use the Pittaja herbs if Pitta is predominant in the Vikriti (imbalance) with a Pitta Vikriti diet / lifestyle.

Use the Kaphaja herbs if Kapha is predominant in the Vikriti (imbalance) with a Kapha Vikriti diet / lifestyle.

# Worms

| Dosha | Code | Common Name | Latin Name |
|-------|------|-------------|------------|
| Vataja | 209 | Punarnava | Boerhaavia diffusa |
| | 407 | Turmeric | Curcuma longa |
| | | Barberry | Berberis vulgaris |
| | | Dandelion | Taraxacum officinale |
| | 401 | Cumin | Cumimum cyminum |
| | | Fennel | Foeniculum vulgare |
| | | Cardamom | Elettaria cardamomum |
| Pittaja | 209 | Punarnava | Boerhaavia diffusa |
| | 407 | Turmeric | Curcuma longa |
| | | Barberry | Berberis vulgaris |
| | | Dandelion | Taraxacum officinale |
| | 402 | Coriander | Coriandrum sativum |
| | | Cumin | Cumimum cyminum |
| | | Fennel | Foeniculum vulgare |
| Kaphaja | 209 | Punarnava | Boerhaavia diffusa |
| | 407 | Turmeric | Curcuma longa |
| | | Barberry | Berberis vulgaris |
| | | Dandelion | Taraxacum officinale |
| | 403 | Ginger | Zingiber officinale |
| | | Cumin | Cumimum cyminum |
| | | Fenugreek | Trigonella foenum-graecum |

| Dosha | Low Dose | High Dose |
|-------|----------|-----------|
| Vata | 1 of each X2 per day before meals | 2 of each X2 per day before meals |
| Pitta | 1 of each X2 per day with meals | 2 of each X2 per day with meals |
| Kapha | 2 of each X2 per day after meals | 3 of each X2 per day after meals |

## Description:

Intestinal worms are caused by a group of parasitic worms, most commonly hookworm, roundworm (*ascariasis*) and whipworm (*trichuriasis*) that are either transmitted through contaminated soil or by ingesting parasite eggs. Direct person-to-person transmission of intestinal worm eggs is not needed, they mature in soil. Intestinal worms are therefore transmitted by parasite eggs that are passed in the feces of infected individuals through the soil.

While hookworm infection is primarily caused by walking barefoot on contaminated soil, both roundworm and whipworm infections are caused by ingesting infective parasitic eggs. Once inside the body, adult worms live in the intestines and produce thousands of eggs a day. Though symptoms vary, they include: anemia, malnutrition, vitamin A deficiency, swelling of the abdomen, weight loss, diarrhea, and inflammation of the intestines. Studies have shown that children infected with hookworm have a twenty-three percent drop in school attendance.

In North America worms are most common in children who eat earth, or in families that have poor hygiene. Adults can also get worms from poorly washed salads, or by contamination during travel in countries such as India.

These herbal blends are symptomatic to remove the parasites from the intestines. For very chronic infections these herbs may not be strong enough, in which case add 30 drops of Golden Seal (*Hydrastis canadensis*) mother tincture X3 per day in a little water. Treatment of these herbal blends should continue for one month after all symptoms have disappeared in order to kill any eggs left in the liver or intestines.

Use the Vataja herbs if Vata is predominant in the Vikriti (imbalance) with a Vata Vikriti diet / lifestyle.

Use the Pittaja herbs if Pitta is predominant in the Vikriti (imbalance) with a Pitta Vikriti diet / lifestyle.

Use the Kaphaja herbs if Kapha is predominant in the Vikriti (imbalance) with a Kapha Vikriti diet / lifestyle.

## Yeast infections (thrush)

| Dosha | Code | Common Name | Latin Name |
|---|---|---|---|
| Vataja | 211 | Shatavari | Asparagus racemosus |
| | 212 | Pau d'arco | Tabebuia impetiginosa |
| | 401 | Cumin | Cumimum cyminum |
| | | Fennel | Foeniculum vulgare |
| | | Cardamom | Elettaria cardamomum |
| | 407 | Turmeric | Curcuma longa |
| | | Barberry | Berberis vulgaris |
| | | Dandelion | Taraxacum officinale |
| Pittaja | 211 | Shatavari | Asparagus racemosus |
| | 212 | Pau d'arco | Tabebuia impetiginosa |
| | 402 | Coriander | Coriandrum sativum |
| | | Cumin | Cumimum cyminum |
| | | Fennel | Foeniculum vulgare |
| | 407 | Turmeric | Curcuma longa |
| | | Barberry | Berberis vulgaris |
| | | Dandelion | Taraxacum officinale |
| Kaphaja | 212 | Pau d'arco | Tabebuia impetiginosa |
| | 403 | Ginger | Zingiber officinale |
| | | Cumin | Cumimum cyminum |
| | | Fenugreek | Trigonella foenum-graecum |
| | 406 | Myrrh | Commiphora myrrha |
| | | Elecampane | Inula helenium |
| | | Yellow dock | Rumex crispus |
| | 407 | Turmeric | Curcuma longa |
| | | Barberry | Berberis vulgaris |
| | | Dandelion | Taraxacum officinale |

| Dosha | Low Dose | High Dose |
|---|---|---|
| Vata | 1 of each X2 per day before meals | 2 of each X2 per day before meals |
| Pitta | 1 of each X2 per day with meals | 2 of each X2 per day with meals |
| Kapha | 2 of each X2 per day after meals | 3 of each X2 per day after meals |

## Description:
These herbal blends can be used for all types of Yeast infections, Thrush, or Leucorrhea. This is basically Kapha Roga disorder that can be caused by Vata, Pitta or Kapha. Verify that there is not a chronic digestive problem. An imbalance in the colon will provoke leucorrhea; in other words, this is usually an Ama condition in the colon that causes an increase in bacteria, vaginal or intestinal. Often

chronic or reoccurring cases of thrush are due to an intestinal imbalance of the Candida yeasts that migrate to the vagina. This disrupts the vaginal flora and promotes the manifestation of vagina candida or thrush. If this is the case begin with herbal blends under 'Ama' to lower the Ama in the digestive system before beginning with this formula. Excessive sexual intercourse, or poor hygiene can also be a factor if there is no Ama present. These herbal blends can be used for a period of one to three months.

The diet should be changed to an anti-Ama diet appropriate for the Prakriti of the person. Coffee, carbonated drinks, alcohol and sugar should be removed from the diet as well as red meat. A vegan diet would be the best if possible. Lifestyle and diet should follow the Vikriti of the patient after the Anti-Ama diet has been completed.

Use the Vataja herbs if Vata is predominant in the Vikriti (imbalance) with a Vata Prakriti diet and Vikriti lifestyle.

Use the Pittaja herbs if Pitta is predominant in the Vikriti (imbalance) with a Pitta Prakriti diet and Vikriti lifestyle.

Use the Kaphaja herbs if Kapha is predominant in the Vikriti (imbalance) with a Kapha Prakriti diet and Vikriti lifestyle.

# Chapter Five
# Key to Disorders

Here is a quick reference guide in table form of all of the herbal blends used for each disorder listed in this book.

## KEY TO LIST OF DISEASES & FORMULAS

| Disorder | Vataja | Pittaja | Kaphaja |
|---|---|---|---|
| Abdominal distention | 401+407 | 402+407 | 403+407 |
| Abdominal pain | 404+301 | 405+301 | 405+301 |
| Acidity (heart burn) | 211+210+201 | 405+201 | 407+201 |
| Acne | 401+407+408 | 402+208+405 | 403+408+209 |
| Adrenal weakness | 301+409+205 | 402+409+208+205 | 403+409+209+208 |
| Agni (imbalanced) | 401+404 | 402+405 | 403+406 |
| AIDS | 301+203+206+212 | 301+201+206+212 | 301+206+209+212 |
| Alzheimer's | 301+203+206+211 | 301+203+206+208 | 301+203+206+209 |
| Ama | 401+407 | 402+407 | 403+407 |
| Amenorrhea (deficient) | 401+408+211 | 402+405+408+208 | 403+406+408+208 |
| Anemia | 301+404+209 | 301+405+208 | 301+406+209 |
| Angina | 401+202+203 | 402+202+208 | 403+202+209 |

| | | | |
|---|---|---|---|
| Anorexia | 401+404+211 | 402+201+211 | 403+203 |
| Anxiety | 207+210+404+410 | 402+410+204 | 403+410+204 |
| Aphrodisiac | 301+203+205+211 | 402+201+203+211 | 403+201+203+206 |
| Arteriosclerosis | 401+202+207 | 402+202+407 | 403+202+407 |
| Arthritis | 401+404+407 | 402+405+407 | 403+406+407 |
| Asthma | 401+410+210 | 402+410+201 | 403+406+209 |
| Atheroma | 301+202+404 | 301+202+405+407 | 301+202+209+407 |
| Atherosclerosis | 301+202+404 | 301+202+405+407 | 301+202+209+407 |
| Autoimmune disorders | 301+203+206+212 | 301+201+206+212 | 301+206+209+212 |
| Bacterial infections | 407+207 | 407+201 | 407+406 |
| Blood clots | 208+407+205+403 | 208+407+405+402 | 208+407+202+403 |
| Blood disorders | 301+208+404+407 | 301+208+405+407 | 301+208+406+407 |
| Boils | 208+212+407+404 | 208+212+407+405 | 208+212+407+406 |
| Brain tonic | 204+210+301 | 204+210+402+407 | 204+210+403+407 |
| Breast disorders | 401+407+408+211 | 402+405+407 | 403+406+407 |
| Bronchitis | 406+407+211 | 406+407+402 | 406+407+403 |
| Candida | 401+407+211+207 | 402+407+211+212 | 403+407+207+212 |
| Cardiac edema | 202+209+404 | 202+209+405 | 202+209+406 |
| Cardiovascular Disease (CVD) | 301+202+404 | 301+202+405+407 | 301+202+209+407 |
| Cholesterol | 301+202+404 | 301+202+405+407 | 301+202+209+407 |
| Chronic Fatigue Syndrome (CFS) | 301+203+206+212 | 301+201+206+212 | 301+206+209+212 |
| Cirrhosis | 401+407 | 402+405+407 | 403+407+208 |
| Colds | 405+406+401 | 405+406+402 | 405+406+403 |
| Colic | 401+404+207 | 402+407+201 | 403+407+207 |
| Colitis | 301+407+211 | 301+407+206 | 301+407+206 |

384

| | | | |
|---|---|---|---|
| Congestive heart disorders | 301+202+404 | 301+202+405+407 | 301+202+209+407 |
| Constipation | 301+207 | 301+407 | 403+207+406 |
| Convalescence | 301+203+206+211 | 301+201+206+211 | 301+206+209+212 |
| Convulsions | 210+204+401 | 210+204+402 | 210+204+403 |
| Coronary artery disorders | 301+202+404 | 301+202+405+407 | 301+202+209+407 |
| Cough | 403+406+407+409 | 403+406+407+402 | 403+406+407+209 |
| Cramps | 210+408+403 | 210+408+402 | 210+408+403 |
| Cystitis | 205+405+402+409 | 205+405+402+409 | 205+209+405+402 |
| Cysts | 401+406+407+408 | 402+405+407+408 | 403+406+407+408 |
| Debility | 301+203+206+212 | 301+201+206+212 | 301+206+209+212 |
| Deficiency / Wasting diseases | 301+203+206+211 | 301+201+206+211 | 301+203+206+209 |
| Dehydration | 401+409+211 | 402+409+211 | 403+409+211 |
| Delayed menstruation | 403+408+211 | 402+407+408+211 | 403+407+408+208 |
| Depression | 204+210+401+404 | 204+210+402+410 | 204+403+406+410 |
| Diabetes, type II | 205+208+407+401 | 205+208+407+402 | 205+208+407+403 |
| Diarrhea | 401+407+409 | 402+407+409 | 403+407+409 |
| Digestive problems | 301+401+407 | 402+407 | 403+407 |
| Digestive stimulant | 401+404 | 402+405 | 403+406 |
| Diverticulitis | 404+407+401+409 | 404+407+402+409 | 404+407+403 |
| Duodenal ulcers | 201+211+401+404 | 201+211+402+405 | 201+211+402+404 |
| Dysentery | 207+212+407+401 | 207+212+407+402 | 207+212+407+403 |
| Dysmenorrhea | 208+408+401+404 | 208+408+402+405 | 208+408+403+406 |
| Dyspepsia | 401+404+207 | 402+407+201 | 403+407+207 |
| Eczema | 407+410+401+404 | 407+410+402+405 | 407+410+403+405 |

| | | | |
|---|---|---|---|
| Edema | 209+409+205+401 | 209+409+205+402 | 209+406+403 |
| Emaciation | 203+211+301 | 203+211+301 | 203+211+301 |
| Endometriosis | 407+408+206+406+401 | 407+408+206+405+402 | 407+408+206+406+403 |
| Enlarged liver | 205+206+208+401 | 205+206+208+402 | 205+206+208+403 |
| Enlarged spleen | 205+206+208+401 | 205+206+208+402 | 205+206+208+403 |
| Epilepsy | 204+210+410+401 | 204+210+410+402 | 204+210+410+403 |
| Epstein bar | 206+212+401+404 | 206+212+402+407 | 206+212+403+407 |
| Eye disorders | 301 | 301 | 301 |
| Fatigue | 203+211+407+401 | 203+211+407+402 | 203+211+407+403 |
| Fever | 206+212+407+401+207 | 206+212+407+402+405 | 206+212+407+403+405 |
| Fertility Male | 203+205+211+401 | 203+205+211+402 | 203+205+211+403 |
| Fertility Female | 203+211+408+401+301 | 201+203+211+408+402 | 203+211+408+403+301 |
| Fibroids | 406+407+408+207+404 | 406+407+408+201+405 | 406+407+408+207 |
| Flatulence | 401+404+207 | 402+407+201 | 403+407+207 |
| Flu | 212+206+403 | 212+206+403 | 212+206+403 |
| Food allergies | 207+404+407+401+409 | 405+407+402 | 207+404+407+403 |
| Frequent urination | 409+401 | 409+402 | 409+403 |
| Frigidity | 203+211+408+401 | 201+203+211+408+402 | 203+207+211+408+403 |
| Fungal infections | 207+212+401+404 | 212+402 | 207+212+403 |
| Gall bladder stones | 208+405+401+404 | 208+405+402+407 | 208+405+403+407 |
| Gas | 401+404+207 | 402+407+201 | 403+407+207 |
| Gastric ulcers | 201+211+401+404 | 201+211+402+405 | 201+211+402+404 |
| Gastritis | 404+407+401+409 | 405+407+402+409 | 404+407+403 |

| | | | |
|---|---|---|---|
| General debility | 301+203+206+211 | 301+201+206+211 | 301+206+209+212 |
| Genital herpes | 207+208+212+401 | 207+208+212+402 | 207+208+212+403 |
| Glaucoma | 301+404 | 301+405 | 301+406 |
| Goiter | 203+206+401+404 | 203+206+402+405 | 203+206+403+406 |
| Gout | 207+208+401+404 | 201+208+402+405 | 207+208+403+406 |
| Hay fever | 212+409+401 | 212+407+402 | 212+209+403 |
| Headaches | 401+404+407 | 402+405+407 | 403+406+407 |
| Heartburn (acidity) | 211+210+201 | 405+201 | 407+201 |
| Hemorrhoids | 206+207+403+404 | 206+207+402+407 | 206+207+403+407 |
| Hepatitis | 206+207+407+401 | 206+207+407+402+405 | 206+207+407+403+405 |
| Herpes (I & II) | 207+208+212+401 | 207+208+212+402 | 207+208+212+403 |
| Hiatus hernia | 403+409 | 403+409 | 403+409 |
| High blood pressure | 401+202+203+210 | 402+405+202 | 403+405+407+202 |
| High blood sugar | 205+208+301+401 | 205+208+407+402 | 205+208+407+403 |
| High Kapha | 0 | 0 | 403+406+209 |
| High Pitta | 0 | 402+405+201 | 0 |
| High Vata | 401+404+207 | 0 | 0 |
| HIV | 301+203+206+212 | 301+201+206+212 | 301+206+209+212 |
| Hodgkin's disease | 203+206+212+401 | 203+206+212+402 | 203+206+212+403 |
| Hormonal deficiency | 407+408+409+401+404 | 407+408+409+402 | 407+408+409+403 |
| Hormone related headaches | 404+408+301 | 208+408+301 | 404+408+301 |
| Hot flashes | 211+408+409+401 | 211+408+409+402 | 408+409+403 |
| Hyperacidity | 211+210+201 | 405+201 | 406+201 |
| Hyperglycemia | 205+210+407+401 | 205+208+407+402 | 205+208+407+403 |

| Hypertension | 401+202+203+210 | 402+405+202 | 403+405+407+202 |
|---|---|---|---|
| Hypoglycemia | 401+404+407 | 402+405+407 | 403+405+407 |
| Hysteria | 204+210+401 | 204+210+402 | 204+210+403 |
| Impotence | 203+205+211+403 | 203+205+211+301 | 203+205+211+403 |
| Incontinence | 401+407+409 | 402+407+409 | 403+407+409 |
| Indigestion | 401+404+207 | 402+407+201 | 403+407+207 |
| Infection of urethra | 205+206+409 | 205+206+409 | 205+206+409 |
| Infertility Male | 203+205+211+401 | 203+205+211+402 | 203+205+211+403 |
| Infertility Female | 203+211+408+401+301 | 201+203+211+408+402 | 203+211+408+403+301 |
| Inflammation (intestines) | 201+206+407 | 201+206+407 | 201+206+407 |
| Inflammation (prostrate) | 205+407+409+401 | 205+407+409+402+405 | 205+407+409+403+406 |
| Inflammation (skin) | 405+407+409+401 | 405+407+409+402 | 405+407+409+403 |
| Inflammation (urinary system) | 205+405+402+409 | 205+405+402+409 | 205+209+405+402 |
| Insomnia | 210+410+401 | 210+410+402 | 210+410+403 |
| Irregular menstruation | 404+408+211+403 | 405+408+211+402 | 404+408+211+403 |
| Irritable bowel syndrome (IBS) | 404+407+401+409 | 404+407+402+409 | 404+407+403 |
| Kidney disorders | 205+407+409+401 | 205+407+409+402+208 | 205+407+409+403+208 |
| Kidney stones | 205+407+409+401 | 205+407+409+402+208 | 205+407+409+403+208 |
| Lactation (lack of) | 211+401 | 211+402 | 211+401 |
| Leucorrhea | 212+407+408+404+401 | 212+407+408+405+402 | 212+407+408+406+403 |
| Liver disorders | 206+207+407+401 | 206+207+407+402+405 | 206+207+407+403+405 |
| Low appetite | 401+404 | 402+405 | 403+406 |
| Low immunity | 301+203+206+211 | 301+201+206+211 | 301+203+206+209 |
| Low Ojas | 301+203+206+211 | 301+201+206+211 | 301+203+206+209 |

| | | | |
|---|---|---|---|
| Lumbago | 401+406+410 | 402+406+410 | 403+406+410 |
| Lung congestion | 403+406 | 402+406 | 403+406 |
| Lung disorders | 211+403+406 | 211+402+406 | 211+403+406 |
| Lupus | 207+208+212+ 401 | 207+208+212+ 402 | 207+208+212+ 403 |
| Lymphatic congestion | 401+405+407 | 402+405+407 | 403+405+407 |
| Malabsorption syndrome | 202+207+301 | 202+301 | 202+207+301 |
| Memory loss | 204 | 204 | 204 |
| Menopause | 211+408+401+ 404 | 208+211+408+ 402 | 211+408+403+ 404 |
| Menorrhagia | 202+407+401 | 202+407+402 | 202+407+403 |
| Menstrual cramps | 211+408+401+ 404 | 208+211+408+ 402 | 211+408+403+ 404 |
| Menstrual disorders | 208+211+408+ 404+401 | 208+211+408+ 402 | 202+208+404+ 408+403 |
| Mental debility | 204+210+410+ 401 | 204+210+410+ 402 | 204+210+410+ 403 |
| Migraines | 401+404+407 | 402+405+407 | 403+406+407 |
| Migrating joint pain | 404+408+401 | 404+408+402 | 404+408+403 |
| Multiple scleroses | 203+205+401+ 404 | 203+205+402+ 405 | 203+205+403+ 405 |
| Muscle cramps | 408+410+401 | 408+410+402 | 408+410+403 |
| Nausea | 401+404+207 | 402+407+201 | 403+407+207 |
| Nephritis | 209+407+409+ 401 | 205+407+409+ 402 | 209+407+409+ 403 |
| Nerve pain | 203+204+401+ 404 | 203+204+402+ 410 | 203+204+403+ 410 |
| Nervous disorders | 204+207+210+ 410+301 | 201+204+210+ 410+301 | 204+209+210+ 410+301 |
| Neuralgia | 203+204+401+ 404 | 203+204+402+ 410 | 203+204+403+ 410 |
| Obesity | 209+406+401+ 407 | 209+406+402+ 405 | 209+403+406+ 407 |
| Oedema (Edema) | 209+409+403 | 209+409+402 | 209+409+403 |
| Old age | 203+204+211+ 301 | 203+204+211+ 301 | 203+204+211+ 301 |
| Osteoarthritis | 401+404+407 | 402+405+407 | 403+406+407 |

| | | | |
|---|---|---|---|
| Osteoporosis | 203+207+401+404 | 203+207+402+405 | 203+207+403+404 |
| Overwork | 203+204+211+401 | 203+204+211+402 | 203+204+211+403 |
| Palpitations | 202+203+210+301 | 201+202+210+301 | 202+209+210+301 |
| Paralysis | 204+210+401 | 204+210+402 | 204+210+403 |
| Parkinson's disease | 203+204+211+301 | 203+204+211+301 | 203+204+211+301 |
| Peptic ulcers | 201+211+401+404 | 201+211+402+405 | 201+211+402+404 |
| Pleurisy | 406+211+403 | 406+211+402 | 406+211+403 |
| PMS | 404+408+211+403 | 404+408+211+402 | 404+408+211+403 |
| Pneumonia | 406+211+403 | 406+211+402 | 406+211+403 |
| Poisoning | 204+206+212+301 | 204+206+212+301 | 204+206+212+301 |
| Post-natal care | 211+301 | 211+301 | 211+301 |
| Premature ejaculation | 203+211+301+401 | 203+211+301+402 | 203+211+301+403 |
| Premenstrual disorders | 404+408+211+403 | 404+408+211+402 | 404+408+211+403 |
| Prostate disorders | 205+407+409+401 | 205+407+409+402+405 | 205+407+409+403+406 |
| Prostatitis | 205+407+409+401 | 205+407+409+402+405 | 205+407+409+403+406 |
| Psoriasis | 212+407+409+401+404 | 212+407+409+402+405 | 212+407+409+403+405 |
| Raynaud's disease | 206+403+407+404 | 206+403+407+405 | 206+403+407+406 |
| Reproductive disorders | 203+205+211+301 | 203+205+211+301 | 203+205+211+301 |
| Respiratory allergies | 212+409+401 | 212+409+402 | 212+409+403 |
| Rheumatic pain | 206+212+407+401+404 | 206+212+407+402+405 | 206+212+407+403+406 |
| Rheumatism | 206+212+407+401+404 | 206+212+407+402+405 | 206+212+407+403+406 |
| Rheumatoid arthritis | 206+212+407+401+404 | 206+212+407+402+405 | 206+212+407+403+406 |
| Sciatica | 210+410+301 | 210+410+301 | 210+410+301 |

| | | | |
|---|---|---|---|
| Senility | 203+204+211+301 | 203+204+211+301 | 203+204+211+301 |
| Sexual debility | 203+207+211+401 | 203+207+211+402 | 203+207+211+403 |
| Shingles | 207+208+212+401 | 207+208+212+402 | 207+208+212+403 |
| Sinus congestion | 405+406+401 | 405+406+402 | 405+406+403 |
| Sinusitis | 405+406+401 | 405+406+402 | 405+406+403 |
| Skin disorders | 407+410+401+404 | 407+410+402+405 | 407+410+403+405 |
| Skin inflammations | 407+410+401+404 | 407+410+402+405 | 407+410+403+405 |
| Sore breasts | 211+408+404+401 | 211+408+404+402 | 211+408+404+403 |
| Spermatorrhea | 203+204+205+301 | 203+204+205+301 | 203+204+205+301 |
| Staphylococcus | 207+211+401+407 | 207+211+402+407 | 207+211+403+407 |
| Stomach cramps | 401+404+207 | 402+407+201 | 403+407+207 |
| Stress | 204+210+410+401 | 204+210+410+402 | 204+210+410+403 |
| Thrombosis | 208+407+401+404 | 208+407+402+405 | 208+407+403 |
| Thyroid | 203+407+410+401 | 203+407+410+402 | 203+407+410+403 |
| Tinnitus | 203+204+401 | 203+204+402 | 203+204+403 |
| Toxic blood | 207+208+403 | 207+208+402+405 | 207+208+403+405 |
| Tuberculosis | 212+406+401+211 | 212+406+402+211 | 212+406+403 |
| Tumors | 204+208+212+401 | 204+208+212+402 | 204+208+212+403+406 |
| Ulcers | 201+211+401+404 | 201+211+402+405 | 201+211+402+404 |
| Ulcers of the mouth | 201+208+401 | 201+208+402+405 | 201+208+403 |
| Urinary disorders | 205+405+402+409 | 205+405+402+409 | 205+209+405+402 |
| Uterine fibroids | 406+407+408+401+404 | 406+407+408+402+405 | 406+407+408+403 |
| Vaginitis | 206+211+301+ | 206+211+301+ | 206+211+301+ |

|  | 401 | 402 | 403 |
|---|---|---|---|
| Varicose veins | 208+407+401 | 208+407+402+405 | 208+407+403+406 |
| Wasting / Deficiency diseases | 301+203+206+211 | 301+201+206+211 | 301+203+206+209 |
| Water retention | 209+204+409+403 | 209+204+409+402 | 209+204+409+403 |
| Worms | 209+407+401 | 209+407+402 | 209+407+403 |
| Yeast infections | 401+211+212+407 | 402+407+211+212 | 403+406+407+212 |

This section lists the ingredients for each product code by common name and Latin name.

**Code**
**Common name**     **Latin name**

## CODE 200

| | | |
|---|---|---|
| 201 | Amalaki | Emblica officinalis |
| 202 | Arjuna | Terminalia arjuna |
| 203 | Ashwagandha | Withania somnifera |
| 204 | Bramhi | Bacopa monnieri |
| 205 | Gokshura | Tribulus terrestris |
| 206 | Guduchi | Tinospora cordifolia |
| 207 | Haritaki | Terminalia chebula |
| 208 | Manjishta | Rubia cordifolia |
| 209 | Punarnava | Boerhaavia diffusa |
| 210 | Shankhpushpi | Convolvulus pluricaulis |
| 211 | Shatavari | Asparagus racemosus |
| 212 | Pau d'arco | Tabebuia impetiginosa |

## CODE 300

| | | |
|---|---|---|
| 301 | Triphala | |
| | Amalaki | Emblica officinalis |
| | Bibhitaki | Terminalia belerica |
| | Haritaki | Terminalia chebula |

## CODE 400

| | | |
|---|---|---|
| 401 | Cumin | Cumimum cyminum |
| | Fennel | Foeniculum vulgare |
| | Cardamom | Elettaria cardamomum |
| 402 | Coriander | Coriandrum sativum |
| | Cumin | Cumimum cyminum |
| | Fennel | Foeniculum vulgare |
| 403 | Ginger | Zingiber officinale |
| | Cumin | Cumimum cyminum |
| | Fenugreek | Trigonella foenum-graecum |
| 404 | Angelica | Angelica archangelica |
| | Wild yam | Dioscorea villosa |
| | Valerian | Valeriana officinalis |

405 Burdock        Arctium lappa
    Yellow dock    Rumex crispus
    Milk Thistle   Silybum marianum

406 Myrrh          Commiphora myrrha
    Elecampane     Inula helenium
    Yellow dock    Rumex crispus

407 Turmeric       Curcuma longa
    Barberry       Berberis vulgaris
    Dandelion      Taraxacum officinale

408 Vitex          Vitex agnus-castus
    Black cohosh   Cimicifuga racemosa
    Cramp bark     Viburnum opulus

409 Marshmallow    Althaea officinalis
    Gotu kola      Centella asiatica
    Stinging nettles Urtica dioica

410 Passion flower Passiflora incarnata
    Skullcap       Scutellaria lateriflora
    Gotu kola      Centella asiatica

# BIBLIOGRAPHY

## Bibliography of Classical Texts

*Astanga Hrdayam*, vols.; I - III, trans. Murthy, Prof. K.R. Srikantha, Varanasi, India; Krishnadas Academy, 3rd ed. 1996

*Astanga Samgraha*, vols.; I - III, trans. Murthy, Prof. K.R. Srikantha, Varanasi, India; Chaukhamba Orientalia, 8th ed. 2004

*Bhavaprakaśa*, vols.; I - II, trans. Murthy, Prof. K.R. Srikantha, Varanasi, India; Krishnadas Academy, 1998

*Caraka Samhita*, vols.; I - VII, trans. Dash, Vaidya Bhagwan & Sharma, Dr. R.K., Varanasi, India; Chowkhamba Series Office, 1992-2002.

*Caraka Samhita*, vols.; I - IV, trans. Sharma, Prof. P.V., Varanasi, India; Chowkhamba, 1987-2002.

*Madhava Nidanam*, trans. Murthy, Prof. K.R. Srikantha, Varanasi, India; Chaukhamba Orientalia, 4th ed. 2004

*Suśruta Samhita*, vols.; I - III, trans. K.K. Bhishagratna, Varanasi, India; Chaukhamba Sanskrit Pratishthan, 1998- 2002

## Bibliography

Chunekar, Prof. K.C., *Plants of the Bhāva Prakāśa*, New Delhi, India; National Academy of Āyurveda, 1999

_____, *Medicinal Plants of Suśruta Samhitā*, Varanasi, India; EIVS 2005

*Database on Medicinal Plants Used in Ayurveda*, vols.; I - VII, New Delhi, India, Central Council for Research in Ayurveda, Ministry of Health & Family Welfare, 2000.

Gogte, Vaidya V.M., *Ayurvedic Pharmacology*, Bombay, India; Bharatiya Vidya Bhāvan, 2000

Grieve, M., *A Modern Herbal*, London, UK; Tiger Books, 1931 (1994 ed.)

Kamat, Dr. S.D., *Dhanvantri-Nighantu*, Delhi, India; Chaukhamba Sanskrit Pratishthan, 2002

Pandey, Dr. Gyanendra, *Dravyaguna Vijñāna*, Varanasi, India; Krishnadas Academy, 3rd ed. 2002

Riggs BL, Melton LJ III. *Involutional osteoporosis*. N Engl J Med 1986; 314: 1676-84.

Smith, Vaidya Atreya, Ayurvedic Medicine for Westerners, Vol. 1; *Anatomy and Physiology in Ayurveda*, CreateSpace, 2013

_____, Ayurvedic Medicine for Westerners, Vol. 2; *Pathology & Diagnosis in Ayurveda*, CreateSpace, 2014

_____, Ayurvedic Medicine for Westerners, Vol. 3; *Clinical Protocols & Treatments in Ayurveda*, CreateSpace, 2015

_____, Ayurvedic Medicine for Westerners, Vol. 4; *Dravyaguna for Westerners*, CreateSpace, 2013

_____, Ayurvedic Medicine for Westerners, Vol. 5; *Application of Ayurvedic Treatments Throughout Life*, CreateSpace, 2016

*The Ayurvedic Pharmacopoeia of India*, vols.; I - V, New Delhi, India, Ministry of Health & Family Welfare, 2nd Edition 2001

*The Ayurvedic Formulary of India*, vols.; I-II, New Delhi, India, Ministry of Health & Family Welfare, 1st Edition 2000

# GLOSSARY

**Agni**: first of three cosmic principals; god of fire; digestive fire of which there are three classifications – Jathar Agni (1), Pancha Bhuta Agni (5) and the Dhatva Agni (7) – this makes 13 categories of Agni in the body, but as each cell has Agni there are over 37 trillion

**Allopathy**: western medicine, modern medicine

**Apana Vayu**: one of the five forms of Vata Dosha; the Vayu that controls all evacuation, called the downward breath; resides in the lower abdomen

**Aphrodisiac**: any substance that promotes health to the reproductive organs

**Ayurveda**: the part of the Vedas dealing with health; the science of life: longevity

**Caraka Samhita**: the oldest surviving text of Ayurveda

**Chit**: consciousness

**Constitution**: an individual's unique mix of the three Doshas or Prakriti

**Dosha**: Sanskrit for intelligent manager of the body; lit: 'that which stains'

**Dhatu:** tissue; there are seven different tissue levels in Ayurveda (Rasa, Rakta, Mamsa, Meda, Asthi, Majja, Shukra) - plasma, red blood cells, muscle, fat, bone, bone marrow and nerve tissue, and reproductive fluids

**Five elements**: see Five States of Matter

**Five States of Matter**: commonly called the Five Elements; the five states of matter are: mass, liquidity, transformation, movement, and the field in which they function; also called: earth, water, fire, air & ether

**Guna**: quality or attribute; there are three Maha Gunas: Sattva, Rajas, and Tamas; and there are twenty Gurvadi Gunas

**Kapha**: one of the three Doshas; controls water and earth elements; there are five sub-types: Tarpaka Kapha, Bodhaka Kapha, Kledaka Kapha, Avalambaka Kapha, Shleshaka Kapha

**Marma**: the acupressure and acupuncture points of Ayurveda

**Nadishodhana pranayama:** alternate breathing between two nostrils; see 'pranayama'

**Ojas**: there are two kinds, 1) the essence of food metabolized by the seen Dhatus; 2) humans are born with eight drops of Ojas in the heart; together they form the basis of basic vitality and the immune system by storing Prana; it is reputed to be white or golden in color

**Pitta**: one of the three Doshas; controls fire and water elements; there are five sub-types: Sadhaka Pitta, Alochaka Pitta, Pachaka Pitta, Ranjaka Pitta, Bhrajaka Pitta

**Prakriti**: the dynamic energy of consciousness; nature in general; as used in Ayurveda, the natal constitution

**Prana**: pra = before, ana = breath; the vital force; it arises from substratum of pure consciousness with intelligence, Agni, and love, together they create the individualized consciousness

**Prana Vayu:** chief of the five Pranas in the body, called the outward going breath, it resides in the head and the heart; one of the five forms of Vata Dosha

**Pranayama**: awareness of breath; method of breath observation used to regulate the mind, thereby the physical and mental health

**Purusha**: the inert aspect of consciousness; Sat Chit Ananda

**Rajas**: one of the three Maha Gunas; action, movement, bright, energy, aggression, aggravated mind, achievement, and strong emotions

**Rasa**: lit. taste, juice; first Dhatu

**Samana Vayu:** one of the five Pranas in the body; called the equalizing Prana it resides in the navel region; one of the five forms of Vata Dosha

**Sattva**: one of the three Maha Gunas; purity, peace, calm, beauty, happiness, quite obedient mind, and stable emotions

**Srotas or Srotamsi:** channels in the Ayurvedic system

**Sushruta Samhita:** one of the three ancient Ayurvedic texts of medicine

**Tamas**: one of the three Maha Gunas; inertia, dull, depressed, void, stupid, lazy, despair, and self-destructive emotions

**Udana Vayu**: one of the five Pranas in the body; called the upward moving breath, it is seated in the throat; one of the five forms of Vata Dosha

**Utvartana or Udvartana:** dry powder massage to stimulate the body and reduce Kapha Dosha

**Vikriti**: lit. that which covers Prakriti; pathology in the body

**Vata**: that which moves; one of the three Doshas; controls wind (air) and ether elements; there are five forms in the body, Prana, Apana, Samana, Udana and Vyana

**Vayu**: God of the Wind; another name for Vata; another name for Prana

**Vedas**: Literally it means knowledge, but used here to mean the Book of Knowledge, the oldest book in the world; there are four Vedas

**Vyana Vayu**: one of the five Pranas in the body; called the equalizing breath it unifies all the other Pranas and the body, it is defused throughout the body; one of the five forms of Vata Dosha

**Yoga**: Union; methodology which leads one back to the original Source; generally understood to mean a path or a practice leading to the Divine

# INDEX - GENERAL

# S

# T

# U

# V

# W

# Y

# INDEX - DISORDERS

405

# INDEX – HERBS BY LATIN NAMES

83, 85, 87, 88, 92, 93, 97, 98, 101, 103,
110, 116, 119, 121, 124, 126, 128, 139,
144, 148, 154, 157, 158, 162, 164, 166,
169, 171, 174, 178, 182, 183, 195, 198,
200, 215, 217, 219, 223, 232, 234, 236,
240, 242, 243, 247, 261, 265, 279, 284,
286, 295, 297, 301, 311, 314, 316, 318,
323, 325, 327, 336, 338, 340, 342, 353,
359, 361, 363, 365, 367, 368, 370, 374,
381, 394

# S

Salvia officinalis                                      89
Scutellaria lateriflora        58, 63, 110, 124,
132, 158, 221, 240, 259, 268, 274, 275,
277, 329, 340, 342, 351, 355, 394
Serenoa serrulata                                  313
Silybum marianum  42, 43, 44, 46, 53, 55,
61, 64, 66, 70, 72, 74, 76, 82, 83, 85,
87, 88, 92, 97, 101, 103, 116, 119, 121,
124, 128, 139, 144, 148, 154, 157, 158,
162, 164, 166, 169, 171, 174, 178, 183,
195, 198, 200, 215, 217, 219, 223, 232,
234, 236, 247, 261, 265, 279, 284, 286,
295, 311, 314, 316, 318, 323, 325, 327,
336, 338, 340, 342, 353, 359, 365, 367,
368, 370, 374, 394

# T

Tabebuia impetiginosa  47, 67, 74, 80, 86,
94, 105, 120, 134, 139, 147, 153, 160,
161, 168, 176, 185, 187, 232, 245, 303,
316, 321, 323, 325, 327, 334, 347, 361,
363, 381, 393
Taraxacum officinale     41, 43, 44, 51, 60,
61, 64, 66, 69, 70, 72, 74, 75, 76, 77,
78, 80, 83, 85, 87, 90, 91, 92, 93, 97,
98, 103, 108, 112, 113, 115, 117, 120,
123, 124, 128, 134, 138, 139, 144, 146,
148, 154, 156, 158, 168, 169, 171, 172,
174, 178, 180, 189, 197, 198, 200, 205,
207, 214, 215, 217, 225, 227, 229, 232,
234, 247, 253, 261, 270, 272, 279, 284,
311, 314, 316, 318, 323, 325, 327, 340,

342, 347, 349, 353, 355, 370, 374, 379,
381, 394
Terminalia arjuna     56, 60, 64, 66, 70, 82,
83, 85, 92, 97, 178, 198, 199, 249, 253,
257, 289, 393
Terminalia belerica  42, 45, 47, 49, 55, 59,
64, 66, 67, 72, 75, 83, 85, 86, 91, 92,
93, 94, 97, 105, 106, 115, 127, 136,
142, 160, 162, 180, 185, 191, 203, 211,
237, 239, 249, 275, 282, 289, 293, 303,
305, 307, 320, 329, 331, 346, 372, 376,
393
Terminalia chebula  42, 45, 47, 49, 55, 58,
59, 60, 64, 66, 67, 69, 72, 75, 80, 83,
85, 86, 90, 91, 92, 93, 94, 97, 105, 106,
115, 120, 123, 127, 136, 139, 142, 144,
146, 148, 151, 153, 156, 160, 161, 162,
166, 172, 174, 176, 180, 184, 185, 191,
203, 207, 211, 234, 237, 239, 245, 249,
270, 275, 282, 286, 289, 293, 303, 305,
307, 320, 329, 331, 333, 334, 346, 347,
349, 359, 372, 376, 393
Thymus vulgaris                        79, 89, 339
Tinospora cordifolia     47, 49, 59, 67, 86,
91, 94, 105, 106, 128, 130, 131, 134,
139, 147, 160, 164, 172, 174, 185, 187,
208, 214, 234, 237, 239, 303, 318, 323,
325, 327, 372, 376, 393
Tribulus terrestris     45, 59, 70, 101, 112,
126, 130, 131, 141, 180, 197, 203, 208,
209, 215, 219, 227, 229, 265, 272, 311,
314, 320, 346, 368, 393
Trigonella foenum-graecum     31, 41, 44,
45, 46, 51, 53, 56, 57, 58, 59, 60, 61,
63, 70, 75, 76, 78, 80, 87, 88, 90, 93,
95, 98, 100, 103, 107, 108, 110, 112,
113, 115, 116, 117, 120, 121, 123, 124,
126, 128, 130, 131, 132, 134, 138, 139,
141, 142, 146, 147, 148, 150, 151, 153,
154, 156, 158, 161, 164, 166, 168, 169,
172, 174, 176, 177, 178, 180, 182, 187,
189, 193, 197, 198, 200, 202, 203, 205,
207, 209, 211, 215, 217, 221, 223, 225,
227, 229, 232, 234, 236, 240, 242, 243,
245, 247, 251, 253, 255, 257, 259, 261,
263, 265, 268, 270, 272, 274, 277, 279,

281, 284, 286, 288, 291, 297, 299, 301,
307, 309, 311, 314, 316, 318, 321, 323,
325, 327, 333, 334, 336, 338, 340, 342,
344, 347, 349, 351, 353, 355, 357, 359,
361, 363, 367, 370, 372, 374, 378, 379,
381, 393

## U

Urtica dioica  45, 98, 101, 107, 113, 117,
126, 148, 150, 168, 177, 189, 193, 205,
208, 215, 217, 219, 225, 227, 229, 272,
281, 311, 314, 316, 321, 368, 378, 394

## V

Valeriana officinalis 42, 46, 55, 57, 58, 61,
64, 66, 72, 74, 82, 83, 85, 90, 92, 97,
110, 116, 117, 119, 121, 123, 124, 134,
144, 146, 148, 153, 154, 156, 157, 158,
162, 164, 166, 169, 172, 184, 189, 191,
200, 207, 223, 225, 232, 236, 251, 255,
257, 261, 263, 265, 270, 274, 277, 284,
286, 295, 299, 309, 316, 318, 323, 325,
327, 340, 342, 344, 349, 353, 365, 370,
393
Viburnum opulus    44, 53, 76, 100, 103,
108, 121, 128, 142, 144, 151, 189, 191,
193, 211, 223, 232, 251, 255, 257, 263,
268, 299, 309, 344, 370, 371, 394
Vitex agnus-castus    44, 53, 76, 100, 103,
108, 121, 128, 142, 144, 151, 189, 191,
193, 211, 223, 231, 232, 251, 255, 257,
263, 268, 299, 309, 344, 370, 394

## W

Withania somnifera 47, 49, 56, 57, 59, 67,
86, 94, 105, 106, 127, 138, 141, 142,
151, 160, 164, 178, 185, 187, 198, 203,
209, 211, 237, 239, 265, 274, 277, 282,
286, 288, 289, 293, 307, 320, 331, 333,
346, 355, 357, 376, 393

## Z

Zingiber officinale  41, 44, 45, 46, 51, 53,
56, 57, 58, 59, 60, 61, 63, 70, 75, 76,
78, 80, 87, 88, 90, 93, 95, 98, 100, 103,
107, 108, 110, 112, 113, 115, 116, 117,
120, 121, 123, 124, 126, 128, 130, 131,
132, 134, 138, 139, 141, 142, 146, 147,
148, 150, 151, 153, 154, 156,158, 161,
164, 166, 168, 169, 172, 174, 176, 177,
178, 180, 182, 187, 189, 193, 197, 198,
200, 202, 203, 205, 207, 209, 211, 215,
217, 221, 223, 225, 227, 229, 232, 234,
236, 240, 242, 243, 245, 247, 251, 253,
255, 257, 259, 261, 263, 265, 268, 270,
272, 274, 277, 279, 281, 284, 286, 288,
291, 297, 299, 301, 307, 309, 311, 314,
316, 318, 321, 323, 325, 327, 333, 334,
336, 338, 340, 342, 344, 347, 349, 351,
353, 355, 357, 359, 361, 363, 367, 370,
372, 374, 378, 379, 381, 393

# INDEX – HERBS BY COMMON NAMES

# C

# D

# V

# W

# Y

# ABOUT THE AUTHOR

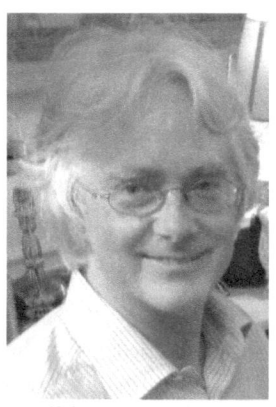 Born in Santa Monica, California in 1956, Vaidya Atreya Smith is the author of fourteen books published in nine different languages on the art of Indian medicine and healing. Since 1998 he founded and directs the European Institute of Vedic Studies, Switzerland. Atreya began to meditate at the age of 17 and moved into an ashram at the age of 25. Passionate about Vedanta he was a member of the American Vedanta Society at the age of 19 until he moved to India in 1987 to study Vedanta and Ayurveda in depth. Since 1987 he has studied with a number of Indian professors of Ayurveda in India. He continues his studies on Ayurveda with his teachers in India. He has a BSc in Biology and in 2005 was awarded the title of 'Vaidya' in Varanasi for his work in Ayurveda. Atreya has been a professional in health care since 1987 and has worked with thousands of patients in countries all over the world. He is a professional herbalist and the member of several professional organizations. Atreya is the author of a series of textbooks for Western students of Ayurveda called 'Ayurvedic Medicine for Westerners'; Vol. 1, *Anatomy and Physiology in Ayurveda*; Vol. 2, *Pathology & Diagnosis in Ayurveda*; Vol. 3, *Clinical Protocols & Treatments in Ayurveda*; Vol. 4, *Dravyaguna for Westerners;* and Vol 5, *Application of Ayurvedic Treatments Throughout Life*. He is one of the most sought after teachers of Ayurveda in Europe. Atreya and his Institute are affiliated with a number of institutes throughout the world for the promotion of Ayurveda and other Indian sciences. Atreya is the founder of Ayur-Vidya™. He currently lives with his wife in Switzerland near Lake Geneva.

Since 2010 Vaidya Atreya Smith offers a three-level training program to anyone who is interested in learning Āyurveda online. The first part of the program is offered by Atreya using the latest technology on an e-learning platform. This program lasts one school year. After completion of the first part (e-learning) students qualify for the second level - a three-week clinical studies program with Dr. Sunil V. Joshi, MD(ayu) in Nagpur, India. The third level is on Dravyaguna for Westerners and is taught by Atreya through e-learning. This program also lasts one school year. For students who have diplomas from other schools it is possible to join our Part Two program in India or our Part Three program on medicinal plants and treatments. For further information look at our websites.

www.atreya.com
www.ayurvedicnutrition.com

To insure the preservation of medicinal plants around the world Vaidya Atreya Smith has started several projects to actively protect this important natural resource. Information on the vision and how to support it can be found on this website:

www.eivs.org

www.ingramcontent.com/pod-product-compliance
Lightning Source LLC
Chambersburg PA
CBHW021418170526
45164CB00001B/7